FOLIC ACID

Biochemistry and Physiology in Relation to the Human Nutrition Requirement

Proceedings of a Workshop on
Human Folate Requirements

Washington, D.C.
June 2–3, 1975

Food and Nutrition Board
National Research Council

NATIONAL ACADEMY OF SCIENCES
Washington, D.C.   1977

NOTICE: The project that is the subject of this report was approved by the Governing Board of the National Research Council, whose members are drawn from the Councils of the National Academy of Sciences, the National Academy of Engineering, and the Institute of Medicine. The members of the Committee responsible for the report were chosen for their special competences and with regard for appropriate balance.

This report has been reviewed by a group other than the authors according to procedures approved by a Report Review Committee consisting of members of the National Academy of Sciences, the National Academy of Engineering, and the Institute of Medicine.

This workshop conference was supported by NIAMD Grant 1 R13 AM 17546-01 and grants from Miles Laboratories, Inc., and The Nutrition Foundation, Inc.

Library of Congress Cataloging in Publication Data

Workshop on Human Folate Requirements, Washington,
    D.C., 1975.
    Folic acid.

    1. Vitamin M—Metabolism—Congresses. 2. Vitamin M in human nutrition—Congresses. I. National Research Council. Food and Nutrition Board. II. Title.
QP772.F6W67   1975   612'.399   77-8182
ISBN 0-309-02605-9

Available from:

Printing and Publishing Office
National Academy of Sciences
2101 Constitution Avenue, N.W.
Washington, D.C. 20418

Printed in the United States of America

Acknowledgments

The Food and Nutrition Board gratefully acknowledges the editorial contributions of Harry P. Broquist, Vanderbilt University School of Medicine; Charles E. Butterworth, Jr., University of Alabama Medical Center; and Conrad Wagner, Vanderbilt University School of Medicine.

Contents

v

1

Introduction

C. E. BUTTERWORTH, JR.

I am sure that all of you would agree that there has been a rapid expansion of knowledge and information about folic acid during the 30 years since it was first synthesized. The pace seems to be quickening; thus, we feel that it is appropriate to have a workshop such as this.

Our purposes are to take stock of where we stand, try to establish areas of agreement, determine what we *know* or *do not know*, and try to make some practical, useful application of this knowledge.

In particular, one of our aims is to determine the role of folate in human nutrition and to recommend dietary allowances for it. This seems simple, but I would like to offer it as one of our principal objectives.

I think it is ironic that when the Ten-State survey was completed, in spite of all the information that has been assembled over the past 30 years, it was exceedingly difficult to make a meaningful analysis of the folate data. Perhaps we should try to come to some agreement on how our knowledge can be applied in evaluating survey data.

I have drawn up a list of seven questions that I think are crucial— questions for which it would be most desirable to have answers. I have tried to word these carefully. Some of them will seem very simple. I hope they will have more meaning than the simple words imply.

First, what do we recommend as the dietary allowances for folate?
Second, how does one assess nutritional status with regard to folate?
Third, what is the effect of folate deficiency, and, as a corollary, what is the effect of folic acid excess on man?
Fourth, what can be done to standardize methodology and techniques for folate assays so that we can uniformly exchange information?
Fifth, is there a need to standardize procedures for determining total folate? For example, how uniform and accurate are the methods for enzymic release of folic acid polyglutamates?
Sixth, is there a need for a system of equivalents? For example, is a molecule of polyglutamyl folate nutritionally equivalent to a molecule of pteroylmonoglutamate?
Seventh, with tongue in cheek, are we entirely satisfied with the presently available tables of folate content in food?

These are just a few topics. I am sure that there are many more that will emerge as the discussion goes on, but I hope this will serve as a starting point.

2

Folic Acid Biochemistry: Present Status and Future Direction

RAYMOND L. BLAKLEY

To review even superficially the many investigations of folic acid biochemistry published over the past 5 years would be a task impossible to encompass within the scope of this paper. Instead, I propose to choose four lines of work that I think may be representative of important trends or foci in research effort in this general area. In doing so, I must necessarily ignore a large body of excellent and important research on such subjects as serine hydroxymethyl transferase, formyl-tetrahydrofolate synthetase, and the glycine decarboxylating system, to mention but a few. No value judgment is implied by my choices, which actually reflect my own idiosyncratic interests.

NEW METABOLIC REACTIONS

New reactions of folate metabolism are a natural focus of attention, but relatively few new reactions involving folic acid or its derivatives have come to light over the past few years, and those that have been reported do not open up any radically different functions of these

3

coenzymes. What was purported to be new methyl transfer reactions from 5-methyltetrahydrofolate (methylTHF) to dopamine (Laduron, 1972) and to other biogenic amines (Banerjee and Snyder, 1973; Hsu and Mandell, 1973; Laduron *et al.*, 1974) have subsequently been shown (Leysen and Laduron, 1974) to be more likely due to oxidation of methylTHF to methylenetetrahydrofolate (methyleneTHF), hydrolysis of the latter to yield formaldehyde, followed by nonenzymic combination of formaldehyde with the amines (Figure 2-1). It has been proposed that formaldehyde formation is catalyzed by methyleneTHF reductase, which is localized in the soluble fraction of brain together with methylTHF:homocysteine methyltransferase, whereas serine hydroxymethyltransferase and the glycine cleavage complex are located in the mitochondria (Burton and Sallach, 1975). This route for generation of formaldehyde is surprising, since Kutzbach and Stokstad (1971) have confirmed that the equilibrium is very unfavorable for methyleneTHF formation. They calculated that, although the equilibrium constant for methyleneTHF formation is 8×10^3 with the artificial electron acceptor menadione, the constant is 10^{-7} when NADP is the electron acceptor. They confirmed this calculation by showing that, in the presence of enzyme purified more than 300-fold from pig or rat liver, very little methyleneTHF is formed from methylTHF when NADP + FAD is substituted for menadione or menadione + FAD (Table 2-1).

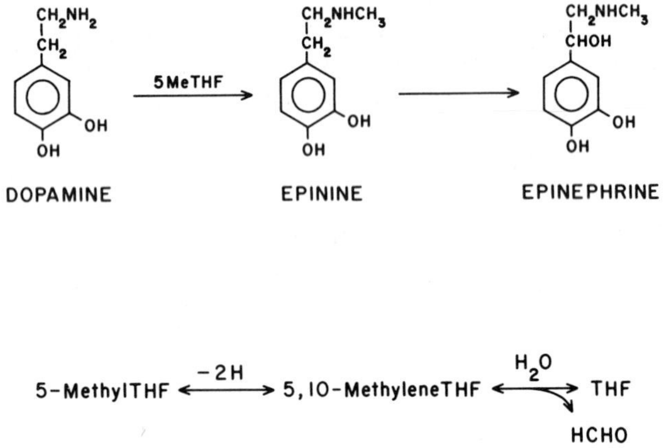

FIGURE 2-1 Proposed pathway for methylation of dopamine. The upper series of reactions shows the proposed transmethylation from 5-methytetrahydrofolate to dopamine. The lower series shows the pathway for formaldehyde generation from 5-methyltetrahydrofolate.

TABLE 2-1   Reversibility of MethyleneTHF Reductase Reaction[a]

Electron Acceptors	Formaldehyde Formed, nmol/mg enzyme
FAD, menadione	2,050
Menadione	850
FAD	75
FAD, NADP$^+$	53
FAD, NADP$^+$, NADP$^+$ regenerating system	97

SOURCE: Kutzbach and Stokstad (1971).
[a]Reaction mixture contained [^{14}CH₃] methylTHF (0.55 mM; 330 nmol), 8 mM ascorbate, 0.166 M K phosphate buffer (pH 6.3), 1.6 mM EDTA, 8 mM FAD, and enzyme. NADP$^+$ at 3.3 mM or menadione at 3.5 mM was added as indicated. Formaldehyde was isolated as dimedone complex.

However, only fractions of a nanomole of labeled amine were formed per hour with the brain preparations, and such small amounts of formaldehyde may well be derived from methylTHF by the proposed pathway.

Another function of tetrahydrofolate derivatives that has recently come to light is the methylation of uracil residues in tRNA. Ribosylthymine is a minor constituent of tRNA in both procaryotes and eucaryotes, and until recently it was assumed that, like other minor bases of RNA, it received its methyl group from *S*-adenosylmethionine. However, Delk and Rabinowitz (1975) have shown that, although *Escherichia coli* derives the methyl of tRNA thymine from methionine, in *Streptococcus faecalis* [methyl-^{14}C]methionine does not label thymine of tRNA—[^{14}C]formate does. Furthermore, ribosylthymine is not present in tRNA of *S. faecalis* grown on folate-free medium, and Arnold and Kersten (1975) have been able to show that trimethoprim, an inhibitor of bacterial dihydrofolate reductase, prevents synthesis of ribosylthymine in tRNA of *Bacillus subtilis* and *Micrococcus lysodeikticus*.

Delk and Rabinowitz (1975) also demonstrated that *S. faecalis* is able to use this dependence on folate derivatives for ribosylthymine synthesis in a curiously advantageous manner (Table 2-2). Procaryotes initiate protein synthesis with fMet-tRNA^{fMet}, which is formed by transformylation from 10-formylTHF to Met-tRNA^{fMet}. In the presence of trimethoprim, which causes a deficiency in tetrahydrofolate derivatives, *E. coli* supplied with purines, thymidine, and amino acids still cannot grow normally because of an inability to inititate protein synthesis. However, in folate-deficient medium *S. faecalis* does not suffer in the same way. Under these conditions *S. faecalis* makes an altered

TABLE 2-2   Changes in tRNA and Initiation of Protein Synthesis in *S. faecalis* in Folate Deficiency

Culture Conditions	tRNA for Initiation of Protein Synthesis	
	Charged State for Initiation	Structure of Loop IV
Normal	fMet-tRNA^{fMet}	GTψC
Folate-deficient	Met-tRNA^{*fMet}	GUψC

SOURCE: Delk and Rabinowitz (1974, 1975).

tRNA (tRNA^{*fMet}) that can initiate protein synthesis as unformylated Met-tRNA^{*fMet} (Samuel *et al.*, 1970, 1972; Samuel and Rabinowitz, 1974). The tRNA^{*fMet} with this capacity has a single modification (Delk and Rabinowitz, 1974)—in loop IV it has GUψC instead of GTψC—and this modification automatically results from the inability to methylate uracil when folate is deficient. A similar situation probably exists in *B. subtilis* and *M. lysodeikticus* (Arnold and Kersten, 1975). Whether any comparable situation exists in eucaryotic organisms is unknown.

REGULATION OF FOLATE METABOLISM

Although feedback inhibition and end product repression of bacterial enzymes involved in folate metabolism has been known for many years (Silber and Mansouri, 1971), evidence for the regulation of such enzymes in mammals has been obtained only in recent years. The activities of several enzymes of folate metabolism have been shown to rise and fall during the growth of cultured mammalian cells (Rosenberg *et al.*, 1971; Conrad, 1971; Conrad and Ruddle, 1972; Hillcoat *et al.*, 1973; Rosenblatt and Erbe, 1973). The activities of dihydrofolate reductase, thymidylate synthetase, serine hydroxymethyltransferase, and 10-formyltetrahydrofolate synthetase all increase 4- to 20-fold as the cultures pass from lag phase to logarithmic phase, and they decline again as the stationary phase is entered. In the case of some enzymes it has been shown that puromycin and cycloheximide prevent the increases (Conrad and Ruddle, 1972; Hillcoat *et al.*, 1973) so that *de novo* protein synthesis is probably involved. However, methyleneTHF reductase and 5-methylTHF:homocysteine methyltransferase apparently do not increase in human fibroblasts during log phase (Rosenblatt and Erbe, 1973). In Chinese hamster cells synchronized with colcemid, thymidylate synthetase rose during S phase and fell during G_2, M, and G_1 phases (Conrad, 1971), but there is little information on how other enzymes of folate metabolism behave during the cell cycle.

The mechanism for regulation of the levels of the four enzymes of folate metabolism during cell culture remains uncertain but, as suggested some time ago (Bertino and Hillcoat, 1968; Nichol, 1968), the concentration of folate derivatives may be one factor of importance. One of the first observations suggesting this view was the "induction" of dihydrofolate reductase in the red and white cells of patients receiving methotrexate (Bertino *et al.*, 1963b); most of the rise in reductase level was due to an increase in methotrexate-bound enzyme (Bertino *et al.*, 1965a). Similarly when methotrexate was added to an established human hematoblastoid cell line, total dihydrofolate reductase rose to twice the level in the control; the increase was due to methotrexate-enzyme complex, which appeared to have been stabilized against normal proteolytic breakdown (Hillcoat *et al.*, 1967). Hillcoat and co-workers (1973) have shown that the addition of 0.1 mM folate to cultures of this cell line also doubled the rise in dihydrofolate reductase during log phase (Figure 2-2), although whether folate also acts by retarding the rate of breakdown of the enzyme is not clear. The latter seems unlikely since the destruction of folate derivatives in the medium of cultured cells by carboxypeptidase G_1 results in a decrease in dihydrofolate reductase activity (Chello and Bertino, 1972).

Although administered folic acid does not increase dihydrofolate reductase levels in human subjects (Bertino *et al.*, 1963a), presumably because high enough serum levels are not readily achievable, it has been reported that in rats a high-folate diet increases the level in jejunum of glutamate formimino-transferase, serine hydroxymethyltransferase, and methyleneTHF dehydrogenase (Stifel *et al.*, 1970). A low-protein diet increases the level of hepatic methylTHF:homocysteine methyltransferase in rats (Finkelstein *et al.*, 1971).

It has been proposed that the inhibition by folate derivatives of serine hydroxymethyltransferase (Schirch and Ropp, 1967), dihydrofolate reductase, methyleneTHF, dehydrogenase, and methyleneTHF cyclohydrolase (Rowe and Lewis, 1973) may serve to regulate pathways of folate metabolism. Inhibition constants are mostly in the range 10^{-5} to 10^{-4} M (Table 2-3), which seems rather high considering the low concentrations of folate derivatives in tissues, and there is the further problem that specific feedback inhibition of these enzymes would be difficult to achieve because of the close interactions and interconversions of the various folate cofactors (Bertino and Hillcoat, 1968). Nevertheless, this possibility cannot be dismissed without further evidence.

A further suggestion along these lines has been prompted by the

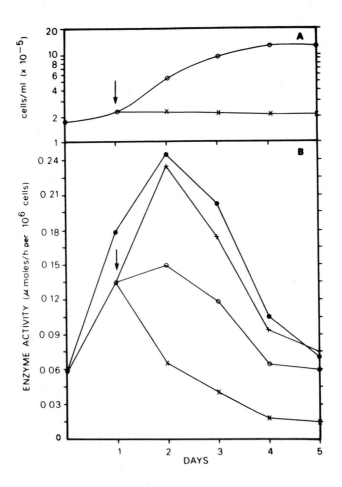

FIGURE 2-2   Response of dihydrofolate reductase activity in the human cell line RPMI 4265 to addition of folate and cycloheximide. (A) ○, Growth curve of cells with no addition of folate or addition of 0.1 mM folate at zero time or at 24 h (arrow); ×, growth curve when 0.1 mM folate and 1 mM cycloheximide were added together (arrow). (B) Variation in enzyme activity under the conditions in (A): ○, Control; ●, folate added at zero time; +, folate added at 24 h (arrow); ×, folate and cycloheximide added at 24 h (arrow) (reproduced with the permission of B. L. Hillcoat and Biochim. Biophys. Acta *293*:282, 1973, Amsterdam, the Netherlands).

TABLE 2-3   Inhibition of Some Enzymic Reactions by Folate Derivatives

Enzyme	K_i, M $\times$ 10^5				
	5-MethylTHF	5-FormylTHF	MethyleneTHF	THF	DHF
Serine CH_2OH-transferase	9.2	130			
DHF reductase		12	1.2		
MethyleneTHF dehydrogenase	20	20		36	24
MethyleneTHF cyclohydrolase	3.0	0.86	0.2	0.7	0.88

SOURCE: Rowe and Lewis (1973); Schirch and Ropp (1967).

discovery that rat liver slices form 10-formylfolic acid when incubated with folic acid (Urso-Scott *et al.*, 1974). Rauen (1957) observed many years ago that 10-formylfolic acid is formed from folic acid by homogenates of rat liver or pig liver and that the conversion was increased by the presence of ATP, pyridoxine, and a one-carbon donor such as serine. Recently, 10-formylfolate has also been shown to be produced in the serosal fluid by everted sacs of rat gut exposed to folate on the mucosal side (Perry and Chanarin, 1973). These indications of the biological formation of formylfolate are of interest because this derivative has been found to act as a powerful inhibitor of dihydrofolate reductase of Ehrlich ascites cells with a K_i of 6.1 $\times$ 10^{-9} M (Bertino *et al.*, 1965b). If, as suggested by the evidence of Urso-Scott and his co-workers (1974), formylation proceeds without reduction, a new reaction of folic acid awaits characterization. On the other hand, if formylfolate arises by oxidation of 10-formyltetrahydrofolate, the inhibitory effect of formylfolate on dihydrofolate reductase might serve to shut off the pathway to 10-formyltetrahydrofolate when the latter accumulates to such an extent that it undergoes significant degradation to 10-formylfolate (Figure 2-3).

Regulation of folate metabolism by cobalamines will be discussed in later chapters. However, possible regulation by some other nonfolate compounds should be mentioned. Conrad and Ruddle (1972) observed that methotrexate added in log phase to cultures of Don Chinese hamster cells causes a three- to fourfold *increase* above control values in the specific activity of thymidylate synthetase (Figure 2-4). They interpret their results to mean that the control of this enzyme in log phase may involve thymidine triphosphate, presumably as a repressor of thymidylate synthetase synthesis. Another metabolite that may be involved in regulation of a folate-dependent pathway is

RAYMOND L. BLAKLEY

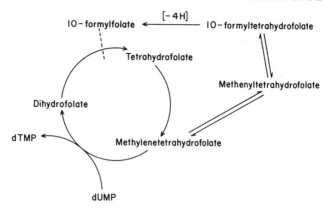

FIGURE 2-3 Postulated regulation of dihydrofolate by 10-formylfolate.

S-adenosylmethionine. This has been shown to produce 50 percent inhibition of 5-methylTHF:homocysteine transmethylase activity at concentrations of 2–8 μM and to fulfill many of the criteria of a metabolic regulator (Kutzbach and Stokstad, 1971).

THYMIDYLATE SYNTHETASE

This enzyme has attracted attention second only to that given dihydrofolate reductase. Its purification from insects (Carpenter, 1974), bacteria (Crusbert et al., 1970; Dunlap et al., 1971; Leary and Kisliuk, 1971; Whiteley et al., 1974a, 1974b; McCuen and Sirotnak, 1975), phage-infected bacteria (Capco and Mathews, 1973; Capco et al., 1973; Galivan et al., 1974), and mammalian cells (Fridland et al., 1971; Danenberg and Heidelberger, 1974) has been reported together with descriptions of the properties of the enzyme from these sources, particularly susceptibility to inhibition by various antifolates and analogs of dUMP. There have been preliminary reports on the structure of the enzyme (Dunlap et al., 1971; Loeble and Dunlap, 1972; Capco et al., 1973; Galivan et al., 1974; Aull et al., 1974a) that indicate that from bacteria the enzyme is composed of two identical subunits, each with a molecular weight of about 30,000, but subunits were not detected in the case of the synthetase from Ehrlich ascites cells (Fridland et al., 1971).

The formation of a relatively stable complex between the enzyme

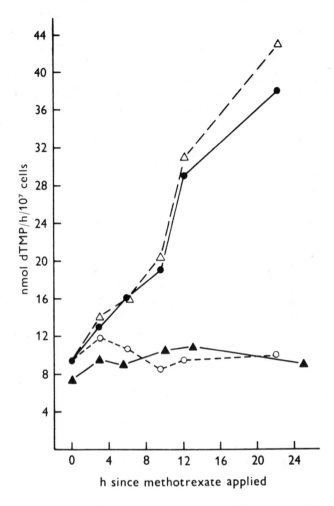

FIGURE 2-4 Effect of methotrexate on thymidylate synthetase activity in log-phase cultures of Don Chinese hamster cells. Methotrexate (10^{-6} M) was added to cultures in log phase (24 h after subculture). Puromycin (10 μg/ml) was also added at this time to some cultures, and 5 h later actinomycin D (5 μg/ml) was added to others. Thymidylate synthetase activity was determined in extracts of the cells. ○, Controls; ●, with methotrexate; ▲, with methotrexate + puromycin; △, with methotrexate + actinomycin D (reproduced with the permission of A. H. Conrad and F. H. Ruddle and J. Cell Sci. *10*:471–486, Figure 8, 1972, England).

and the inhibitor 5-fluoro-2'-deoxyuridine-5'-phosphate (FdUMP) in the presence of the substrate 5,10-methylenetetrahydrofolate has been reported by several groups. Aull *et al.* (1974b) have shown that both a 1:1:1 complex and a 2:2:1 complex of FdUMP, methylenetetrahydrofolate, and *Lactobacillus casei* enzyme could be isolated by polyacrylamide gel electrophoresis or by ion-exchange. A 1:1:1 complex of the enzyme from Ehrlich ascites cells has also been reported (Danenberg *et al.*, 1974). The stability of the ternary complex formed by the *L. casei* enzyme is illustrated by maintenance of stoichiometry during this isolation procedure, as well as during ultrafiltration (Santi *et al.*, 1974a). It has also been reported that 6 M urea or 6 M guanidine hydrochloride does not increase the rate of dissociation of the ternary complex (Santi and McHenry, 1972; Santi *et al.*, 1974b), which suggests covalent attachment of the ligands to the enzyme. A similar ternary complex formed by the enzyme from Ehrlich ascites cells is not disrupted upon denaturation of the enzyme with urea or sodium dodecyl sulfate or on precipitation with trichloroacetic acid (Langenbach *et al.*, 1972). Digestion of the ternary complex of the *L. casei* enzyme with pronase yields most of the FdUMP attached to peptide fragments, one of which has the composition Thr, His, Ala, Leu, Pro$_2$ (Sommer and Santi, 1974). The ultraviolet and excitation spectra (Figures 2-5 and 2-6) indicate that the peptide also has attached a tetrahydrofolate derivative in equimolar amounts with FdUMP. The spectra suggest that this derivative is a 5-alkyltetrahydrofolate.

The possibility that a nucleophilic group of the enzyme adds to the 6 position of FdUMP in the formation of the ternary complex, and to the 6 position of dUMP in the formation of an intermediate of the

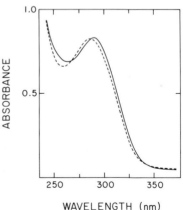

FIGURE 2-5 Ultraviolet spectra of 24 μM purified FdUMP–peptide–methylenetetrahydrofolate complex (————) and 24 μM 5-methyltetrahydrofolate (--------) in 25 mM ammonium acetate–10 mM 2-mercaptoethanol (pH 7.0) (Sommer and Santi, 1974).

FIGURE 2-6 Fluorescence spectra of 4 μM purified FdUMP–peptide–methylenetetrahydrofolate complex (———) and 4 μM 5-methyltetrahydrofolate (- - - - - -) in 25 mM ammonium acetate–10 mM 2-mercaptoethanol (pH 7.0). For excitation spectra, emission wavelength was 360 nm; for emission spectra, excitation was 300 nm for the complex and 298 nm for 5-methyltetrahydrofolate. Band width was 10 nm, and fluorescence intensity is reported in arbitrary units (Sommer and Santi, 1974).

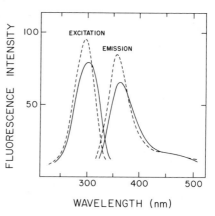

normal reaction, has been suggested by the study of various model reactions. These include the hydrolysis of *N*-alkylated 5-*p*-nitrophenoxymethyluracil (Pogolotti and Santi, 1974) and base-catalyzed 5-hydrogen exchange and 5-hydroxymethylation of 1-substituted uracils (Santi and Brewer, 1973). These authors conclude that a threonine or histidine residue provides the nucleophilic group.

Attachment of the folate derivative via the methylene group to the 5 position of the pyrimidine ring is in agreement with the spectroscopic properties (Santi and McHenry, 1972; Sommer and Santi, 1974), the relative stability of the tetrahydrofolate derivative to oxidation (Sommer and Santi, 1974), the requirement for the methylene group in the folate derivative (Danenberg et al., 1974; Santi *et al.*, 1974b), and the probable potential for iminium cation formation by methylenetetrahydrofolate (Kallen and Jencks, 1966).

Essentially similar conclusions about the structure of the stable ternary complex have been reached by Danenberg and his co-workers (1974), except for indications that the nucleophile in the Ehrlich ascites enzyme may be cysteine, a view also proposed by Kalman (1972).

The mechanism to which these conclusions lead is shown in Figure 2-7. Reaction within the ternary complex is initiated by attack of the enzyme nucleophilic group on position 5 of dUMP with formation of a reactive carbanion. This reacts with the iminium cation of methylenetetrahydrofolate to give the covalent ternary complex (II). It is unlikely that free thymidylyl-tetrahydrofolate (IV) would be formed; it is more likely that III undergoes a β-elimination to produce the highly reactive exocyclic methylene intermediate (V) and tetrahydrofolate bound in close proximity. Intermolecular hydride transfer from tet-

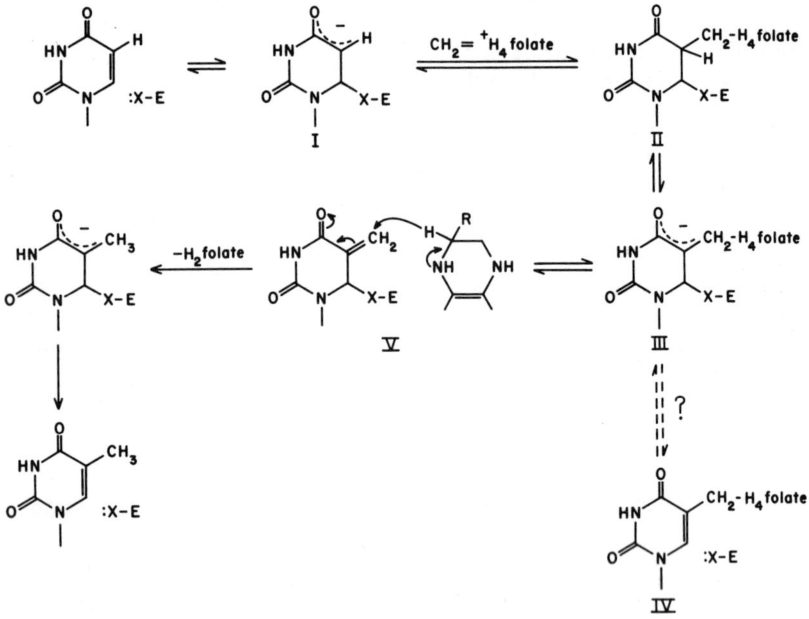

FIGURE 2-7   Proposed reaction mechanism for thymidylate synthetase (Pogolotti and Santi, 1974).

rahydrofolate to V would yield dTMP, dihydrofolate, and the native enzyme.

DIHYDROFOLATE REDUCTASE

Since more research effort has been expended in the past few years on this enzyme than any other involved in folate metabolism, it is appropriate to mention a few of the major lines of investigation.

A number of laboratories are involved in structural studies of the reductase from a variety of sources. Chemical modification of reductase has resulted in loss of activity when tryptophan, histidine, cysteine, or methionine residues were modified (Warwick et al., 1972; Greenfield, 1974; Liu and Dunlap, 1974; Gleisner and Blakley, 1975; Warwick and Freisheim, 1975; Williams, 1975), but only in two cases was evidence produced indicating that the modified residue was at the binding site for one specific substrate (Table 2-4). The determination of the primary sequence of the enzyme from methotrexate-resistant strains of E. coli

TABLE 2-4 Modification of Residues in Dihydrofolate Reductase Causing Loss of Activity

Enzyme Source	Residue Modified	Reagent	Reference
S. faecium	Trp	*N*-Bromosuccinimide	Warwick *et al.* (1972)
L. casei	Trp[a]	*N*-Bromosuccinimide	Liu and Dunlap (1974)
E. coli MB 1428	His, Trp	*N*-Bromosuccinimide	Williams (1975)
E. coli MB 1428	His	Ethoxyformic anhydride	Greenfield (1974)
S. faecium	Cys	DTNB	Warwick and Freisheim (1975)
S. faecium	Met[b]	Iodoacetate	Gleisner and Blakley (1975)

[a]Postulated to be at NADPH-binding site.
[b]Postulated to be at DHF-binding site.

(Bennett, 1974) and of *Streptococcus faecium* var. *Durans* (Gleisner *et al.*, 1974) has revealed considerable homology between the structures in two regions that we consider as contributors of residues involved in the binding of DHF and NADPH, respectively. In the sequence of the *S. faecium* enzyme the methionine residue completely modified by iodoacetate, but protected by aminopterin, is Met 28, which lies within one of the domains of homology and identifies this domain as contributing the DHF-binding region (Table 2-5). Work on the sequence of enzyme from mammalian sources is progressing, and we have been able to compare (Peterson *et al.*, 1975) the amino-terminal regions of the two bacterial enzymes with that of the beef liver enzyme (Figure 2-8). It may be seen that rather more homology exists than might have been expected from the much tighter binding of antifolates like trimethoprim to the bacterial enzyme than to the mammalian enzyme. In fact, in this region of the sequence as much homology exists between the beef liver and *S. faecium* structures as between the structure of the two bacterial enzymes.

The structure of this enzyme, and particularly the perturbation of it on binding substrate or inhibitor, has also been studied by various physical–biochemical methods such as those involving the use of circular dichroism (D'Souza and Friesheim, 1972; Greenfield *et al.*, 1972), protein nuclear magnetic resonance (Pastore *et al.*, 1974; Roberts *et al.*, 1974), fluorescence (Williams *et al.*, 1973a, 1973b), and ultraviolet difference spectroscopy (Poe *et al.*, 1974). In the latter study, evidence was obtained suggesting that at least one tryptophan residue is involved in the binding of NADPH.

One of the unusual features of dihydrofolate reductase from certain

TABLE 2-5 Distribution of Labeled Methionine Residues

Conditions of Carboxymethylation	^{14}C-Carboxymethyl Groups on Specific Methionine Residues[a]						Total,[b] groups/mol	Intact Protein, groups/mol
	1 and 5	28	36	42[c]	50	163		
No inhibitor	NS[d]	0.92	0.46	<0.01	0.48	0.19	2.15	2.22
Presence of 1 mM aminopterin	NS	0	0.44	<0.02	0.10	0.27	0.82	0.81
Differential labeling	NS	0.93	0.31	<0.01	0.37	0.14	1.75	1.83
		(0)[e]	(0.45)		(0.09)	(0.18)	(0.72)	

SOURCE: Gleisner and Blakley (1975).

[a]Observed ratio: μmol labeled peptide/μmol labeled + μmol unlabeled.
[b]Sum of carboxymethyl groups found in positions 28, 36, 50, and 163.
[c]Estimated from the radioactivity present in LT 4-T1.
[d]Not significant.
[e]Values in parentheses are for unlabeled carboxymethyl groups.

```
       1    2    3    4    5    6    7    8    9   10   CYS  12   13   14   15
A    VAL-ARG-PRO-LEU-ASN-ALA-ILE-VAL-ALA-VAL-SER-GLU-ASP-MET-GLY-
B    MET-PHE-ILE-SER-MET-TRP-            ALA-GLN-ASP-LYS-ASN-GLY-LEU-
C    MET-ILE-SER-LEU-ILE-ALA-            ALA-LEU-ALA-VAL-ASP-ARG-VAL-


      16   17   18   19   20   21   22   23   24   25   26   27   28   29   30
     ILE-GLY-LYS-ASP-GLY-TYR-LEU-PRO-TRP-PRO-PRO-LEU-———-———-ASX-GLU-
     ILE-GLY-LYS-ASP-GLY-LEU-LEU-PRO-TRP-ARG-LEU-PRO-ASN-ASP-MET-
     ILE-GLY-MET-GLU-ASN-ALA-MET-PRO-TRP-ASN-LEU-PRO-ALA-ASP-LEU-


      31   32   33   34   35   36   37
     PHE-GLU-TYR-PHE-———-———-GLU
     ARG-PHE-PHE-ARG-GLU-HIS-THR
     ALA TRP PHE  LYS  ARG  ASN  THR
```

FIGURE 2-8   Amino-terminal sequence of dihydrofolate reductase from bovine liver (top), *S. faecium* (middle) and *E. coli* (bottom) (Peterson *et al.*, in press).

sources is its capacity to form stable complexes with NADPH, with the result that multiple forms that differ in the presence or absence of tightly bound NADPH can be detected (Table 2-6). Huennekens and his co-workers (Gundersen *et al.*, 1972; Otting and Huennekens, 1972) have demonstrated that the reductase of a methotrexate-resistant strain of *L. casei* could be separated into two principal forms by electrophoresis. One of these forms could be converted to the other by incubation with NADPH. The NADPH-containing form could be converted to the NADPH-free form by incubation with dihydrofolate. Reductase from a methotrexate-resistant subline of L1210 leukemia also showed multiple forms (Harding *et al.*, 1970) that could be separated by electrophoresis in the presence of NADPH or by ion-exchange chromatography. Although in this case the nature of the difference between the forms was not demonstrated, it was assumed to be due to tight binding of NADPH. However, the nature of the multiple forms observed on electrophoresis of dihydrofolate reductase from

TABLE 2-6   Types of Multiple Forms of Dihydrofolate Reductase

Source	Difference Between Forms	Reference
L. casei	NADPH complex formation	Gundersen *et al.* (1972)
L1210	(NADPH complex formation?)	Harding *et al.* (1970)
Cell cultures	Buffer complex formation	Gauldie *et al.* (1973)
Hamster cells	(Primary structure?)	Hänggi and Littlefield (1974)
S. faecium	Primary structure	Nixon and Blakley (1968)

mammalian cells is a complex one. Gauldie *et al.* (1973) found that multiple forms that they observed in reductase isolated from various established lines of mammalian cells did not appear to be due to binding of NADPH but rather to interaction with the buffer. On the other hand, Hänggi and Littlefield (1974) found two forms of reductase from methotrexate-resistant hamster cells, which apparently were not related, by complexing NADPH or aggregation. Although tryptic peptide maps were not distinguishable, the authors favor a difference in primary structure, such as has been demonstrated for the isoenzymes of *S. faecium* (Nixon and Blakley, 1968). We have not observed multiple forms during electrophoresis of the homogeneous beef liver enzyme (Peterson *et al.*, 1975).

It has not been completely clarified whether the NADPH bound tightly to the reductase of *L. casei* is in the normal substrate site or whether a second molecule can bind at some other site. The former seems likely, because dihydrofolate converts the NADPH complex to the free enzyme as NADP is formed and dissociates. On the other hand, Williams and her co-workers (1973a) have obtained evidence from fluorescence and ultrafiltration experiments that the reductase from an *E. coli* mutant does have two binding sites for NADPH. This is surprising when the small size of this protein (161 residues; Delk and Rabinowitz, 1975) relative to the size of the substrates is considered.

It seems likely that research on the biochemistry of folate derivatives is likely to continue in these general areas for some time to come. Perhaps some undiscovered reactions of folate metabolism still remain to be elucidated, but if so they are unlikely to be many, and they will almost certainly be variations of the presently known functions of folate derivatives. In the brain, where folates play an important but little understood role, it is most likely that additional roles of folate remain to be discovered. The control of one-carbon metabolism by regulation of the synthesis of enzymes metabolizing folate derivatives and by feedback control of enzymic reactions is an important aspect of cellular metabolism with considerable clinical implications, and it will undoubtedly receive further attention. The nature of the regulatory response to folate deficiency or excess is of special interest. Much also remains to be clarified about the reaction mechanisms of many enzyme-catalyzed reactions of folate, and future studies in this area will be closely linked to the growing interest in the structure of the active sites of folate-metabolizing enzymes. Additional work is already in progress in this area and will culminate in the elucidation of three-dimensional structures of the complexes of several of these enzymes with their folate substrates.

DISCUSSION

HERBERT: Can the formation of different buffer complexes in cell cultures explain apparent differences in stability of folate derivatives?

BLAKLEY: I do not think we have data at the moment to answer that, but, if several folate enzymes complex with the buffer, it is a possibility. Multiple complexes were found at low buffer concentrations, whereas at high buffer concentrations only one form was present. It is conceivable that some folate derivatives might have different microbiological activity at different concentrations of buffer. This might be a pitfall in assaying folate derivatives microbiologically.

ROSENBERG: In the development of studies on coenzyme–enzyme interactions in the folate area, are we learning anything about what the advantage is (if there is an advantage) for the coenzyme to have a polyglutamate chain?

BLAKLEY: Little that I can see. Dr. Bertino's group has published K_m and K_i values for a series of polyglutamates with dihydrofolate reductase. Additional glutamate residues have some effect. As more glutamates are attached, the binding to the dihydrofolate reductase becomes greater. But it is not as great as I would have expected. To increase binding only a fewfold, much effort is expended by the cell.

SCOTT: 10-Formylfolic acid is nutritionally active for *Lactobacillus casei*. It has also been reported to be nutritionally active in man. I had always assumed, perhaps naively, that dihydrofolate reductase caused the reduction of 10-formylfolic acid to 10-formyltetrahydrofolic acid. That does not fit in with its being an inhibitor of dihydrofolate reductase. It would fit in with its being a substrate, but not an inhibitor. We recently found that, if 10-formyltetrahydrofolic acid is oxidized under mild conditions, it does not break at the 9–10 bond; it goes quantitatively to 10-formylfolic acid. Dr. Butterworth has shown that 10-formyltetrahydrofolate is a very substantial constituent of food. Now, if the cell contains something like 30 or 40 percent of its folate as 10-formyltetrahydrofolic acid, which goes to 10-formylfolic acid, then whether the latter is utilizable is of great nutritional consequen .

WAGNER: Could the discrepancy between the inhibitory effect and the need to act as a substrate be the result of these multiple forms that Dr. Blakley has talked about? Perhaps some forms are inhibited by 10-formylfolate.

SCOTT: Well, it is apparent that some agency in microorganisms and also in man is able to return 10-formylfolic acid to the metabolic pool. I just wonder if in fact it is the reductase, as I have always assumed it is, or is there some other mechanism?

BLAKLEY: I think there are three pieces of evidence that would be valuable in regard to this problem. One is what happens to labeled 10-formyltetrahydrofolate *in vivo*? Does it, in fact, break down to formylfolate? I do not think that is available. The second is how common is this inhibition of dihydrofolate reductase? The work I quoted was with Ehrlich ascites dihydrofolate reductase. I do not think that similar inhibition has been demonstrated with reductase from most other sources. The third is what do cells do with formylfolate supplied to them? I do not think we know any of these things.

CHANARIN: We looked at 10-formyltetrahydrofolate in everted rat gut. It was very rapidly converted into 5-methyltetrahydrofolate. The other thing that interested me very much was your data on the reversibility of 5,10-methylenetetrahydrofolate to 5-methyltetrahydrofolate. We have all been brought up in the belief that this is irreversible. Is there any other evidence in the mammalian tissue that this can be reversed?

BLAKLEY: I have some data from Dr. Stokstad's work that give the micromoles of formaldehyde formed from ^{14}C-labeled methyltetrahydrofolate by a rat liver preparation. If one puts in menadione, which is a good electron acceptor in the system, there is quite a substantial amount of formaldehyde formed. These are micromole quantities, but, nevertheless, the reaction does go in that direction. Also, very much less is formed with NADP and FAD. It is increased somewhat with an NADP-regenerating system. The amounts therefore are small, but they are measurable. In the work on the biogenic amines, as I mentioned, tracer methods were used to measure apparent incorporation into the amines, so that it would only take such micromole amounts to account for their observation.

HERBERT: I think the point is that the reaction only goes in the presence of menadione, and this is only true in bacteria. We tried to make this reaction go in a study with Friedkin and found that menadione could not make the reaction, that is the reversal from methyltetrahydrofolate back to 5,10-methylenetetrahydrofolate, go in a human system.

BLAKLEY: The results I quoted are for a rat liver system.

LITERATURE CITED

Arnold, H. H., and Kersten, H. 1975. Inhibition of the tetrahydrofolate-dependent biosynthesis of ribothymidine in tRNAs of *B. subtilis and M. lysodeikticus* by trimethoprim. FEBS Lett. *53*:258–261.

Aull, J. L., Loeble, R. B., and Dunlap, R. B. 1974a. The carboxypeptidase-dependent inactivation of thymidylate synthetase. J. Biol. Chem. *249*:1167–1172.

Aull, J. L., Lyon, J. A., and Dunlap, R. B. 1974b. Separation, identification, and stoichiometry of the ternary complexes of thymidylate synthetase. Arch. Biochem. Biophys. *165*:805–808.

Banerjee, S. P., and Snyder, S. H. 1973. Methyltetrahydrofolic acid mediates N- and O-methylation of biogenic amines. Science *182*:74–75.

Bennett, C. D. 1974. Similarity in the sequence of *Escherichia coli* dihydrofolate reductase with other pyridine nucleotide-requiring enzymes. Nature *248*:67–68.

Bertino, J. R., and Hillcoat, B. L. 1968. Regulation of dihydrofolate reductase and other folate-requiring enzymes. Adv. Enzyme Regul. *6*:335–349.

Bertino, J. R., Donohue, D. M., Simmons, B., Gabrio, B. W., Silber, R., and Huennekens, F. M. 1963a. The "induction" of dihydrofolic reductase activity in leukocytes and erythrocytes of patients treated with amethopterin. J. Clin. Invest. *42*:466–475.

Bertino, J. R., Silber, R., Freeman, M., Alenty, A., Albrecht, A., Gabrio, B. W., and Huennekens, F. M. 1963b. Studies on normal and leukemic leukocytes. IV. Tetrahydrofolate-dependent enzyme systems and dihydrofolic reductase. J. Clin. Invest. *42*:1899–1907.

Bertino, J. R., Cashmore, A., Fink, M., Calabresi, P., and Lefkowitz, E. 1965a. The "induction" of leukocyte and erythrocyte dihydrofolate reductase by methotrexate. II. Clinical and pharmacologic studies. Clin. Pharmacol. Ther. *6*:763–770.

Bertino, J. R., Perkins, J. P., and Johns, D. G. 1965b. Purification and properties of dihydrofolate reductase from Ehrlich ascites carcinoma cells. Biochemistry *4*:839–846.

Burton, E. G., and Sallach, H. J. 1975. Methylenetetrahydrofolate reductase in the rat central nervous system: intracellular and regional distribution. Arch. Biochem. Biophys. *166*:483–494.

Capco, G. R., and Mathews, C. K. 1973. Bacteriophage-coded thymidylate synthetase. Evidence that the T4 enzyme is a capsid protein. Arch. Biochem. Biophys. *158*:736–743.

Capco, G. R., Krupp, J. R., and Mathews, C. K. 1973. Bacteriophage-coded thymidylate synthetase: characteristics of the T4 and T5 enzymes. Arch. Biochem. Biophys. *158*:726–735.

Carpenter, N. J. 1974. Properties and inhibition of thymidylate synthetase in *Drosophila melanogaster*. J. Insect Physiol. *20*:1389–1401.

Chello, P. L., and Bertino, J. R. 1972. Effect of carboxypeptidase G_1 on levels of dihydrofolate reductase and N_{10} formyltetrahydrofolate synthetase in human 4265 leukemia cells in tissue culture. Proc. Am. Assoc. Cancer Res. *13*:89. (Abstract)

Conrad, A. H. 1971. Thymidylate synthetase activity in cultured mammalian cells. J. Biol. Chem. *246*:1318–1323.

Conrad, A. H., and Ruddle, F. H. 1972. Regulation of thymidylate synthetase activity in cultured mammalian cells. J. Cell. Sci. *10*:471–486.

Crusberg, T. C., Leary, R., and Kisliuk, R. L. 1970. Properties of thymidylate synthetase from dichloromethotrexate-resistant *Lactobacillus casei*. J. Biol. Chem. *245*:5292–5296.

Danenberg, P. V., and Heidelberger, C. 1974. Purification of thymidylate synthetase with 2'-deoxyuridylate-agarose. Methods Enzymol. *34*:520–523.

Danenberg, P. V., Langenbach, R. J., and Heidelberger, C. 1974. Structures of reversible and irreversible complexes of thymidylate synthetase and fluorinated pyrimidine nucleotides. Biochemistry *13*:926–933.

Delk, A. S., and Rabinowitz, J. C. 1974. Partial nucleotide sequence of a prokaryote initiator tRNA that functions in its non-formylated form. Nature *252*:106–109.

Delk, A. S., and Rabinowitz, J. C. 1975. Biosynthesis of ribosylthymine in the transfer RNA of *Streptococcus faecalis*: a folate-dependent methylation not involving S-adenosylmethionine. Proc. Natl. Acad. Sci. U.S.A. *72*:528–530.

D'Souza, L., and Friesheim, J. H. 1972. Circular dichroic studies of the interaction of dihydrofolate reductase with substrates, coenzymes, and inhibitors. Biochemistry *11*:3770–3774.

Dunlap, R. B., Harding, N. G. L., and Huennekens, F. M. 1971. Thymidylate synthetase from amethopterin-resistant *Lactobacillus casei*. Biochemistry *10*:88–97.

Finkelstein, J. D., Kyle, W. E., and Harris, B. J. 1971. Methionine metabolism in mammals. Regulation of homocysteine methyltransferases in rat tissue. Arch. Biochem. Biophys. *146*:84–92.

Fridland, A., Langenbach, R. J., and Heidelberger, C. 1971. Purification of thymidylate synthetase from Ehrlich ascites carcinoma cells. J. Biol. Chem. *246*:7110–7114.

Galivan, J., Maley, G. F., and Maley, F. 1974. Purification and properties of T2 bacteriophage-induced thymidylate synthetase. Biochemistry *13*:2282–2289.

Gauldie, J., Marshall, L., and Hillcoat, B. L. 1973. Purification and properties of dihydrofolate reductase from cultured mammalian cells. Biochem. J. *133*:349–356.

Gleisner, J. M., and Blakley, R. L. (In press). Eur. J. Biochem.

Gleisner, J. M., and Blakley, R. L. 1975. The structure of dihydrofolate reductase. I. Inactivation of bacterial dihydrofolate reductase concomitant with modification of a methionine residue at the active site. J. Biol. Chem. *250*:1580–1587.

Gleisner, J. M., Peterson, D. L., and Blakley, R. L. 1974. Amino-acid sequence of dihydrofolate reductase from a methotrexate-resistant mutant of *Streptococcus faecium* and identification of methionine residues at the inhibitor binding site. (dehydrogenases/homology/pyridine nucleotides.) Proc. Natl. Acad. Sci. U.S.A. *71*:3001–3005.

Greenfield, N. J. 1974. The effect of histidine modification on the activity of dihydrofolate reductase from a methotrexate-resistant strain of *Escherichia coli* B. Biochemistry *13*:4494–4500.

Greenfield, N. J., Williams, M. N., Poe, M., and Hoogsteen, K. 1972. Circular dichroism studies of dihydrofolate reductase from a methotrexate-resistant strain of *Escherichia coli*. Biochemistry *11*:4706–4711.

Gundersen, L. E., Dunlap, R. B., Harding, N. G. L., Freisheim, J. H., Otting, F., and Huennekens, F. M. 1972. Dihydrofolate reductase from amethopterin resistant *Lactobacillus casei*. Biochemistry *11*:1018–1023.

Hänggi, U. J., and Littlefield, J. W. 1974. Isolation and characterization of the multiple forms of dihydrofolate reductase from methotrexate-resistant hamster cells. J. Biol. Chem. *249*:1390–1397.

Harding, N. G., Martelli, M. F., and Huennekens, F. M. 1970. Amethopterin-induced changes in the multiple forms of dihydrofolate reductase from L1210 cells. Arch. Biochem. Biophys. *137*:295–296.

Hillcoat, B. L., Swett, V., and Bertino, J. R. 1967. Increase of dihydrofolate reductase activity in cultured mammalian cells after exposure to methotrexate. Proc. Natl. Acad. Sci. U.S.A. *58*:1632–1637.

Hillcoat, B. L., Marshall, L., and Patterson, J. 1973. Dihydrofolate reductase induced by folic acid in cultured human cells. Biochim. Biophys. Acta *293*:281–284.

Hsu, L. L., and Mandell, A. J. 1973. Multiple N-methyltransferases for aromatic alkylamines in brain. Life Sci. *13*:847–858.

Kallen, R. G., and Jencks, W. P. 1966. The mechanism of the condensation of formaldehyde with tetrahydrofolic acid. J. Biol. Chem. *241*:5851–5863.

Kalman, T. I. 1972. Inhibition of thymidylate synthetase by showdomycin and its 5'-phosphate. Biochem. Biophys. Res. Commun. *49*:1007–1013.

Kutzbach, C., and Stokstad, E. L. R. 1971. Mammalian methylenetetrahydrofolate reductase. Partial purification properties, and inhibition by S-adenosylmethionine. Biochim. Biophys. Acta *250*:459–477.

Laduron, P. M. 1972. N-methylation of dopamine to epinine in brain tissue using N-methyltetrahydrofolic acid as the methyl donor. Nature New Biol. *238*:212–213.

Laduron, P. M., Gommeren, W. R., and Leysen, J. E. 1974. *N*-methylation of biogenic amines. I. Characterization and properties of an *N*-methyltransferase in rat brain using 5-methyltetrahydrofolic acid as the methyl donor. Biochem. Pharmacol. *23*:1599–1608.

Langenbach, R. J., Danenberg, P. V., and Heidelberger, C. 1972. Thymidylate synthetase: mechanism of inhibition by 5-fluoro-2'-deoxyuridylate. Biochem. Biophys. Res. Commun. *48*:1565–1571.

Leary, R. P., and Kisliuk, R. L. 1971. Crystalline thymidylate synthetase from duchloromethotrexate resistant *Lactobacillus casei*. Prep. Biochem. *1*:47–54.

Leysen, J., and Laduron, P. 1974. Characterization of an enzyme yielding formaldehyde from 5-methyltetrahydrofolic acid. FEBS Lett. *47*:299–303.

Liu, J. K., and Dunlap, R. B. 1974. Implication of a tryptophyl residue in the active site of dihydrofolate reductase. Biochemistry *13*:1807–1814.

Loeble, R. B., and Dunlap, R. B. 1972. Characterization of the subunits of thymidylate synthetase. Biochem. Biophys. Res. Commun. *49*:1671–1677.

McCuen, R. W., and Sirotnak, F. M. 1975. Thymidylate synthetase from diplococcus pneumoniae. Properties and inhibition by folate analogs. Biochim. Biophys. Acta *384*:369–380.

Nichol, C. A. 1968. Studies on dihydrofolate reductase related to the drug sensitivity of microbial and neoplastic cells. Adv. Enzyme Regul. *6*:305–322.

Nixon, P. F., and Blakley, R. L. 1968. Dihydrofolate reductase of *Streptococcus faecium*. II. Purification and some properties of two dihydrofolate reductases from the amethopterin-resistant mutant, *Streptococcus faecium* var. *Durans* strain A. J. Biol. Chem. *243*:4722–4731.

Otting, F., and Huennekens, F. M. 1972. TPNH-dependent binding of amethopterin by dihydrofolate reductase from *Lactobacillus casei*. Arch. Biochem. Biophys. *152*:429–431.

Pastore, E. J., Kisliuk, R. L., Plante, L. T., Wright, J. M., and Kaplan, N. O. 1974. Conformational changes induced in dihydrofolate reductase by folates, pyridine nucleotide coenzymes, and methotrexate (220 MHz proton magnetic resonance/antifolates/ligand binding). Proc. Natl. Acad. Sci. U.S.A. *71*:3849–3853.

Perry, J., and Chanarin, I. 1973. Formylation of folate as step in physiological folate absorption. Br. Med. J. *2*:588–589.

Peterson, D. L., Gleisner, J. M., and Blakley, R. L. (In press). Biochemistry.

Poe, M., Greenfield, N. J., and Williams, M. N. 1974. Dihydrofolate reductase from a methotrexate-resistant *Escherichia coli*. Binding of pyridine nucleotides as monitored by ultraviolet difference spectroscopy. J. Biol. Chem. *249*:2710–2716.

Pogolotti, A. L., Jr., and Santi, D. V. 1974. Model studies of the thymidylate synthetase reaction. Nucleophilic displacement of 5-*p*-nitrophenoxymethyluracils. Biochemistry *13*:456–466.

Rauen, H. M. 1957. Transformylierungen und Transoxymethylierungen. I. Allgemeine Reaktionsbedingungen und Formyldonatoren der aeroben N¹⁰-Formyl ierung der Pteroylglutaminsäure. Biochem. Z. *328*:562–575.

Roberts, G. C. K., Feeney, J., Burgen, A. S. V., Yuferov, V., Dann, J. G., and Bjur, R. 1974. Nuclear magnetic resonance studies of the binding of substrate analogs and coenzyme to dihydrofolate reductase from *Lactobacillus casei*. Biochemistry *13*:5351–5357.

Rosenblatt, D. S., and Erbe, R. W. 1973. Reciprocal changes in the levels of functionally related folate enzymes during the culture cycle in human fibroblasts. Biochem. Biophys. Res. Commun. *54*:1627–1633.

Rosenberg, R. N., Vandeventer, L., Francesco, L. D., and Friedkin, M. E. 1971. Regulation of the synthesis of choline-O-acetyltransferase and thymidylate synthetase in mouse neuroblastoma in cell culture (confluent cells/rapidly-dividing cells/specific activity). Proc. Natl. Acad. Sci. U.S.A. *68*:1436–1440.

Rowe, P. B., and Lewis, G. P. 1973. Mammalian folate metabolism. Regulation of folate interconversion enzymes. Biochemistry *12*:1962–1969.

Samuel, C. E., and Rabinowitz, J. C. 1974. Initiation of protein synthesis by folate-sufficient and folate-deficient *Streptococcus faecalis* R. Biochemical and biophysical properties of methionine transfer ribonucleic acid. J. Biol. Chem. *249*:1198–1206.

Samuel, C. E., D'Ari, L., and Rabinowitz, J. C. 1970. Evidence against the folate-mediated formylation of formyl-accepting methionyl transfer ribonucleic acid in *Streptococcus faecalis* R. J. Biol. Chem. *245*:5115–5121.

Samuel, C. E., Murray, C. L., and Rabinowitz, J. C. 1972. Methionine transfer ribonucleic acid from folate-sufficient and folate-deficient *Streptococcus faecalis* R. J. Biol. Chem. *247*:6856–6865.

Santi, D. V., and Brewer, C. F. 1973. Model studies of thymidylate synthetase. Intramolecular catalysis of 5-hydrogen exchange and 5-hydroxymethylation of 1-substituted uracils. Biochemistry *12*:2416–2424.

Santi, D. V., and McHenry, C. S. 1972. 5-fluoro-2'-deoxyuridylate: covalent complex with thymidylate synthetase (affinity labeling/enzyme mechanism/inhibition/ fluorinated pyrimidines). Proc. Natl. Acad. Sci. U.S.A. 69:1855–1857.

Santi, D. V., McHenry, C. S., and Perriard, E. R. 1974a. A filter assay for thymidylate synthetase using 5-fluoro-2'-deoxyuridylate as an active site titrant. Biochemistry *13*:467–470.

Santi, D. V., McHenry, C. S., and Sommer, H. 1974b. Mechanism of interaction of thymidylate synthetase with 5-fluorodeoxyuridylate. Biochemistry *13*:471–480.

Schirch, L., and Ropp, M. 1967. Serine transhydroxymethylase. Affinity of tetrahydrofolate compounds for the enzyme and enzyme-glycine complex. Biochemistry *6*:253–257.

Silber, R., and Mansouri, A. 1971. Regulation of folate-dependent enzymes. Ann. N.Y. Acad. Sci. *186*:55–69.

Sommer, H., and Santi, D. V. 1974. Purification and amino acid analysis of an active site peptide from thymidylate synthetase containing covalently bound 5-fluoro-2'-deoxyuridylate and methylenetetrahydrofolate. Biochem. Biophys. Res. Commun. *57*:689–695.

Stifel, F. B., Herman, R. H., and Rosensweig, N. S. 1970. Dietary regulation of glycolytic enzymes. VII. Effect of diet and oral folate upon folate-metabolizing enzymes in rat jejunum. Biochim. Biophys. Acta *208*:381–386.

Urso-Scott, M. D., Uhoch, J., and Bertino, J. R. 1974. Formation of 10-formylfolic acid, a potent inhibitor of dihydrofolate reductase, in rat liver slices incubated with folic acid (folate metabolism/folate coenzymes/natural folate enzyme inhibitors/regulation). Proc. Natl. Acad. Sci. U.S.A. *71*:2736–2739.

Warwick, P. E., and Freisheim, J. H. 1975. Modification of the cysteine residue of streptococcal dihydrofolate reductase. Biochemistry 14:664.

Warwick, P. E., D'Souza, L., and Freisheim, J. H. 1972. Role of tryptophan in dihydrofolate reductase. Biochemistry *11*:3775–3779.

Whiteley, J. M., Jerkunica, I., and Deits, T. 1974a. Affinity chromatography of thymidylate synthetases using 5-fluoro-2'-deoxyuridine 5'-phosphate derivatives of sepharose. Adv. Exp. Med. Biol. *42*:135–146.

Whiteley, J. M., Jerkunica, I., and Deits, T. 1974b. Thymidylate synthetase from amethopterin-resistant *Lactobacillus casei*. Purification by affinity chromatography. Biochemistry *13*:2044–2050.

Williams, M. N. 1975. Effect of N-bromosuccinimide modification on dihydrofolate reductase from a methotrexate-resistant strain of *Escherichia coli*. Activity, spectrophotometric, fluorescence, and circular dichroism studies. J. Biol. Chem. *250*:322–330.

Williams, M. N., Greenfield, N. J., and Hoogsteen, K. 1973a. Evidence for two reduced triphosphopyridine nucleotide binding sites on dihydrofolate reductase from a methotrexate-resistant strain of *Escherichia coli*. J. Biol. Chem. *248*:6380–6386.

Williams, M. N., Poe, M., Greenfield, N. J., Hirshfield, J. M., and Hoogsteen, K. 1973b. Methotrexate binding to dihydrofolate reductase from a methotrexate-resistant strain of *Escherichia coli*. J. Biol. Chem. *248*:6375–6379.

3

Studies on the
Biological Role of Folic
Acid Polyglutamates

CARLOS L. KRUMDIECK, PHILLIP E. CORNWELL,
RONALD W. THOMPSON, *and* WILLIAM E. WHITE, JR.

The biological importance of the polyglutamyl side chain of the folates is indicated by the universality of its occurrence and by the fact that during evolution the ability to synthesize the peptide side chain has been retained, even by organisms that have lost the machinery for folic acid synthesis. Loss of the polyglutamate-synthesizing system indeed represents a serious survival handicap—as recently demonstrated by McBurney and Whitmore (1974a, 1974b). These authors have produced mutants of Chinese hamster ovary cells that have a requirement for purines, glycine, and thymidine and have demonstrated that the metabolic lesion resulting in these abnormalities resides in an inability to make folyl-polyglutamates. The way in which the absence of the polyglutamates results in impaired purine, glycine, and thymidine synthesis is, however, not clearly understood. We thus have compelling evidence of the importance of the biological role of the polygluta- mates but an incomplete understanding of what the role itself may be.

Some years ago we postulated that the peptide chain of naturally occurring folates serves a role in the regulation of one-carbon metabolism. At least three mechanisms by which the peptidyl side chain could effect a regulatory action were envisioned:

1. By affecting the passage of the coenzymes across biological membranes. The presence of the proper folate coenzyme, at the necessary concentration and at a given moment inside a cell or subcellular organelle, could be determined by the ability of the coenzymes to permeate the required membranes. Since the length of the polyglutamyl chain affects the passage of folates across cell membranes, a key regulatory function is proposed for the conjugases (pteroyl–polyglutamyl–carboxy peptidases) as likely modifiers of coenzyme distribution and transport.

2. By determining enzyme–coenzyme specificity. The recognition by a given enzyme of its proper coenzyme–one-carbon-fragment complex may be dictated by the length of the polyglutamyl chain and/or modifications of it.

3. By exerting activating or inhibitory effects (allosteric?) on enzymes directly or indirectly related to one-carbon metabolism.

There is now considerable evidence in support of each of these three possible mechanisms, which, it must be noted, are not mutually exclusive and may indeed operate simultaneously. The point to emphasize here is that whatever the mechanisms involved, if regulation of one-carbon metabolism is indeed the role of the polyglutamates, it should be possible to demonstrate changes occurring *in vivo* in the composition of folate polyglutamates and in the activities of the enzymes responsible for their degradation and synthesis under circumstances that require alterations in the steady state of one-carbon metabolism.

We wish to report here the results of experiments designed to detect such *in vivo* changes.

The first experimental model we examined was the normally cycling rat uterus. The choice of model was based on a number of reported observations suggesting that the regulation of cellular proliferation in the uterus, brought about by steroid hormones, may be mediated through systems involving folate coenzymes. Whitehead *et al.* (1973) described "megaloblastic" abnormalities in cervico–vaginal cells in a significant number of women taking progestogens for the purpose of fertility control. These abnormalities, which are thought to represent an impairment in DNA synthesis, were corrected by administration of folic acid. None of the affected individuals had any evidence of folate or B_{12} deficiency, which led the authors to postulate a *localized* interference with folate metabolism at the target-organ level. A number of recent reports from Italy have appeared concerning the nature of the folate coenzymes in rat uterus and their relation to hormonal stimulation. Laffi *et al.* (1972) observed that castration produced a decrease in the N^{10}-formyltetrahydrofolate content of the uterus, and they were able to prevent this effect by the administration of estradiol 17β. Tolomelli *et al.* (1972) and Bovina *et al.* (1971) extended these studies to show that castration produced a reduction in the activity of several liver enzymes requiring folate cofactors and that this effect could be partially reversed by estrogen administration.

In all of these studies, no attention was given either to the poly-γ-glutamyl side chain of these coenzymes or to the activity of the conjugases. This seemed an important omission since there is now considerable evidence that coenzyme activity is influenced greatly by the length of the gamma glutamyl side chain of folates and not only by the nature of the substituents in the pteroyl moiety. For example, Friedkin *et al.* (1971) have shown that 5-formyl tetrahydropteroyl-polyglutamate is one hundred times as inhibitory as 5-formyl tetrahydropteroyl-monoglutamate for a purified preparation of *E. coli* thymidylate synthetase, and Kisliuk *et al.* (1974) have shown that unsubstituted oxidized, dihydro, and tetrahydro forms of pteroyl-polyglutamates are powerful inhibitors of *L. casei* thymidylate synthetase. One can envision that the activity of thymidylate synthetase could be subjected to tight regulation by the ratio of two forms of folates, one being the N^{5-10}-methylenetetrahydrofolate, the required coenzyme, and the other an inhibitory polyglutamyl derivative whose removal would enhance the enzyme's activity. The latter role would be assigned to the conjugases.

Finally, the fact that estrogens stimulate resting cells in target tissues to initiate DNA synthesis, whereas progestogens tend to inhibit further progress through the mitotic cycle in estrogen-stimulated cells (O'Malley and Means, 1974), led us to the idea that the normally cycling uterus, with its alternating periods of cell division and arrest, would provide a good model to test the hypothesis that polyglutamates of folic acid and the conjugases may participate in the regulation of cell multiplication. Consequently, we determined conjugase activity (Krumdieck and Baugh, 1970) and folate levels before and after conjugase treatment in uteri obtained at various states of the estrous cycle.

As shown in Figure 3-1, there is a pronounced elevation of conjugase activity during proestrus, the time of maximal estrogen secretion. The total activity in the organ reaches values approximately three times as great as those observed at any other stage in the cycle. The increase in

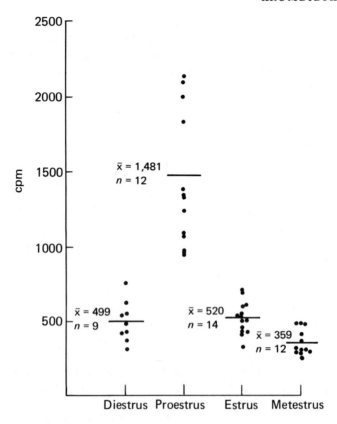

FIGURE 3-1 Conjugase activity (per half organ) in rat uteri at various stages of the estrous cycle. Expressed as radioactivity liberated by enzyme action from a synthetic substrate: pteroyl-(γ-glutamyl)$_2$-U-^{14}C glutamic acid. Specific activity, 0.35 μCi/μmol in 10-min incubations. Probability of difference between activity at proestrus and all other stages <0.001.

conjugase activity is not due to an increase in plasma conjugase resulting from the marked vascular congestion of the organ at that stage, nor is it due to the presence of conjugase activity in the fluid filling the uterine cavity during proestrus, since there is no activity in this fluid. The highest conjugase activity found in plasma could not account for the increase in uterine activity at proestrus, even assuming that the total weight gained by the organ in passing from metestrus to proestrus was due to plasma alone. Furthermore, we have shown that the conjugase activity of the uterus of castrated rats is significantly increased some 12 to 20 h after the administration of physiologic doses of estradiol 17β, (Krumdieck *et al.*, 1975).

Coinciding with the elevation of conjugase activity, there is an increase in the folate content of the organ (Figure 3-2). It was also observed that the concentration of "free folate" (assayable prior to conjugase treatment) reached its highest value during proestrus, together with the peak of conjugase activity. However, this observation is subject to revision since it may be an artifact resulting from the action of the uterine conjugase itself during the process of extraction of the folates and may not therefore represent the levels of free folates occurring *in vivo* (Krumdieck *et al.*, 1975).

A key question posed by these experiments is whether or not the changes observed are general and occur in other systems whenever there is a cycle of cell multiplication. In attempting to answer this question, we realized that the outstanding characteristic of the normally cycling uterus model is that it contains a population of cells that, almost in synchrony, goes through rapid periods of growth and arrest. Tissues that grow continuously in a nonsynchronous fashion would not

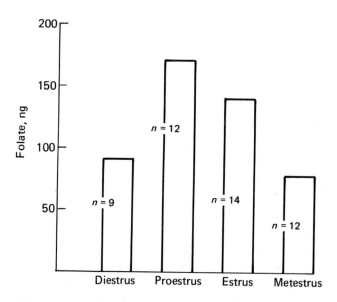

FIGURE 3-2   Total folates (nanograms per half organ) in rat uteri at various stages of the estrous cycle. (*L. casei* assays after hog kidney conjugase treatment).

be suitable models since the chain length of the polyglutamates and the levels of conjugase activity at any one time would be a constant composite of the patterns present in cells at many stages of their life cycle. It thus seemed necessary to study synchronous biological systems or to introduce experimental changes such that all (or most) of the cells in the system would abruptly be put to a new task requiring a shift in direction of one-carbon metabolism.

One of us, P. E. Cornwell, suggested the use of the acellular slime mold *Physarum polycephalum.* This organism posesses a complex life cycle that includes a macroplasmodial stage during which it grows as a synchronous syncytium where all the nuclei (about 100×10^6 in a large macroplasmodium) undergo mitosis within 5 to 10 min approximately every 8 h. Furthermore, the organism can be made to differentiate into two different resting stages, sporangia and sclerotium; the former leads to spore formation and a cycle of sexual reproduction, and the latter represents a partition of the syncytium into multiple, discrete, fully walled fragments containing one or a few nuclei. *P. polycephalum* does not require folic acid in the culture medium, but it does efficiently incorporate labeled folate.

To study the folates during the periods of synchronous growth and differentiation, we have adopted the experimental design shown in Figure 3-3. The nonsynchronous microplasmodia are grown in the presence of $[2\text{-}^{14}C]$folic acid, washed, and coalesced into synchronous macroplasmodia (Guttes and Guttes, 1964), which are then allowed to go through two synchronous mitoses (in medium with no radioactive folate) before harvesting. The stage of the cell cycle is determined with a phase-contrast microscope following the morphological changes of the nucleus, as described by Guttes and Guttes (1964). At the appropriate time, the plasmodia are harvested, and an aliquot is homogenized in water for protein and conjugase activity determinations, while the rest of the organisms are dropped in 1% ascorbate (pH 6.0) at 95° C and extracted for 10 min. An aliquot of the extract is bioassayed before and after hog kidney conjugase treatment, and another aliquot is chromatographed in a DEAE–BioGel A column eluted with a linear gradient of 0.01 M 2-mercaptoethanol to 0.5 M NaCl in 0.01 M 2-mercaptoethanol (1 liter each). The resulting fractions are counted and bioassayed with *L. casei* and *S. faecalis* before and after conjugase treatment. Essentially the same approach was followed with the differentiated forms (sclerotia and sporangia) that were obtained by starvation and starvation-plus-illumination respectively, as described by Daniel and Baldwin (1964). Preliminary results (See Figures 3-4 and 3-5) indicate that during periods of growth (micro- and macroplas-

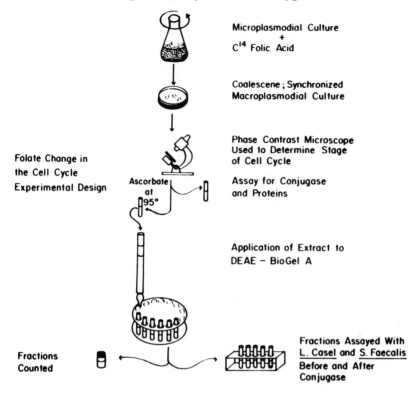

FIGURE 3-3 Changes in folates during the cell cycle of *Physarum polycephalum*. Experimental design (see text).

modia) the folates of *P. polycephalum* are predominantly pteroyl-mono- (or perhaps di-) glutamates capable of supporting both *L. casei* and *S. faecalis* before conjugase treatment. A smaller peak of poly-glutamates (fractions 200–220) is always found in the extracts of the nonsynchronous microplasmodia and in macroplasmodial extracts obtained shortly before or after mitosis. In mid-interphase (about 4 h after mitosis), however, the polyglutamyl peak is greatly reduced in size. In keeping with the chromatographic patterns, the ratios of *L. casei* activity (after/before conjugase treatment) of the crude extracts vary from a low of 1.002 at interphase to a maximum of 1.66 shortly before the onset of prophase.

In marked contrast with the low proportion of polyglutamates found during the growth stages, both of the differentiated survival forms contain mostly polyglutamates. In fact, sporangia contain extremely

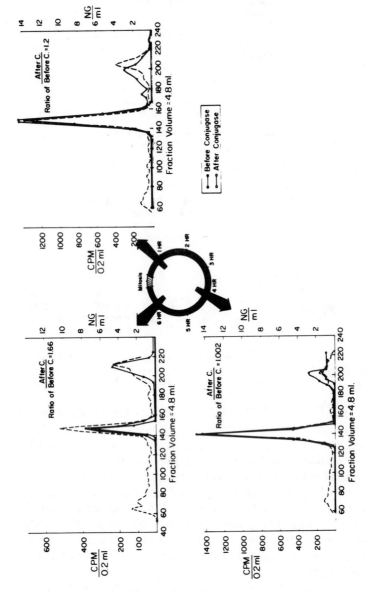

FIGURE 3-4 Folate changes during the cell cycle in synchronous macroplasmodia of *Physarum polycephalum*. – – –, Radioactivity; ●, microbiological activity before hog kidney conjugase; O, microbiological activity after hog kidney conjugase. Ratios of after conjugase/before conjugase were determined in the crude extracts prior to chromatography.

32

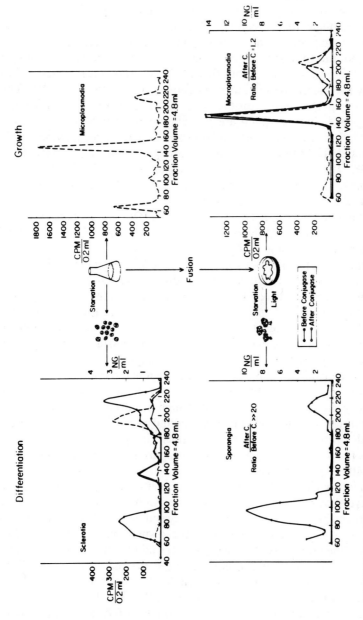

FIGURE 3-5 Folate patterns during growth (micro- and macroplasmodia) and differentiation (sclerotia and sporangia) of *Physarum polycephalum*. Symbols are as in Figure 3-4. No radioactive label was present in the sporangia experiment.

33

low amounts of free folates. Most of the polyglutamates of both sclerotia and sporangia occur in a peak that elutes from the column before the free folates together with a large peak of uv-absorbing material thought to be protein. If the material in this peak is treated with conjugase and rechromatographed, the biological activity separates from the uv-absorbing material and elutes in the position of free folate. It is interesting to note that in the sclerotia most of the radioactivity is concentrated in one peak eluting in fractions 185 to 210. The microbiological activity, on the other hand, appears in at least three major peaks, two of which are polyglutamates (fractions 60–100 and 208–228) that must have been synthesized *de novo* since they bear little or no label. The same applies to the monoglutamate eluted in fractions 130–148. The levels of conjugase activity seem to be lowest in the sporangia. However, with the limited data available we cannot yet discern any pattern of variation during the cell cycle.

The above experiments indicate that some major changes in the polyglutamyl chain of folates accompany the events of cell multiplication and differentiation in *Physarum polycephalum*. In both of these fundamental cellular processes, the synthesis of nucleic acids constitutes an essential component emphasizing the need to study the role of the polyglutamates as coenzymes of purine biosynthesis—an aspect of folate biochemistry that has been sorely neglected. Elucidation of the role of the polyglutamates in purine biosynthesis will undoubtedly require cell-free work; we feel, however, that considerable insight can be gained by studying changes in the composition of tissue folates under circumstances capable of producing a marked increase in purine biosynthesis. Such an increase can be produced in the liver of an uricotelic animal by feeding it a diet high in nitrogen, thereby forcing the synthesis of uric acid. Featherston and Scholz (1968) have demonstrated an approximate fivefold increase in uric acid production in chicks fed a 75 percent protein diet compared to a control group fed a diet with 25 percent protein.

Similar experiments using Japanese quail (*Coturnix coturnix japonica*) have shown that this species tolerates well a diet having as much as 88 percent protein (Featherston and Freedland, 1973). This fact, together with the ease of handling of these small birds, led us to select them for the present study. Two groups of adult male quail were fed for two weeks with a "low protein" (25 percent) and "high protein" (88 percent) isocaloric diet as described by Featherston and Freedland (1973). Two days prior to sacrifice, each animal received an intramuscular injection of 3′, 5′, 9(n) ^{3}H-labeled folic acid (8 μCi/100g; specific activity, 26 Ci/mmol). At sacrifice, the livers were rapidly removed and weighed, and an aliquot was set aside for conjugase and protein determinations. The remaining tissue was sliced and dropped into a homogenizer containing 1% ascorbate (pH 6.0) at 95° C. The extracts were assayed as in the Physarum experiments and chromatographed on a DEAE–cellulose column (1.0 × 92 cm) eluted with a linear gradient of NaCl in 0.01 M 2 mercaptoethanol (0.0 → 1.0 M NaCl, 1 liter each). Figure 3-6 shows the *L. casei* activity/milligram of wet weight before and after conjugase treatment of the livers of the high and low protein groups. The folate content/milligram of liver approximately doubles. All the change is due to an increase in the polyglutamates. Since there is also a considerable increase in the weights of the livers of the high protein group (2,411 ± 136 mg versus 1.993 ± 344 mg) a comparison of the total folate content of the livers makes the difference even larger. The conjugase activities of the two groups is shown in Figure 3-7. Although a two-tailed "t" test comparison of the means gave a relatively high P value (<0.1), the difference in conjugase activity is probably real. Nearly all of the folates were active for *S. faecalis*, indicating a low content of N^5-methyl forms in the liver of this species. These results are in contrast with those of Noronha and Silverman (1962), who found that chicken liver folates are made up

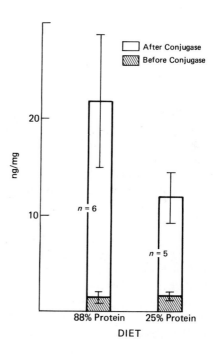

FIGURE 3-6 *L. casei* activity before and after conjugase treatment of liver extracts ($\bar{x} \pm \sigma$) of Japanese quail maintained for 2 weeks on a "high" (88%) and "low" (25%) protein intake (see text).

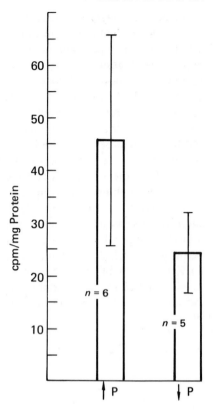

FIGURE 3-7 Conjugase activity (per milligram of protein) in liver homogenates of Japanese quail maintained for 2 weeks on a "high" (88% ↑ P) and "low" (25% ↓ P) protein intake (see text). $\bar{x} \pm \sigma$; P < 0.10.

predominantly of N^5-methylpolyglutamates. It is interesting to consider that, if a significant fraction of the liver folates is committed to purine (uric acid) synthesis, *S. faecalis* active forms should predominate.

The tritium-labeled folic acid was used to allow degradation of the folyl polyglutamates to polyglutamates of *p*-amino benzoic acid and estimation of chain length. These results are not yet available for presentation.

The above experiments show that conditions leading to increased purine synthesis result in elevations of both conjugase and the polyglutamyl fraction of liver folates. We are very much aware, however, that the changes observed may not be solely due to the increased requirement for purine biosynthesis but must also reflect the overloading of pathways of amino acid metabolism involving one-carbon fragments. Regardless, the fact remains that adaptation to a high protein intake, which must imply some drastic changes in the steady state of one-carbon metabolism, *does* result in changes in the polyglutamates and in conjugase activity.

Finally we wish to report on the inhibitory effect of folate polygluta- mates on the enzyme glutamate dehydrogenase (1.4.1.2). This ubiqui- tous enzyme plays a central role in amino acid metabolism and is notorious for the large number of effectors that modify its activity. Some years ago Vogel *et al.* (1964) reported that folic acid, as well as aminopterin and methotrexate, was an inhibitor of glutamic dehydro- genase, but they did not report whether the inhibition results from binding of the pteridine ring, the *p*-aminobenzoyl moiety, or the terminal glutamate. We have examined these questions as well as the role of the poly-γ-glutamyl chain using synthetic polyglutamates (Krumdieck and Baugh, 1969). Lineweaver–Burke plots showed that folic acid and methotrexate are competitive inhibitors of the glutamate site with K_i values of 5×10^{-4} and 7×10^{-4} M, respectively. No inhibition was observed for pteroic acid up to a concentration of 3×10^{-4} M, suggesting that folate binding occurs from the glutamyl end of the molecule. The number of glutamic acid residues in the poly- glutamates significantly affects inhibition (see Figures 3-8 and 3-9). The inhibitory activity increases with chain length up to three to five residues. Secondary effects due to binding of the pteridine ring are demonstrated by the lesser inhibitory activity of the polyglutamates of *p*-amino benzoic acid as well as by the difference in inhibition observed between oxidized and tetrahydrofolates.

The biological significance of these findings is unknown. However, it is interesting that the activity of this important enzyme, which does not require a folate coenzyme, is affected in varying degrees by folyl- polyglutamates of different chain lengths.

In summary, we have presented evidence that conjugase activity increases *in vivo* as a result of physiologically or experimentally induced hormonal stimulation of a target tissue, as well as by the institution of dietary changes necessitating at least a quantitative readjustment in the steady state of one-carbon metabolism. Coinciding with this, we have observed marked elevations of the folate content of the tissues examined.

Studies of the folates of *Physarum polycephalum* at various stages of its life cycle indicate a marked predominance of free folates in the exponentially growing stages with a drastic change to a preponderance of polyglutamyl forms accompanying differentiation to dormant stages. Furthermore, during synchronous growth, subtle changes occur in the ratio of free to polyglutamyl forms; the latter increase shortly before

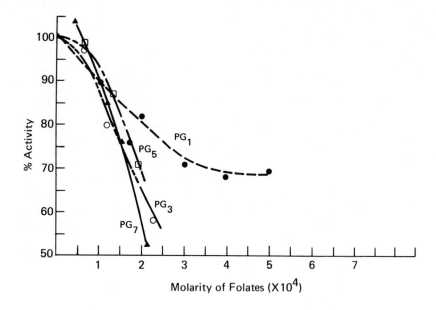

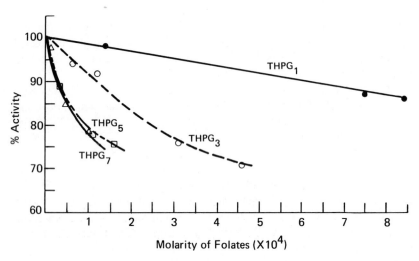

FIGURE 3-8   Inhibition of glutamic dehydrogenase by polyglutamates of folic acid (top) and tetrahydrofolic acid (bottom).

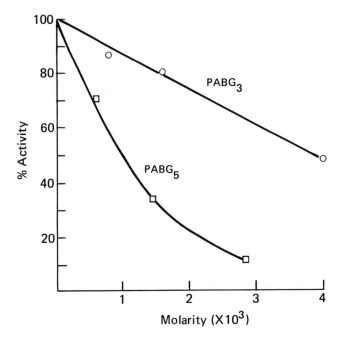

FIGURE 3-9   Inhibition of glutamic dehydrogenase by polyglutamates of *p*-aminobenzoic acid.

mitosis and diminish at mid-interphase. An inhibitory effect of folyl-
polyglutamates on the non-folate-requiring enzyme glutamate dehydrogenase has been observed.

These *in vitro* effects and *in vivo* changes of the folate polyglutamates and of the activity of the enzyme effecting their degradation
provide support for the hypothesis that the peptide chain of the
naturally occurring folates serves a role in the regulation of one-carbon
metabolism.

ACKNOWLEDGMENTS

The technical assistance of Jeannette Krumdieck is gratefully acknowl-
edged.

This work was supported by NIH grant 5-RO1-AM-08644 and NSF grant
BMS 74-17348.

TABLE 3-1   Rat Uterine Folates (*L. casei* Assay), ng/half organ

Phase	Free	Total	Total[a]/Free
Diestrus (n[b] = 9)	11.5	111.21	9.76
Proestrus (n = 15)	20.17	149.6	7.44
Estrus (n = 9)	15.4	134.8	8.88
Metestrus (n = 10)	12.08	102.42	8.63

[a]Significance of differences in ratios: diestrus versus proestrus, $P < 0.01$; estrus versus proestrus, $P < 0.02$; diestrus versus estrus, not significant; proestrus versus metestrus, $P < 0.02$; diestrus versus metestrus, $P < 0.05$; estrus versus metestrus, not significant.
[b]n = number of animals.

ADDENDUM

Since submission of this manuscript, a series of experiments has been concluded indicating that the ratio of total/free folates (*L. casei* activity after/before hog kidney conjugase treatment) decreases during proestrus. In these experiments stringent precautions were taken to inactivate rapidly the uterine conjugase and avoid an artifactual elevation of the "free" folates. The results obtained are summarized in Table 3-1.

These results suggest that the conjugases do act *in vivo* to modify the chain length of the polyglutamates. Furthermore, it must be noted that the ratios of total/free folates determined by *L. casei* assay before and after conjugase treatment would not be altered by shortening of the polyglutamate chain from, for example, seven to five glutamyl residues.

DISCUSSION

HOFFBRAND: In your rat uterus preparation do you note other lysosomal enzymes increase proestrus? Are there other lysosomal enzymes? Your folic conjugase might be something specific for folate metabolism, but it might also be just an increase in lysosomes at that stage of the cell cycle, and this is a lysosomal enzyme. You might just get a rise, as you would with any other massive hydrolase.

KRUMDIECK: I do not know. We have not looked at other enzymes. One thing is important. The duration of the proestrus is rather brief, about 10 h. So, it is hard to imagine that very large changes in the number of cells are taking place. We think it is primarily a change in the activity of the enzyme of the cells that are there at the time.

HOFFBRAND: Do you think that the folate conjugase increase is in fact regulating the size of the polyglutamates? If this is true, it would have to mean that either the conjugase is coming out of the lysosome to do it, or that the folates were going into the lysosomes to be deconjugated in a viable cell. Is there any evidence that that could take place? That there could be movement inside the cell while it is still viable?

KRUMDIECK: I have no idea.

ROSENBERG: I think that perhaps a word of caution is worthwhile here. Much of the work indicating a lysosomal location for conjugase has been limited to studies which may not be necessarily generalizable to all tissues. There has also been evidence of folic conjugase in the cytosol that may or may not have originated from the lysosome. Certainly, there are plenty of precedents where one could suggest a possibility that there might be enzymes in lysosomes, e.g., cathepsins, peptidases, etc. I think it is a very important issue, in terms of regulation of cellular polyglutamate, as to where the enzymes may be, and I do not think that we should lock ourselves into the notion that all these enzymes are lysosomal.

LITERATURE CITED

Bovina, C., Tolomelli, B., Rovinetti, C., and Marchetti, M. 1971. Effect of estradiol on folate coenzymes in the rat. Int. J. Vitam. Nutr. Res. *41*:453.

Daniel, J. W., and Baldwin, H. H. 1964. Methods of culture for plasmodial myxomycetes, p. 9, *in* Methods in cell physiology, H. M. Prescott, ed., Vol. I. Academy Press Inc., New York.

Featherston, W. R., and Freedland, R. A. 1973. "Influence of dietary protein and carbohydrate levels on liver enzyme activities in quail. J. Nutr. *103*:625.

Featherston, W. R., and Scholz, R. W. 1968. Changes in liver xanthine dehydrogenase and uric acid excretion in chicks during adaptation to a high protein diet. J. Nutr. *95*:393.

Freidkin, M., Crawford, E. J., and Plante, L. T. 1971. Empirical vs. rational approaches in cancer chemotherapy. Ann. N.Y. Acad. Sci. *186*:209.

Guttes, E., and Guttes, S. 1964. Mitotic synchrony in the plasmodia of *Physarum polycephalum* and mitotic synchronization by coalescence of microplasmodia, p. 43, *in* Methods in Cell Physiology, H. M. Prescott, ed., Vol. I. Academic Press Inc., New York.

Kisliuk, R. L., Gaumont, Y., and Baugh, C. M. 1974. Polyglutamyl derivatives of folate as substrates and inhibitors of thymidylate synthetase. J. Biol. Chem. *249*:4100.

Krumdieck, C. L., and Baugh, C. M. 1969. The solid-phase synthesis of polyglutamates of folic acid. Biochemistry *8*:1568.

Krumdieck, C. L., and Baugh, C. M. 1970. Radioactive assay of folic acid polyglutamate conjugase(s). Anal. Biochem. *35*:123.

Krumdieck, C. L., Boots, L. R., Cornwell, P. E., and Butterworth, C. E., Jr. 1975. Estrogen stimulation of conjugase activity in the uterus of ovariectomized rats. Am. J. Clin. Nutr. *28*:530.

Laffi, R., Tolomelli, B., Bovina, C., and Marchetti, M. 1972. Influence of short-term treatment with estradiol-17β on folate metabolism in the rat. Int. J. Vitam. Nutr. Res. *42*:196.

McBurney, M. W., and Whitmore, G. F. 1974a. Characterization of a Chinese hamster cell with a temperature-sensitive mutation in folate metabolism. Cell *2*:183.

McBurney, M. W., and Whitmore, G. F. 1974b. Isolation and biochemical characterization of folate deficient mutants of Chinese hamster cells. Cell 2:173.

Noronha, J. M., and Silverman, M. 1962. Distribution of folic acid derivatives in natural material. J. Biol. Chem. 237:3299.

O'Malley, B. W., and Means, A. R. 1974. Female steroid hormones and target cell nuclei. Science 183:610.

Tolomelli, B., Bovina, C., Rovinetti, C., and Marchetti, M. 1972. Folate coenzyme metabolism in the castrated rat and treated with 17β-estradiol. Proc. Soc. Exp. Biol. Med. 141:436.

Vogel, W. H., Snyder, R., and Schulman, M. P. 1964. The inhibition of dehydrogenases by folic acid and several of its analogues. Biochem. Biophys. Res. Commun. 10:97.

Whitehead, N., Reyner, F., and Lindenbaum, J. 1973. Megaloblastic changes in cervical epithelium; association with oral contraceptive therapy and reversal with folic acid. J. Am. Med. Assoc. 226:1421.

4

Folate Polyglutamyl Chain Length of Mammalian and Bacterial Cells

JOHN M. SCOTT

In the course of characterization of one of the original folate* isolates, it became apparent that yeast folate, although it was active as an antianaemia factor in the chick, was not active for *Lactobacillus casei* or *Streptococcus faecalis* (Binkley *et al.*, 1944). Further studies explained this discrepancy, showing that yeast folate, when isolated, existed "conjugated" to a polyglutamyl chain. Deconjugation with γ-glutamyl-carboxypeptidase ("conjugase") resulted in the loss of some of the glutamyl residues, and a microbiologically active vitamin was the product (Pfiffner *et al.*, 1946). Since these early studies, this approach of showing increase in microbiologically assayable folate after conjugase treatment has been used to demonstrate the presence of folate polyglutamates in a vast range of cell types. However, these studies give no information as to the number of glutamyl residues

---

*The name folate is used according to the IUPAC–IUB rules (Biochim. Biophys. Acta 107:11–12, 1965). It is the general term for any form of the vitamin without reference to state of reduction, degree of substitution, or number of glutamates. Thus folate heptaglutamate in this context would have a *total* of seven glutamyl residues attached.

43

present, merely that folates made active for *S. faecalis* had originally more than one glutamyl residue and those made active for *L. casei* had originally more than three. The finding by Tamura *et al.* (1972) that tetra-, penta-, and hexafolate polyglutamates have some, albeit decreased, activity for *L. casei* makes conclusions drawn by this approach even less definitive. Claims that intracellular folates are monoglutamates can probably be explained by endogenous conjugase activity changing the folate polyglutamates originally present in the cells to lower homologues (Chanarin *et al.*, 1966; Sotobayashi *et al.*, 1966; Zakrzenski and Grzelakowska-Sztabert, 1973; d'Urso-Scott *et al.*, 1974).

A number of studies have attempted to elucidate the number of glutamyl residues to which the vitamin is attached in different cell types. These studies can be divided into two approaches: isolation and chemical analysis, and chromatographic separation and microbiological or radioactive analysis.

ISOLATION

This approach has been limited by the low levels of the vitamin found in most circumstances. Sufficient folate was isolated from yeast to permit a chemical assessment of the number of glutamyl residues present to be made (Pfiffner *et al.*, 1946). It was concluded that yeast holds all of its folate attached to seven glutamyl residues. A similar study on yeast isolated a *p*-aminobenzoyl polyglutamate attached to 10 or 11 glutamyl residues that may or may not have had a folate origin (Ratner *et al.*, 1946). More recently, the folate isolated from *Clostridium acidi-urici* has been chemically identified as being exclusively the triglutamate (Curthoys *et al.*, 1972).

CHROMATOGRAPHIC SEPARATION

The most widely used approach in the elucidation of folate polyglutamate chain length has been to separate various cellular extracts by a variety of chromatographic methods and following the elution profile either with microbiological assay or radioactive analysis if a radioactive folate has been used to label the folate pool.

One of the first such studies was carried out by Noronha and Silverman (1962). They separated chicken liver extract, which had been protected from endogenous conjugase action, on DEAE–cellulose using microbiological assay to analyze the fractions. Although this study added little information as to the chain length of chicken folates, it was important in that it brought the difficulties into focus. First, it was apparent that, without the use of synthetic standards to calibrate the elution positions of the various folate polyglutamates, one could only guess as to their chain length. Second, it was clear that the problem of resolution was a difficult one, since they were trying to fractionate material according to the number of glutamyl residues present with the full knowledge that these would exist as a complex mixture of differently changed derivatives of the nitrogens and pteridine ring at the other end of the molecule.

Up to this time the only folate polyglutamates that had been synthesized were pteroyltriglutamate and pteroylheptaglutamate (Boothe *et al.*, 1948), and these were not generally available. In 1968 a new synthesis for folate polyglutamates based on the solid-phase peptide synthesis of Merrifield (1963) was devised by Krumdieck and Baugh (1969). Their procedure made folate polyglutamate standards of all chain lengths up to seven available for the first time, and this contribution has completely transformed this area of investigation. The problem of the complexity of the folates to be separated still remained.

Bacteriophage folates

Kozloff and Lute (1965) had isolated a folate component from T-even bacteriophages that, on the basis of comparing its electrophoretic mobility with synthetic pteroyltriglutamate and pteroylglutamic acid, they claimed was a pteroylpentaglutamate. In further studies they attempted to resolve the folate present on the basis of molecular size using P-2 polyacrylamide gel (Kozloff *et al.*, 1970a). They found, however, that the dihydrofolate derivatives that they were chromatographing interacted with the gel and did not elute as predicted by molecular weights. Consequently, they allowed these labile, reduced derivatives to oxidize to the corresponding p-aminobenzoylpolyglutamates, which then behaved as expected on the gel. Using nonfolate polyglutamate markers as standards, they calculated their phage p-aminobenzoylpolyglutamate to have a molecular weight of 1,157 and concluded that it was a penta- or hexapolyglutamate. In a subsequent study (Kozloff and Lute, 1973), they had the advantage of having synthetic standards supplied by Krumdieck and Baugh. However, they separated the folates present, without cleavage, on controlled pore-glass columns according to their molecular size. The resolution of this system was poor, and, while it is clear from metabolic studies by the same group (Kozloff *et al.*, 1970b) that T-even bacteriophages contain a folate hexaglutamate, it would be hard to assert on the basis of their glass-bead separation alone.

Mammalian folates

Stokstad's group and our own, having successfully synthesized the range of folate polyglutamate standards by the method of Krumdieck and Baugh (1969), independently concluded that radioactive folate incorporated into rat liver was converted into a pentaglutamate within 24 h (Houlihan and Scott, 1972; Shin *et al.*, 1972b). The methodological approach in each instance was very different. In this and subsequent studies, Stokstad's group separated the intact folates by a combination of gel filtration chromatography with Sephadex and ion-exchange chromatography with DEAE. On the basis of these studies, they have concluded that rat liver contains exclusively the folate pentaglutamate but that rat red blood cells contain substantial amounts of folate hexaglutamate in addition (Shin *et al.*, 1972a, 1972b, 1974).

As part of our preliminary studies on the determination of folate polyglutamate chain length, as well as synthesizing the standards required, we had evaluated several systems of separation. One such system was Sephadex, by which we had hoped to separate the folates on the basis of size alone. It became apparent that there was substantial and differential interaction with the gel, and we concluded that the only feasible method involved converting the folates to a common derivative. The simplest "common denominator" could be achieved by cleavage of the C-9, N-10 bond. Two well-recognized methods were available to do this: a reductive cleavage under acidic conditions with a zinc catalyst or alkaline permanganate oxidation (Freed, 1966). We made a preliminary study of both procedures. The reductive-acid procedure gave erratic results, indicating that some degradation was occurring—either chemical or enzymatic. Alkaline permanganate oxidation gave good consistent results, possibly because the structures involved may be more stable to alkaline pH or because cell disruption at alkaline pH effectively eliminates all endogenous conjugase activity. Control experiments showed that alkaline permanganate oxidation quantitatively and reproducibly cleaved the C-9, N-10 bond of the following folates: pteroylglutamate, 5-formyltetrahydropteroylglutamate, tetrahydropteroylglutamate, 5-methyltetrahydropteroylglutamate, 5,10-methylenetetrahydropteroylglutamate, 5,10-methenyltetrahydropteroylglutamate, dihydropteroylglutamate, 5-methyldihydropteroylglutamate, 10-formyltetrahydropteroylglutamate, and 10-formylpteroylglutamate. During this procedure there was no detectable destruction of the folates involved, and, in all instances except the latter two, p-aminobenzoylglutamate resulted. Cleavage of the two 10-substituted formyl derivatives gave p-aminobenzoylglutamate and a derivative of p-aminobenzoylglutamate. However, while these compounds resolved on QAE–Sephadex, they do not separate on the DEAE columns used in our folate polyglutamate distribution studies. Further control experiments comparing the folate polyglutamate distribution of 5- and 10-formyl derivatives showed them to be identical. This method gave almost total extraction from mammalian cells in most instances. Similar high extraction values were found with yeast under the appropriate conditions, but some bacterial cells, particularly *S. faecalis*, gave poor extractions. Experiments in which folate polyglutamates were added during the extraction procedure showed endogenous conjugase activity to be zero. Thus the combination of alkaline conditions and vigorous chemical oxidation effectively prevents endogenous conjugase action, quantitatively converts the folate polyglutamates to simpler, easily separable forms without any detectable destruction or cleavage of the peptide bonds, and gives good extraction in most instances.

As mentioned above, our initial studies using this method indicated that, 24 h after intraperitoneal administration of a small quantity of radioactive pteroylglutamate, rat liver had converted it primarily to a pentaglutamate (Houlihan and Scott, 1972). It soon became apparent that, while it was true that this was the major folate present at that time, other folates (principally the hexaglutamate and some tetraglutamate) were also present (Brown et al., 1973). Similar patterns (Figure 4-1) of primarily penta with hexa and some tetra were found by our group with guinea pigs and hamsters (Brown et al., 1974a). It became clear that animal-to-animal variation gave different degrees of equilibration, resulting in slightly different patterns. This lack of total equilibration became more obvious when we compared the exogenous radioactive folate polyglutamate distribution (solid line) with the fully equilibrated endogenous pattern (dotted line) in monkey liver (Figure 4-2) (Brown et al., 1974b). First, it was clear that folate polyglutamate biosynthesis by the monkey was much slower than by the rat. This is also probably true in man since we have found that human marrow cells *in vitro* make no detectable folate polyglutamate in 6 h. After 3 days in the monkey, the radioactive exogenous folate had been converted to a range of folate polyglutamates from the tri to the hepta, with the penta being the predominant form. However, the endogenous, fully

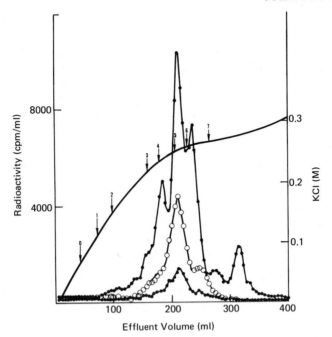

FIGURE 4-1 DEAE–cellulose column chromatography of folate
derivatives synthesized *in vivo* from injected [³H]PteGlu in the liver
of the hamster, guinea pig, and rat. Tritium activity represents
p-amino-[3',5'-³H]benzoylpoly-γ-L-glutamates obtained by KMnO₄/
H₂O₂ oxidation of 50 mM Tris-HCl, pH 9, extracts of liver homogenates prepared 24 h following injection. •, Hamster, 2 g of liver,
12.5-μCi dose; ○, rat, 2 g of liver, 10-μCi dose; ■, guinea pig, 4 g of
liver, 25-μCi dose. Numerals indicate peak elution positions (±5%)
of synthetic standards (*p*-aminobenzoylglutamate$_n$, n = 0,1,2,3,4,
5,6,7) (reproduced with permission: J. P. Brown, G. E. Davidson,
and J. M. Scott. Int. J. Biochem. 5:735–739, 1974).

equilibrated pattern showed a definite shift to higher forms, with the
hexaglutamate now the predominant form and some heptaglutamate
also present.

Using a method similar to our own, involving cleavage of the folate
polyglutamates to the corresponding *p*-aminobenzoylpolyglutamates
but using the zinc reductive method, Baugh and his co-workers (Leslie
and Baugh, 1974) have recently found that rat liver at 24 h contains
primarily folate pentaglutamate with some hexaglutamate. Longer
equilibration periods resulted in increased amounts of hexa- and hep-
tapolyglutamates being formed; and, after very long equilibration,

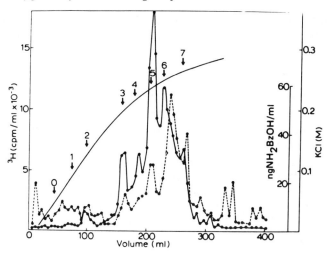

FIGURE 4-2 DEAE–cellulose chromatography of liver extracts, *p*-amino[3′,5′-³H]benzoylpolyglutamates obtained by KMnO₄/ H₂O₂ oxidation of 50 mM K₂HPO₄ extracts of *Cunamolgus* sp. liver. The animals received 230 μCi 72 h prior to extraction. Numerals indicate peak elution positions of synthetic standards (*p*-aminobenzoylglutamate$_n$, $n = 0,1,2,3,4,5,6,7$). Microbiological activity (nanograms of *p*-aminobenzoate/ml of effluent) for *p*-aminobenzoate-requiring mutant of *E. coli* following alkaline hydrolysis of fraction aliquots (reproduced with permission: J. P. Brown, G. E. Davidson, and J. M. Scott. Biochim. Biophys. Acta *343*:78–88, 1974).

although the radioactivity present at that stage makes accurate analysis difficult, the final pattern appeared to be predominantly the hexaglutamate, with about equal amounts of penta and hepta. This is very similar to our own findings with fully equilibrated monkey folate polyglutamates obtained by microbiological assay (Brown *et al.,* 1974b). Our own view is that studies using microbiological assays to determine the final pattern will give the ultimate picture in all cases; however, the organism used for these assays is a mutant of *E. coli* and, while it can be made to work in a satisfactory manner, it is difficult to use because of a tendency to revert.

Thus, for mammalian folates there is good agreement between the studies published by our own and Baugh's groups, showing rapid synthesis of the folate pentaglutamates with a final pattern indicating that the folate hexaglutamate predominates with substantial amounts of the penta and hepta derivative also present. Stokstad's group, on the other hand, has reported only finding folate pentaglutamates (except in rat red blood cells, where they also found the hexaglutamate).

Bacterial folates

While our findings are similar to those of Baugh's group and different from those of Stokstad's group for the mammalian cells discussed above, with the bacterial systems examined by the three groups our results (Brown et al., 1974c) agree with those of Stokstad's group (Buehring et al., 1974) and disagree with those of Baugh's group (Baugh et al., 1974). The former two studies from that S. faecalis contains substantial amounts of tetra and penta derivatives, while Baugh et al. (1974) found that the majority of the folate present exists as the tetra with virtually no penta. There is even sharper disagreement when L. casei is considered. Brown et al. (1974c) and Buehring et al. (1974) found that the folate present is attached to very-long-chain polyglutamates, hexa and greater. Baugh et al. (1974) found mostly tetra and penta. We are confident that under our growth conditions L. casei converts exogenous folate primarily into hexa-, hepta-, octo-, and nonopolyglutamates (Figure 4-3), and it is perhaps significant that Buehring et al. (1974), using a completely different method of analysis, obtained similar results. The explanation may possibly lie in the growth conditions used. Baugh et al. (1974), because of the lower specific activity of their radioactive tracer, used much higher concentrations of folate in their medium.

Yeast

Folate studies carried out by this group on yeast folate indicate that the original report (Pfiffner et al., 1946) showing it to contain exclusively folate heptaglutamate may be incorrect (Figure 4-4). We have found that, while the predominant form present is the heptaglutamate, substantial amounts of penta and octo derivatives also occur and that this was true throughout the growth cycle of the cell. Using the p-aminobenzoate-requiring yeast mutant used in these studies and radioactive p-aminobenzoate, folate polyglutamate markers of high specific activity are easily produced.

Altered folate polyglutamates biosynthesis

Possible alterations to folate polyglutamate biosynthesis under different conditions have been studied. Alcohol, but not phenytoin, was

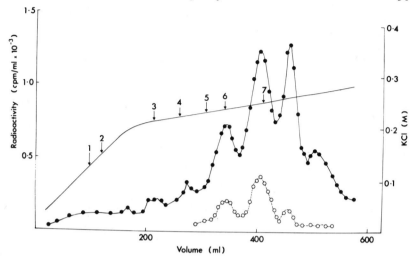

FIGURE 4-3 DEAE–cellulose chromatography of *p*-amino[³H]benzoylpoly-γ-L-glutamate derivatives of the folate requiring strain of *L. casei* (ATCC 7469) obtained by alkaline $KMnO_4$ oxidation of native of extracts of the organism grown on $3',5',9$-[³H]pteroylglutamate$_n$ (●). Numerals indicate the approximate elution positions (±3%) of chemically synthesized standards (*p*-aminobenzoylglutamate$_n$, $n = 0,1,2,3,4,5,6,7$). In addition, *p*-[¹⁴C]aminobenzoylpolyglutamates from yeast prepared as described in the legend to Figure 4-4 were also co-chromatographed for comparative purposes (○).

found to retard the rate of synthesis, but it was not determined if the final pattern that emerged was abnormal (Brown *et al.*, 1973). Human lymphocytes, whether normal or vitamin B_{12} deficient, have been shown to synthesize primarily the pentaglutamate over short periods (Lavoie *et al.*, 1974a). Similar studies found no differences between normal and hepatectomized rat liver (Lavoie *et al.*, 1974b). Developing chicks and developing mice show normal adult patterns of folate polyglutamate biosynthesis (Scott *et al.*, 1975).

SUMMARY

In mammalian cells, absorbed folate monoglutamates are converted to the pentaglutamate derivative comparatively rapidly, with smaller pools of hexapolyglutamates and possibly tetrapolyglutamates also detectable. This process takes about 1 day in rat liver but about 3 days in monkey liver. After prolonged equilibration of several days or

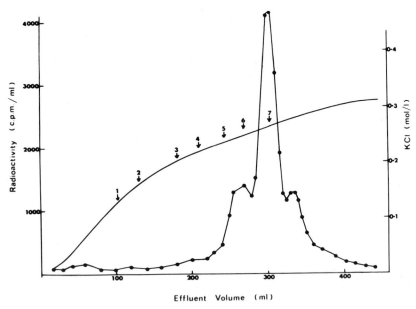

FIGURE 4-4   DEAE–cellulose chromatography of p-amino[^{3}H]benzoylpoly-γ-L-glutamate derivatives obtained by alkaline $KMnO_4$ oxidation of native folates from a p-aminobenzoate-requiring strain of *S. cerevisiae* grown on p-amino[^{3}H]benzoate. Numerals indicate the approximate elution positions ($\pm3\%$) of chemically synthesized standards (p-aminobenzoylglutamate$_n$, n = 0,1,2,3,4,5,6,7).

weeks, the final fully equilibrated pattern in the monkey and possibly in the rat shows predominantly the folate hexaglutamate, with substantial amounts of penta and hepta derivatives also present. Some bacterial cells, *S. faecalis* and *E. coli*, have relatively short-chain folate polyglutamates, although whether these are tri and tetra or tetra and penta is disputed. *L. casei* has been reported by two groups to have very-long-chain folate polyglutamates hexa, hepta, octo, and nono while another group has found only the tetra and penta to predominate in this microorganism. A strain of clostridia has been shown to contain exclusively folate triglutamate. The long-standing claim that yeast contains only folate heptaglutamate appears to be incorrect in that, while this is the predominant form, the hexa and octo derivatives also occur. The tail of T-even bacteriophage contains a structural folate hexaglutamate. Altered conditions of growth for mammalian cells do not appear to cause an altered pattern of distribution to emerge.

DISCUSSION

KRUMDIECK: I would like to make a comment about the procedure of extraction with urea and chloroform (Baugh *et al.,* 1974) as opposed to extraction with your method. We started out using the urea–chloroform procedure of extraction. The urea-chloroform extract gives a considerably lower total amount of folate. We are now pursuing this investigation, because we believe that urea is not indeed an inactive chemical and that probably what we are doing is derivatizing some tetrahydrofolate by reacting it with cyanate, which is a contaminant of all urea solutions. In fact, we now have evidence that a carbon-substituted derivative of tetrahydrofolate is formed. Maybe this is a way of explaining the discrepancies.

SCOTT: Certainly, in Dr. Baugh's work, he goes to a great deal of trouble to preserve the folate with urea and chloroform. If you are going to break the 9,10 bond, I think that such steps would only be useful if they increased extractability or stopped conjugase action. We get very good extractability and no conjugase action by our method. The latter is almost certainly due to the alkaline pH. Our work on red cell haemolysates would also indicate this. If you can get the homogenate away from the optimum pH, and then boil to irreversibly inactivate the conjugase, you get no conjugase action. If you are using an acid extraction (Baugh *et al.,* 1974), it may not be as effective. Removing the extract out of the pH activity range of conjugase is the key. Heating alone is not really the answer; if done without pH alteration, you get a lot of conjugase action before it is destroyed.

ROSENBERG: Do these extraction procedures liberate the folate present from different kinds of protein binding? Is there any systematic way to suggest that ^{14}C-labeled folate is behaving somewhat differently than tritium-labeled folate and that this may explain some of the discrepancies?

SCOTT: In answer to your first question, I think the evidence is that the extraction is adequate. First of all, there is the increased alkalinity, there is the boiling, and then finally the splitting of the 9,10 bond. The extracted folate is not protein bound but a free-folate polyglutamate. One of the difficulties of trying to keep the 9,10 bond intact is that you cannot afford to use the very drastic conditions that we are using. Regarding the second question, Baugh *et al.* use ^{14}C label, while Dr. Stokstad's group and our laboratory use tritium. The differences in the bacterial studies are more likely due to the much lower specific activity used by Baugh *et al.* than to a difference in label.

LITERATURE CITED

Baugh, C. M., Braverman, E., and Nair, M. G. 1974. The identification of poly-γ-glutamyl chain lengths in bacterial folates. Biochemistry *13*:4952–4957.
Binkley, S. B., Bird, O. D., Bloom, E. S., Brown, R. A., Calkins, D. G., Campbell, C. J., Emmett, A. D., and Pfiffner, J. J. 1944. On the vitamin B_c conjugate in yeast. Science *100*:36–37.

Boothe, J. H., Mowat, J. H., Hutchings, B. L., Angier, R. B., Wallace, C. W., Stokstad, E. L. R., Semb, J., Gazzola, A. L., and Subbarow, Y. 1948. Pteroic acid derivatives. II. Pteroyl-γ-glutamylglutamic acid and pteroyl-γ-glutamyl-γ-glutamylglutamic acid. J. Am. Chem. Soc. 70:1099–1102.

Brown, J. P., Davidson, G. E., Scott, J. M., and Weir, D. G. 1973. Effect of diphenylhydantoin and ethanol feeding on the synthesis of rat liver folates from exogenous pteroylglutamate [³H]. Biochem. Pharmacol. 22:3287–3289.

Brown, J. P., Davidson, G. E., and Scott, J. M. 1974a. Comparative biosynthesis of folate polyglutamates in hamster, guinea-pig and rat. Int. J. Biochem. 5:735–739.

Brown, J. P., Davidson, G. E., and Scott, J. M. 1974b. The identification of the forms of folate found in the liver, kidney and intestine of the monkey and their biosynthesis from exogenous pteroylglutamate (folic acid). Biochem. Biophys. Acta 343:78–88.

Brown, J. P., Dobbs, F., Davidson, G. E., and Scott, J. M. 1974c. Microbiol synthesis of folate polyglutamates from labelled precursors. Gen. Microbiol. 84:163–172.

Buehring, K. U., Tamura, T., and Stokstad, E. L. R. 1974. Folate coenzymes of Lactobacillus casei and Streptococcus faecalis. J. Biol. Chem. 249:1081–1089.

Chanarin, I., Hutchinson, M., McLean, A., and Houle, M. 1966. Hepatic folate in man. Br. Med. J. 1:396–399.

Curthoys, N. P., Scott, J. M., and Rabinowitz, J. C. 1972. Folate coenzymes of Clostridium acidi-urici. The isolation of (l)-5,10-methyltetrahydropteroyltriglutamate, its conversion to (l)-tetrahydropteroyltriglutamate and (l)-10-[¹⁴C] formyltetrahydropteroyltriglutamate and the synthesis of (l)-[6,7-³H₂] tetrahydropteroyltriglutamate. J. Biol. Chem. 247:1959–1964.

Davidson, G. E., Weir, D. G., and Scott, J. M. 1975. The metabolic consequences of vitamin B-12/methionine deficiency in rats. Biochem. Biophys. Acta 392:207–215.

Freed, M. 1966. In Methods of vitamin assay, Interscience, London.

Houlihan, C. M., and Scott, J. M. 1972. The identification of pteroylpentaglutamate as the major folate derivative in rat liver and the demonstration of its biosynthesis from exogenous [³H] pteroylglutamate. Biochem. Biophys. Res. Commun. 48:1675–1681.

Kozloff, L. M., and Lute, M. 1965. Folic acid, a structural component of T4 bacteriophage. J. Mol. Biol. 12:780–792.

Kozloff, L. M., and Lute, M. 1973. Bacteriophage tail component. IV. Pteroyl polyglutamate synthesis in T4D-infected Escherichia coli B. J. Virol. 11:630–636.

Kozloff, L. M., Lute, M., Crosby, K. L., Rao, N., Chapman, V. A., and De Long, S. S. 1970a. Bacteriophage tail components. I. Pteroyl polyglutamates in T-even bacteriophages. J. Virol. 5:726–739.

Kozloff, L. M., Lute, M., and Crosby, L. K. 1970b. Bacteriophage tail components. III. Use of synthetic pteroylhexaglutamate for T4D tail plate assembly. J. Virol. 6:754–759.

Krumdieck, C. L., and Baugh, C. M. 1969. The solid-phase synthesis of polyglutamates of folic acid. Biochemistry 8:1568–1572.

Lavoie, A., Tripp, E. and Hoffbrand, A. V. 1974a. The effect of vitamin B₁₂ deficiency on methylfolate metabolism and pteroylpolyglutamate synthesis in human cells. Clin. Sci. Mol. Med. 47:617–622.

Lavoie, A., Tripp, E., Parsa, K., and Hoffbrand, A. V. 1974b. Polyglutamate forms of folate in resting and proliferating mammalian tissues. Clin. Sci. Mol. Med. 48:67–73.

Leslie, G. I., and Baugh, C. M. 1974. The uptake of pteroyl [¹⁴C] glutamic acid into rat liver and its incorporation into the natural pteroyl poly-γ-glutamates of that organ. Biochemistry 13:4957–4961.

Merrifield, R. B. 1963. Solid-phase peptide synthesis. I. The synthesis of a tetrapeptide. J. Am. Chem. Soc. 85:2149–2154.

Noronha, J. M., and Silverman, M. 1962. Distribution of folic acid derivatives in natural material. I. Chicken liver folates. J. Biol. Chem. *237*:3299–3302.

Pfiffner, J. J., Calkins, D. G., Bloom, E. S., and O'Dell, B. L. 1946. On the peptide nature of vitamin B_c conjugate from yeast. J. Am. Chem. Soc. *68*:1392.

Ratner, S., Blanchard, M., Coburn, A. F., and Green, D. E. 1946. Isolation of a peptide of *p*-aminobenzoic acid from yeast. J. Biol. Chem. *155*:689–690.

Scott, J. M., Houlihan, C. M., Bassett, R., and Weir, D. G. 1975. Folate polyglutamates during development in mammalian cells and during the growth cycle in microorganisms. Abstr. Int. Soc. Haematol. London, August 1975.

Shin, Y. S., Buehring, K. U., and Stokstad, E. L. R. 1972a. Separation of folic acid compounds by gel chromatography on Sephadex G-15 and G-25. J. Biol. Chem. *247*:7266–7269.

Shin, Y. S., Willams, M. A., and Stokstad, E. L. R. 1972b. Identification of folic acid compounds in rat liver. Biochem. Biophys. Res. Commun. *47*:35–43.

Shin, Y. S., Buehring, K. U., and Stokstad, E. L. R. 1974. Studies of folate compounds in nature. Folate compounds in rat kidney and rat red blood cells. Arch. Biochem. Biophys. *163*:211–224.

Sotobayashi, Rosen, H. F., and Nichol, C. A. 1966. Tetrahydrofolate cofactors in tissues sensitive and refractory to amethopterin. Biochemistry *5*:3878–3882.

Tamura, T., Shin, Y. S., Willams, M. A., and Stokstad, E. L. R. 1972. *Lactobacillus casei* response to pteroylpolyglutamates. Anal. Biochem. *49*:517–521.

d'Urso-Scott, M., Uhoch, J., and Bertino, J. R. 1974. Formation of 10-formyl folic acid, a potent inhibitor of dihydrofolate reductase in rat liver slices incubated with folic acid. Proc. Natl. Acad. Sci. U.S.A. *71*:2736–2739.

Zakrzenski, S. F., and Grzelakowska-Sztabert, B. 1973. Uptake and metabolism of folate by a folate-utilizing mutant of *Pediococcus cerevisiae* (8081/S) and the parent strain (8081). J. Biol. Chem. *248*:2684–2690.

5

Distribution of Folate
Forms in Food and
Folate Availability

E. L. R. STOKSTAD, Y. S. SHIN, *and* T. TAMURA

This chapter deals with methods for the identification of folic acid conjugates and their derivatives in biological materials and also with a study of factors that affect the availability of folic acid in food for human subjects.

IDENTIFICATION OF FOLIC ACID DERIVATIVES IN BIOLOGICAL MATERIAL

The original attempts to separate the natural folic acid derivative were based on the method of Silverman *et al.* (1961) in which a phosphate gradient was used to elute folic acid from a DEAE–cellulose column. By using this method, Shin *et al.* (1972a) were able to separate folate derivatives in liver into ten major peaks, which are illustrated in Figure 5-1. The identity of these compounds was established by reference to known compounds containing various numbers of glutamic residues that had been prepared by the method of Baugh *et al.* (1970) and is shown in Table 5-1. The binding of folic acid to the

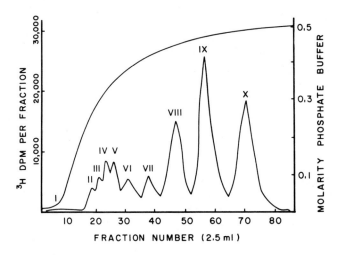

FIGURE 5-1 DEAE–cellulose column chromatography of liver folates. The phosphate concentration gradient is superimposed on the
eluate patterns obtained from chromatography of an equivalent of 1
g of fresh liver.

TABLE 5-1 Identification of Folate Derivatives in Peak Fractions Obtained
by DEAE–Cellulose Chromatography of Liver Extracts

Peak	Fraction No.	Folate Derivative
I	5	Unidentified
II	18	Unidentified
III	21	$10\text{-CHO-}H_4PteGlu$
IV	23	$5\text{-CHO-}H_4PteGlu$, $10\text{-CHO-}H_4PteGlu_2$
V	26	$5\text{-CH}_3\text{-}H_4PteGlu$, $5\text{-CHO-}H_4PteGlu_2$, $10\text{-CHO-}H_4PteGlu_3$
VI	31	$5\text{-CH}_3\text{-}H_4PteGlu_2$, $5\text{-CHO-}H_4PteGlu_3$, $H_4PteGlu$
VII	37	$5\text{-CH}_3\text{-}H_4PteGlu_3$, $10\text{-CHO-}H_4PteGlu_5$,[a] $H_4PteGlu_2$
VIII	46	$5\text{-CHO-}H_4PteGlu_5$[a]
IX	57	$5\text{-CH}_3\text{-}H_4PteGlu_5$[a]
X	70	$H_4PteGlu_5$[a]

SOURCE: Shin *et al.* (1972a).
[a]Major component in liver.

DEAE–cellulose is influenced by the state of reduction (oxidized or tetrahydro form), by the single-carbon constitutent (i.e., 5-methyl or 5-formyl), and by the number of glutamic acid residues. This can result in extensive overlapping of different polyglutamates in a single major peak when different single-carbon substituents are present. For example, it can be seen that peak VII contains three components: 10-formyl-$H_4PteGlu_5$, 5-methyl-$H_4PteGlu_3$, and $H_4PteGlu_2$.

Attempts have also been made to separate folic acid derivatives by means of molecular-sieve chromatography using either G-15 or G-25 Sephadex (Shin *et al.*, 1972b). The behavior of a number of synthetic conjugates has been studied both with water and with various buffer concentrations. When water was used as the eluant, the higher conjugates were apparently excluded from the gel and behaved as if they had much larger molecular sizes, and no separation was possible between the penta- and the heptaglutamates. When 0.1 M phosphate was employed, satisfactory separation was obtained based on the number of glutamic acid residues between 1 and 7. The K_{av} value for certain reference pteroylpolyglutamates and their single-carbon substitutes is shown in Figure 5-2. It will be noted that monoglutamate derivatives have K_{av} values greater than 1, which indicates that they are absorbed by the binding of their aromatic groups to the gel and that their migra-

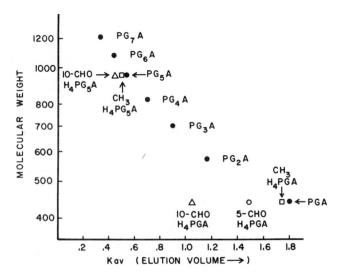

FIGURE 5-2 K_{av} values of polyglutamates on Sephadex G-25. Column, 0.75 × 200 cm; 0.1 M phosphate, pH 7.0.

tion is not based on the principle of sieve-chromatography alone. Furthermore, the K_{av} is influenced by the single-carbon substituent. However, when a higher conjugate such as pentaglutamate is used, the K_{av} values of PteGlu$_5$, 10-CHO-H$_4$PteGlu$_5$, and 5-CH$_3$-H$_4$PteGlu$_5$ are approximately the same. An example of chromatographic separation of liver folates on Sephadex is given in Figure 5-3. Gel chromatography may be quite useful for separating folic acid conjugates of higher molecular weights on the basis of molecular size, but the method is not applicable to the low conjugates.

A combination of chromatography on Sephadex and DEAE has been used to identify folate derivatives in a variety of natural materials. Chromatography was carried out first with Sephadex, and the resulting individual peaks were rechromatographed on DEAE with an appropriate reference marker to establish identity. The nature of the single-carbon substituent could also frequently be established by differential assays using *L. casei*, *S. faecalis*, and *Pediococcus cerevisiae*. The extraction of animal or plant tissue was carried out in such a way that only

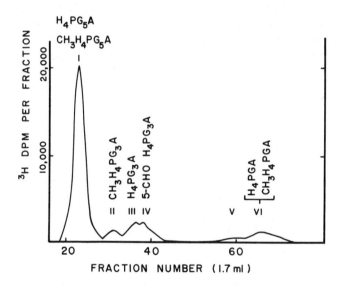

FIGURE 5-3   Sephadex G-15 column chromatography of liver folates. Sample volume, 2.0 ml (0.4 g of fresh liver); bed dimensions, 0.75 × 200 cm; void volume, fraction number 20; flow rate, 7.0 ml/h; eluant, 0.025 M phosphate buffer, pH 7, with 0.2 M mercaptoethanol. Identity of peaks: I, Pentaglutamates; II, 5-CH$_3$-H$_4$PteGlu$_3$; III, H$_4$PteGlu$_3$; IV, 5-CHO-H$_4$PteGlu$_2$; VI, H$_4$PteGlu and CH$_3$-H$_4$PteGlu.

minimal hydrolysis of the conjugates occurred. In the case of liver, this was done by dropping thin slices of the tissue into boiling phosphate buffer containing ascorbic acid. Plant material was cut into small slices and immediately placed in boiling ascorbate buffer, which was then heated for 5 additional min to inactivate conjugases. It was found that certain plant materials such as cabbage contained conjugases that would hydrolyze the natural conjugates present when the plant material was homogenized in a Waring blender and allowed to stand for 15 min before autoclaving.

By the use of these procedures, the distribution of folic acid has been determined for certain representative foods and tissues. The results are given in Tables 5-2 and 5-3.

These results show a wide distribution of general types of folate derivatives. Rat kidney and liver folates are approximately 40 percent methyl derivatives, whereas red cells and milk contain only the methyl form. Plant material also varies in its distribution of folate derivatives. Lettuce, cabbage, and orange juice contain mainly methyl derivative. Soybean contains only 15 percent of this form, and the rest is either the 5- or 10-formyl derivative. Cabbage contains mainly hexa- and heptaglutamates, while soybeans contain 50 percent monoglutamate. Orange juice is approximately 35 percent monoglutamate and 45 percent pentaglutamate. Rat liver and kidney contain mainly pentaglutamates, whereas red cells contain both penta- and hexaglutamates. Milk folate

TABLE 5-2   Identification of Folates in Milk and Soybean[a]

	Percent of Total Folate	
Type of Derivative	Soybean	Milk
Heptaglutamate	–	8
Hexaglutamate	5	6
Pentaglutamate	19	8
Tetraglutamate	3.5	4
Triglutamate	3.5	8
Diglutamate	16	6
Monoglutamate	53	60
$10\text{-CHO-H}_4\text{PteGlu}_n$	20	5
$5\text{-CHO-H}_4\text{PteGlu}_n$	65	3
$5\text{-CH}_3\text{-H}_4\text{PteGlu}_n$	15	92

SOURCE: Shin *et al.* (1975).
[a]Total folate: soybean, 3.0 μg/g; milk, 60 μg/liter.

TABLE 5-3   Distribution of Folic Acid in Various Foods and Tissues

Material	Folate Derivative	Percent	Reference
Lettuce	$5\text{-}CH_3\text{-}H_4PteGlu_5$	34	Batra *et al.* (1973)
	$5\text{-}CHO\text{-}H_4PteGlu_5$	11	
	$5\text{-}CH_3\text{-}H_4PteGlu$	33	
	$5\text{-}CH_3\text{-}H_4PteGlu_{4-2}$	22	
Cabbage	$5\text{-}CH_3\text{-}H_4PteGlu_8$	7.4	Chan *et al.* (1973)
	$5\text{-}CH_3\text{-}H_4PteGlu_7$	51.7	
	$5\text{-}CH_3\text{-}H_4PteGlu_6$	31.7	
	$5\text{-}CHO\text{-}H_4PteGlu_7$	3.0	
Orange juice	$5\text{-}CH_3\text{-}H_4PteGlu_5$	40–50	Tamura *et al.* (in press)
	$5\text{-}CH_3\text{-}H_4PteGlu_{4-2}$	15–30	
	$5\text{-}CH_3\text{-}H_4PteGlu$	30–40	
Rat liver	$10\text{-}CHO\text{-}H_4PteGlu_5$ }	20–30	Shin *et al.* (1972a)
	$10\text{-}CHO\text{-}PteGlu_5$ }		
	$5\text{-}CH_3\text{-}H_4PteGlu_5$	30–40	
	$H_4PteGlu_5$	30–40	
Rat kidney	$10\text{-}CHO\text{-}H_4PteGlu_5$ }	27	Shin *et al.* (1974)
	$10\text{-}CHO\text{-}PteGlu_5$ }		
	$5\text{-}CH_3\text{-}H_4PteGlu_5$	36	
	$H_4PteGlu_5$	15	
	$\chi\text{-}H_4PteGlu$	25	
Red cells	$5\text{-}CH_3\text{-}H_4PteGlu_6$	35	Shin *et al.* (1974)
	$5\text{-}CH_3\text{-}H_4PteGlu_5$	60	

is 60 percent monoglutamate and from 4 to 8 percent each of di- to heptaglutamates.

AVAILABILITY OF FOLIC ACID IN FOOD

The availability of folic acid polyglutamates has been estimated by comparing folate excretion following an oral dose of the test material with that following standard doses of folic acid. Using this method, Swendseid *et al.* (1947) observed that the urinary excretion of folates following oral administration of PteGlu and of $PteGlu_7$ isolated from yeast was about equal. This indicates that the conjugate was absorbed as well as the monoglutamate. However, when $PteGlu_7$ was present in a crude folic acid extract (norite eluate of yeast), the availability of

PteGlu$_7$ was greatly reduced. It was found that this crude extract contained a conjugase inhibitor that was active *in vitro* and that the addition of yeast preparations that contained this inhibitor decreased the absorption of purified preparations of PteGlu$_7$. Similarly, Spray (1952) and Jandl and Lear (1956) found that folate in yeast extracts was about 25 percent available. Similar observations were reported by Schertel *et al.* (1965) with dried crude yeast and by Perry and Chanarin (1968), who used a charcoal eluate of yeast. Thus, there is evidence that, while pure folic acid conjugate from yeast may be utilized as well as folic acid, it has low availability in the presence of conjugase inhibitors that are present in yeast. Estimates of folate availability in various foods have also been made by Retief (1969) using urinary excretion of folic acid as a criterion of absorption. He reported that the availability of folate in liver, spinach, and peas was relatively high, but that in lettuce, cauliflower, and tomato was low.

Tamura and Stokstad (1973) studied the availability of folic acid in foods by measuring folate excretion. In order to increase the excretion following small doses of folic acid, the subjects, which were kept in a metabolic ward, were saturated by a 20-mg dose of folic acid initially and then subsequently by giving 2 mg every other day. The test foods and the reference folic acid standards were given on alternate days. Each metabolic experiment had six subjects and lasted about 6 weeks. Each food sample was fed to all subjects at least once, and four levels of folic acid (0.3, 0.5, 0.7, and 1.0 mg) were given to serve as reference standards. Folic acid was measured in the 8-h collection period following the meal. It had been previously determined that folate excretion has returned to normal by this time. A response curve was constructed for each subject relating the oral dose to the urinary excretion. The response curves for the experiment reported here are given in Figure 5-4. Using this method, Tamura and Stokstad (1973) found that the synthetic tri- and heptaglutamates were absorbed as well as folic acid (PteGlu). Low availability of folates was found in orange juice (31 percent), romaine lettuce (25 percent), and egg yolk (39 percent). Higher availability was found with bananas (82 percent), dried lima beans (70 percent), and frozen lima beans (96 percent).

Experiments were next carried out to determine whether there is an inhibitory factor in certain of these foods that exhibit low folate availability. This was studied first by determining the availability of pure PteGlu$_7$ added to orange juice, romaine lettuce, and egg yolk.

The percentage of availability of folates was calculated by comparing the amount of folate absorbed with the amount of folate in the test materials as measured by microbiological assay after conjugase treat-

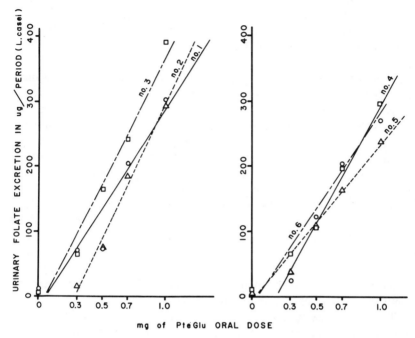

FIGURE 5-4 The individual response curve relating urinary folate excretion to standard PteGlu intake for six subjects.

ment using *L. casei.* Estimation of the availability of PteGlu or PteGlu$_7$ given with orange juice or other foods was made from the estimated absorption due to the added pure derivative. It was calculated as follows:

$$\% \text{ Availability} = \frac{B - C}{A} \times 100$$

where:

   A = Amount of pure folate derivative added to orange juice (equivalent to PteGlu);
   B = Total folate absorbed as calculated from urinary excretion data in reference to response curve; and
   C = Folate absorbed from orange juice alone, calculated from urinary excretion data in reference to response curve.

The results, which are presented in Table 5-4, show that 2.27 mg of PteGlu$_7$ (equivalent to 1.0 mg of PteGlu on a molar basis) given by itself gave a folate excretion of 372 μg. This may be compared with an excretion of 299 μg following 1 mg of PteGlu and would correspond to a calculated availability of 125 percent for PteGlu$_7$. The results also show that, when orange juice concentrate containing 0.61 mg of folate activity was given, the average excretion was 17 μg, which corresponds to an availability of 27 percent. The average excretion following 0.5 μg of PteGlu$_7$ was 108 μg.

The effect of romaine lettuce supplements on the availability of PteGlu$_7$ was also examined. The subjects were given 600 g of romaine lettuce (total folate, 1.1 mg) plus 2.27 mg of synthetic PteGlu$_7$ (equivalent to 1.0 mg of PteGlu). The urinary excretion was 428 μg, which corresponds to an availability of 121 $\pm$ 33 percent for the added PteGlu$_7$. This may be compared with the availability of PteGlu$_7$, when given alone, of 125 $\pm$ 21 percent. Thus romaine lettuce did not show any inhibitory effect. A similar experiment was made with egg yolk, and it was found that the availability of added PteGlu$_7$ was 86 percent. Thus egg yolk does not appear to inhibit the utilization of PteGlu$_7$.

Table 5-5 presents data on the effect of orange juice on the absorption of PteGlu and also on the effect of various components of orange juice on the utilization of PteGlu and PteGlu$_7$. It can be seen from these data that orange juice does not impair the absorption of PteGlu. Folate excretion with orange juice alone was 17 μg, with 1.0 mg of PteGlu

TABLE 5-4   Effect of Orange Juice, Egg Yolk, and Spinach on Absorption of PteGlu$_7$[a]

Supplement	Total Folate Given, mg	Excretion per 8 h, μg	Availability, %
PteGlu (0.5 mg)	0.50	108 (6)	
PteGlu (1.0 mg)	1.00	299 (6)	100
PteGlu$_7$ (1.0 mg)	1.00	371 (6)	125
Orange juice concentrate (600 g)	0.60	17 (6)	27
Orange juice concentrate (600 g) + 1.0 mg PteGlu$_7$	1.6	182 (6)	54
Romaine lettuce (500 g)	0.75	15 (6)	35
Romaine lettuce (600 g) + 1.0 mg PteGlu$_7$	2.1	447 (5)	121
Egg yolk (250 g)[b]	0.34	19 (4)	
Egg yolk (250 g)[b] + 1.0 mg PteGlu$_7$	1.34	300 (4)	86

[a]Data courtesy of Tamura *et al.* (in press).
[b]Data from previous experiment (Tamura and Stokstad, 1973).

TABLE 5-5   Effect of Orange Juice and Its Components on Availability of PteGlu and PteGlu$_7$[a]

Food Supplement	Amount, ml	pH	Total Folate, mg	PteGlu ± SD,[b] %	PteGlu$_7$ ± SD, %
				Availability of Synthetic Folate	
None			1.0	100	125 ± 21 (6)
Orange juice concentrate (no folate added)	600	3.7	0.6	27 ± 14 (6)	
Orange juice concentrate[c]	600	3.7	1.6	121 ± 40 (10)	54 ± 35 (6)
Synthetic orange juice[d]	≈ 600	3.5	1.0		85 ± 31 (6)
K Citrate	≈ 600	3.5	1.0	74 ± 30 (4)	39 ± 26 (9)
K Citrate + sugars	≈ 600	3.7	1.0	104 ± 25 (8)	84 ± 24 (4)
K Citrate	≈ 300	3.7	1.0	87 ± 31 (4)	66 ± 20 (6)
Ca Citrate	≈ 300	4.2	1.0		65 ± 29 (4)
½ Ca · K$_2$ Citrate	≈ 300	6.4	1.0		105 ± 39 (4)

[a]Data courtesy of Tamura *et al.* (in press).
[b]Standard deviation.
[c]Six hundred milliliters of orange juice concentrate (≈ 2,400 ml of fresh orange juice) contains 24 g of citric acid, 120 g of glucose, and 120 g of sucrose.
[d]Contains 24 g of citric acid, 3.6 g of malic acid, 1.2 g of ascorbic acid, 120 g of glucose, and 120 g of sucrose.

alone it was 299 μg, and with a mixture of orange juice (600 ml) plus 1.0 mg of PteGlu it was 389 μg. Since orange juice has no effect on the absorption of PteGlu but does inhibit the absorption of PteGlu$_7$, it appears that orange juice decreases the hydrolysis of folic acid hepta-glutamate to folic acid. A test solution, referred to in Table 5-5 as "synthetic orange juice," was made to contain citric acid, malic acid, ascorbic acid, glucose, and sucrose in the amounts present in 600 ml of orange juice concentrate (≈2,400 ml of fresh juice). The pH of this solution was adjusted to that of orange juice (pH 3.5) using KOH. When this test solution was given to subjects along with PteGlu$_7$, the availability of PteGlu$_7$ was decreased to 82 percent. In order to further examine the mechanism of inhibition, the effect of 12 and 24 g of citric acid alone, after adjusting the pH to 3.7 with KOH, was studied. The availability of PteGlu$_7$ was found to be decreased to 66 percent by 12 g of citric acid and was further decreased to 39 percent by 24 g of citric acid. On the other hand, when PteGlu was given to subjects along with these same amounts of citric acid (12 g and 24 g), the availability of

PteGlu was 87 percent with 12 g of citric acid and 74 percent with 24 g of citric acid.

It was also observed that the mild inhibitory effect of citric acid on the availability of PteGlu (74 percent availability) was eliminated when glucose (120 g) and sucrose (120 g) were added to the citric acid solution, since the availability of PteGlu increased to 104 percent compared to PteGlu alone. However, the addition of the same amount of glucose and sucrose in citric acid solution did not completely reverse the inhibitory effect on the availability of PteGlu$_7$ (84 percent).

Since it is known that citric acid chelates Ca^{++} ion, which is an important cofactor of certain kinds of conjugase, 12 g of citric acid with an equimolar amount of $CaCO_3$ (5.7 g) was given to the subjects along with PteGlu$_7$. This solution (pH 4.2) did not increase the availability of PteGlu$_7$ (65 percent) in comparison with that of citric acid (12 g) alone (66 percent). When the solution containing 12 g of citric acid and 5.6 g of $CaCO_3$ was neutralized to pH 6.4 with KOH (4.2 g), the availability of PteGlu$_7$ was increased to 105 percent. Thus it does not appear that the effect of citric acid in decreasing the availability of PteGlu$_7$ is due to a chelation of calcium ions by citrate.

It appears that the acidity of the citric acid may be a factor in decreased utilization of folic acid conjugates. Neutralizing 12 g of citric acid to pH 6.4 with 4.2 g of KOH (2 equivalents of potassium per mole of citric acid) and one equivalent of calcium permitted 105 percent absorption of PteGlu$_7$, compared with an availability of 66 percent with K citrate at pH 3.7.

It should also be noted that the availability of PteGlu$_7$ seems to be lower in orange juice (54 percent) than it is in mixtures of citric acid and sugars (82 percent and 84 percent, respectively).

These results suggest that the low absorption of folic acid conjugates from orange juice is due to the inhibition of conjugase action by the low pH produced by large amounts of citric acid. It is recognized that the large amounts of orange juice concentrate used (equivalent to 2,400 ml of fresh juice) is much larger than normally consumed in one meal, and that this may not be representative of that which occurs at physiological levels. Methods are needed that can be used to measure availability with lower quantities of food.

DISCUSSION

WAGNER: I was wondering whether the availability of folates might also depend upon whether or not it is protein bound. We know that some of these protein complexes are susceptible to heat, and perhaps there is association between the protein binding and increase in availability.

STOKSTAD: In one of our original experiments we compared cooked cabbage and raw cabbage and found no difference between the two.

ROSENBERG: Absorption of pure monoglutamyl and polyglutamyl folates measured by urinary-excretion techniques are very comparable. But, that does not really get at the question of the impact of binding and intraluminal events on the absorption of folates in food. There is really quite a lot of conjugase activity in the intestine relative to the amount of polyglutamate to be hydrolyzed. If there is a block in the availability of the polyglutamate, it probably is not a block in the amount of conjugase available; rather, it is a block in the ability of the conjugase to act on the polyglutamate or to act upon the polyglutamate–protein association.

ROTHENBERG: With regard to Dr. Rosenberg's comments, the sequence of events would have to be rapid. The problem of folate binding may influence the action of conjugase. For example, virtually all binders of folate will be dissociated with a pH below 5.0 or 4.0. So, if you have a low gastric acidity, you would expect a dissociation of complexes in food. In the duodenum, where the pH is higher, reassociation of the folate–binder complex may occur unless there is rapid tryptic digestion of the protein to permit the polyglutamate to be activated upon by the conjugase.

HOFFBRAND: I would like to ask Dr. Stokstad about the role that conjugase inhibitors in food might play. It has been said that in some food there are conjugase inhibitors, some of which are nucleic acids. I am concerned with detection of these inhibitors by microbiological studies. Several substances we have tested, such as DNA and RNA, inhibit the *L. casei* microbiological assay. In performing absorption studies based on urinary folate excretion, it seems to me that there is a danger that factors that inhibit *L. casei* in food might also be absorbed and appear in the urine, and what might appear to be a low absorption may in fact be something in the urine inhibiting the *L. casei* assay. It is possible that DNA and RNA and other potential conjugase inhibitors actually inhibit conjugase rather than *L. casei* growth?

STOKSTAD: Regarding our microbiological assay, we determined that the folate excreted in the urine was the monoglutamate. We have not experienced any inhibition of the growth of *L. casei* by these conjugase inhibitors.

ROSENBERG: Would we expect with all the nucleases around that ingested DNA and RNA would be excreted?

HOFFBRAND: There have been reports that purines and pyrimidines (and not just intact DNA and RNA) also inhibit the assay.

SCOTT: We have started to do studies in which we are concerned about the autolysis of folate polyglutamates in food, because, if one considers food of mammalian origin, the majority of such food is hung or aged before it is cooked. We have been looking at increasing time to see whether the folate polyglutamates are broken down by the endogenous conjugases that are present. In fact, there is a tremendous amount of polyglutamate hydrolysis in food of mammalian origin before it ever gets cooked. This may not be the case in vegetables, where the conjugases, while they may be present, I do not think are nearly as active.

Our preliminary results show that in food that is hung for a day or a day and a half at ordinary temperatures there is a tremendous amount of autolysis, and the amount of folate present as polyglutamates when such food is eaten is much less than we apparently think.

LITERATURE CITED

Batra, K. K., Wagner, J. R., Stokstad, E. L. R. 1973. Identification of folate coenzyme in romaine lettuce. Fed. Proc. *32*:928.

Baugh, C. M., Stevens, J. C., and Krumdieck, C. L., 1970. Studies on γ-glutamyl carboxypeptidase. I. The solid phase synthesis of analogs of polyglutamates of folic acid and their effects on human liver γ-glutamyl carboxypeptidase. Biochim. Biophys. Acta *212*:116.

Chan, C., Shin, Y. S., and Stokstad, E. L. R. 1973. Studies of folic acid compounds in nature. III. Folic acid compounds in cabbage. Can. J. Biochem. *51*:1617.

Jandl, J. H., and Lear, A. A. 1956. The metabolism of folic acid in cirrhosis. Ann. Int. Med. *45*:1027.

Perry, J., and Chanarin, I. 1968. Absorption and utilization of polyglutamyl forms of folate in man. Br. Med. J. *iv*:546.

Retief, F. P. 1969. Urinary folate excretion after ingestion of pteroylmonoglutamic acid and food folate. Am. J. Clin. Nutr. *22*:352.

Schertel, M. E., Libby, D. A., and Loy, H. W. 1965. Yeast folate availability to man determined microbiologically on human bioassay samples. J. Assoc. Offic. Agric. Chem. *48*:1224.

Shin, Y. S., Williams, M. A., and Stokstad, E. L. R. 1972a. Identification of folic acid compounds in rat liver. Biochem. Biophys. Res. Commun. *47*:35.

Shin, Y. S., Buehring, K. U., and Stokstad, E. L. R. 1972b. Separation of folic acid compounds by gel chromatography on Sephadex G-15 and G-25. J. Biol. Chem. *247*:7266.

Shin, Y. S., Buehring, K. U., and Stokstad, E. L. R. 1974. Studies of folate compounds in nature. Folate compounds in rat kidney and red blood cells. Arch. Biochem. Biophys. *163*:211.

Shin, Y. S., Kim, E. S., Watson, J. E., and Stokstad, E. L. R. 1975. Studies of folic acid compounds in nature. IV. Folic acid compounds in soybeans and cow milk. Can. J. Biochem. *53*:338.

Silverman, M., Law, L. W., and Kaufman, B. 1961. The distribution of folic acid activities in lines of leukemic cells of the mouse. J. Biol. Chem. *236*:2530.

Spray, G. H. 1952. The utilisation of folic acid from natural sources. Clin. Sci. *11*:425.

Swendseid, M. E., Bird, O. D., Brown, R. A., and Bethell, F. H. 1947. Metabolic function of pteroylglutamic acid and its hexaglutamyl conjugate. II. Urinary excretion studies on normal persons. Effect of a conjugase inhibitor. J. Lab. Clin. Med. *32*:23.

Tamura, T., and Stokstad, E. L. R. 1973. The availability of food folate in man. Br. J. Haematol. *25*:513.

Tamura, T., Shin, Y. S., Buehring, K. U., and Stokstad, E. L. R. (In press). The availability of folates in man: Effect of orange juice supplement on intestinal conjugase. Br. J. Haematol.

6

Data on Folacin Activity in Foods: Availability, Applications, and Limitations

K. HOPPNER, B. LAMPI, *and* DOROTHY C. SMITH

The Food and Nutrition Board of the National Academy of Sciences established a recommended dietary allowance (RDA) for folacin in 1968 (FNB, 1968), and since then there has been a widespread demand for information concerning levels of the vitamin in foods.

The subsequent development of nutritional labeling in the United States and completion of nutrition surveys in both the United States and Canada have further encouraged government agencies, food industries, scientists, clinicians, dieticians, nutritionists, and consumers to seek out reliable data on the folacin content of foods.

In the United States, the preparation of tables of food composition has been the responsibility of the Department of Agriculture. Recently, Watt and Murphy (1970) outlined the history of these food tables and detailed areas in which data are needed. In addition, Murphy *et al.* (1973) outlined areas of work being carried out by the Nutrient Data Research Center (NDRC) in the preparation of future publications. A revision of *Handbook 8* (Murphy *et al.,* 1973) is planned, and folacin values will be included in the new edition. This volume will serve as an initial step in the assembly and evaluation of present data on folacin, and it will also provide guidance for future work.

As a prelude to these developments it seems appropriate to review the current availability, application, and limitations of data on folacin content of foods and to discuss possible improvement of future data.

AVAILABILITY AND APPLICATION OF CURRENT DATA

Individual Foods

A survey of studies on folacin content of foods published after 1951 is shown in Table 6-1 (Toepfer *et al.*, 1951; Teply *et al.*, 1953; Burger *et al.*, 1956; Hardinge and Crooks, 1961; Santini *et al.*, 1962; Herbert, 1963; Santini *et al.*, 1964; Hurdle *et al.*, 1968; Henderson, 1969; Hoppner, 1971; Streiff, 1971; Hoppner *et al.*, 1972; Butterfield and Calloway, 1972; Hoppner *et al.*, 1973; Dong and Oace, 1973; Fung-Miller *et al.*, 1973). It begins with a comprehensive review of the folate composition of foods by Toepfer *et al.* (1951) spanning the period from 1941–1951. It is evident from Table 6-1 that, after a period of relative inactivity, there has been a noticeable increase in the number of studies on food folacin content since the beginning of the 1970's. The impetus for this was probably derived from the inclusion of folacin in the 1968 RDA (FNB, 1968).

Prior to our investigation of folacin levels, there were no data on Canadian foods. Several studies on the folacin content of Canadian foods have been completed in our laboratory (Hoppner, 1971; Hoppner *et al.*, 1972, 1973). In addition, the free and total folacin activity of a number of miscellaneous foods that were analyzed to obtain data of folacin intakes for Nutrition Canada are shown in Table 6-2. As expected, the folacin values of foods were markedly affected by the nature and quantity of the components. For example, yeast-leavened donuts provide, as expected, more total folacin than their cake-type counterparts. Similarly, nut-fudge-type chocolate bars provide approximately twice as much free folacin and from three to four times as much total folacin than plain milk-chocolate bars on an equal weight basis.

Diets

Reported data on the daily intake of folacin from various diets are summarized in Table 6-3. (Chung *et al.*, 1961; Butterworth *et al.*, 1963; Read *et al.*, 1965; Lowenstein *et al.*, 1966; Hurdle and Path, 1968; Chanarin *et al.*, 1968; Eichner *et al.*, 1971; Perry, 1971; Van de Mark and Wright, 1972; Moscovitch and Cooper, 1973; Santini and Corcino,

Data on Folacin Activity in Food 71

TABLE 6-1   Available Data on the Folacin Activity in Fresh and Processed Foods

Source	Foods Reported	Remarks[a]
Toepfer et al. (1951)	200 foods—meats, fish, vegetables, fruits, cereals, dairy products— raw, processed, and different market quality (compiled data 1941–1951)	FFA, TFA; *L. casei, S. faecalis;* chicken pancreas, no ascorbate
Tepley et al. (1953)	Various canned foods	TFA; *S. faecalis*
Burger et al. (1956)	30 frozen vegetables, 14 frozen fruits, 7 frozen juices	TFA; *S. faecalis;* chicken pancreas
Hardinge and Crooks (1961)	Compilation of various foods	TFA
Santini et al. (1962)	80 foods—meats, fish, vegetables, fruits, cereals	FFA, TFA; *S. faecalis;* chicken pancreas
Herbert (1963)	Various foods, raw and cooked	FFA, TFA; *L. casei, S. faecalis;* chicken pancreas
Santini et al. (1964)	Various foods	FFA, TFA; *L. casei, S. faecalis;* chicken pancreas, hog kidney
Hurdle et al. (1968)	Various foods, raw and cooked	FFA, TFA; *L. casei;* chicken pancreas
Henderson (1969)	Review—milk data	FFA, TFA; *L. casei, S. faecalis;* chicken pancreas
Hoppner (1971)	40 commercial, strained baby foods	FFA, TFA; *L. casei;* chicken pancreas
Streiff (1971)	Citrus and other juices	FFA, TFA; *L. casei;* chicken pancreas
Hoppner et al. (1972)	162 foods—meats, fish, vegetables, fruits, nuts, cereals, dairy products—raw, processed, and of different market quality	FFA, TFA; *L. casei;* chicken pancreas
Butterfield and Calloway (1972)	Wheat and selected foods	FFA, TFA; *L. casei;* hog kidney
Hoppner et al. (1973)	30 frozen convenience dinners	FFA, TFA; *L. casei;* chicken pancreas
Dong and Oace (1973)	Fruit juices	FFA, TFA; *L. casei, S. faecalis;* hog kidney
Fung-Miller et al. (1973)	Bean products: cooked, canned, and instant powder	FFA, TFA; *L. casei;* hog kidney

[a] FFA, free folacin activity; TFA, total folacin activity.

TABLE 6-2   Free and Total Folacin Activity in Miscellaneous Foods

Food	No. of Samples	Free Folacin Activity,[a] µg/100 g fresh weight		Total Folacin Activity,[a] µg/100 g fresh weight	
		Range	Mean	Range	Mean
Liverwurst	3	16.1–24.7	19.8	25.7– 37.0	29.7
Fish roe, lumpfish	2	3.2– 4.7	4.0	11.6– 12.7	12.2
Bean sprouts, canned	3	5.2– 7.8	6.8	7.5– 11.1	9.7
Beans, baked, in tomato sauce	2	4.4– 4.9	4.7	21.1– 26.7	23.9
Pumpkin, canned	2	1.2– 1.4	1.3	7.0– 9.3	8.1
Brazil nuts, shelled	3	0.4– 0.5	0.5	2.6– 5.5	4.2
Coconut, dried, sweetened	2	0.3– 0.4	0.4	1.4– 1.8	1.6
Cheerios	3	7.3– 9.6	8.5	19.9– 26.8	22.3
Biscuits, arrowroot	3	3.1– 4.4	3.9	6.3– 8.8	7.2
Cake, chocolate with icing	3	3.3– 5.7	4.3	4.9– 8.3	6.4
Cake, white sponge	3	0.8– 6.0	3.1	4.2– 10.8	7.3
Cookies, chocolate chip	3	4.2– 4.9	4.5	8.0– 11.0	9.4
Cookies, sandwich type	3	2.6– 3.9	3.3	4.2– 8.4	6.2
Cookies, shortbread	3	3.5– 4.7	4.0	7.0– 10.0	8.6
Donuts, cake type	3	3.0– 6.0	4.8	6.6– 9.5	8.2
Donuts, yeast leavened	3	3.9– 6.2	4.7	15.5– 26.7	21.6
Pie, apple	3	1.5– 3.4	2.5	2.4– 5.3	3.9
Wheat germ, defatted	2	29.8–35.5	32.7	232.2–252.0	242.1
Wheat germ, whole	1		94.0		178.3
Cream, 10%	3	1.4– 2.1	1.7	2.2– 3.0	2.5
Cream, 18%	3	1.2– 1.6	1.4	2.1– 2.5	2.3
Cream, 32%	3	1.3– 2.2	1.7	3.2– 4.1	3.7
Eggnog	3	0.2– 0.7	0.4	0.8– 1.2	0.9
Cheese spread, processed	3	2.8– 3.8	3.3	6.1– 8.1	7.0
Ice cream, vanilla	2	0.9– 1.1	1.0	1.9– 2.2	2.1
Apricot nectar	2		<0.1	0.6– 0.9	0.8
Barbeque sauce	3	2.4– 3.4	2.9	3.8– 4.3	4.0
Chocolate bar, nut fudge roll	3	7.1–12.3	9.3	17.4– 41.3	31.6
Chocolate bar, plain milk	3	3.3– 5.5	4.2	5.4– 8.4	6.6
Jam, strawberry	2	6.6– 7.8	7.2	7.9– 8.0	8.0
Mayonnaise	3	0.4– 0.6	0.5	1.0– 1.1	1.0
Soup, beef broth	3	1.0– 1.2	1.1	2.5– 5.5	3.9
Soup, clam chowder	3	1.3– 5.0	2.6	5.9– 8.3	7.4
Soup, cream of asparagus	2	4.7– 5.2	5.0	18.0– 19.3	18.7
Soup, cream of mushroom	3	0.7– 0.9	0.8	2.4– 3.6	2.8
Soup, vegetable beef	3	1.7– 2.6	2.1	4.6– 7.6	6.4

SOURCE: Hoppner *et al.* (1972).
[a]Microbiological assay with *L. casei.*

TABLE 6-3 Reported Data on the Daily Intake of Folacin from Various Diets

Source	Folacin, µg		Diet Information
	Free	Total	
Chung *et al.* (1961)	11–33	30–120	Poor to high cost, calculated
	8–172	27–346	Poor to high cost, analyzed
			S. faecalis
Butterworth *et al.* (1963)	24–78	80–308	17 diets, *S. faecalis*
	37–297	379–1,097	4 diets, *L. casei*
Read *et al.* (1965)	–	46–63	Calculated from tables
Lowenstein *et al.* (1966)	–	82–92	Calculated from tables, *L. casei,* uncooked
Hurdle *et al.* (1968)	–	161–297	Young controls
		95–250	Old people at home
		41–190	Old people in hospital
			L. casei
Chanarin *et al.* (1968)	53–296	265–1,615	Home diet, *L. casei*
	34–75	104–492	*S. faecalis*
	33–165	174–1,000	Hospital diet, *L. casei*
Eichner *et al.* (1971)	<5	17–30	Low-folate diets
	163–253	332–429	Control diet, *L. casei*
Perry (1971)	20–104	262–954	Normal diets, *L. casei*
	6–18	43–118	Normal diets, *S. faecalis*
	3–9	24–79	Normal diets, *P. cerevisiae*
Van de Mark and Wright (1972)	–	100–200	Pregnant and nonpregnant teen-agers, calculated
Moscovitch and Cooper (1973)	63–586	69–601	Home diets, *L. casei*
	–	92–656	4-day dietary record
	–	39–138	4-day dietary record, calculated
		183–697	7-day dietary record
		39–224	7-day dietary record, calculated
Santini and Corcino (1974)	37–130	1,588–3,156	High-cost diet
	13–75	152–2,681	Low-cost diet, *L. casei*

1974). Ranges rather than averages have been listed. In most cases, the menus were listed and the folacin content was estimated by analysis of composites. Sometimes the folacin content of the diet was calculated from existing literature values. Only in a few instances were both procedures employed and the results compared. Often, weights and definitions of the individual ingredients were not given.

Recently, an appraisal of the folacin intake of Canadians was taken based on an examination of a composite diet. The diet, originally devised for monitoring pesticide residues (Smith, 1971), was based on the apparent per capita consumption of major foods in Canada (Thompson *et al.*, 1973; Dominion Bureau of Statistics, 1965). The individual foods were divided into 12 groups (Smith, 1971). The group of drinks (group 12) was omitted in this study.

The ingredients, daily per capita consumption, and the alleged average folacin content of fresh foods from published data that were used to calculate the folacin content of the diet are listed in Table 6-4. The prepared composites of each food group were analyzed with *L. casei* (Hoppner *et al.*, 1972). The composites contain 64 percent water

TABLE 6-4   Ingredients of Composite Diet and Their Alleged Mean Folacin Content

Food	Intake,[a] g	Folacin,[b] µg/100 g	
		Free	Total
Group 1			
Butter	23.0	–	–
Cheese, hard	7.5	18.3	18.3
Cheese, processed	2.5	13.2	13.2
Cheese, cottage	1.9	12.1	12.1
Milk, fresh	383.0	5.0	5.0
Evaporated milk	18.8	7.0	7.0
Skim milk	9.5	5.1	5.1
Ice cream	36.2	1.0	2.1
Margarine	11.0	–	–
Group 2			
Beef steak	13.6	4.3	6.0
Beef roast	36.4	3.3	7.4
Hamburger	25.3	2.6	7.7
Pork, bacon	2.7	1.0	2.0
Pork, ham	15.3	0.6	3.7

TABLE 6-4 (Continued)

Food	Intake,[a] g	Folacin,[b] µg/100 g	
		Free	Total
Pork, fresh	4.9	3.8	7.4
Sausage	10.7	1.5	3.7
Liver	6.1	145.0	145.0
Bologna	5.1	2.2	5.1
Chicken	16.2	3.3	7.7
Fish, frozen	9.4	4.5	12.5
Fish, sardines, canned	5.6	5.9	15.5
Eggs	33.2	11.9	21.1
Lamb chops	9.4	1.2	4.9
Group 3			
Bread, white	35.7	8.1	35.6
Bread, brown	33.0	6.5	23.0
Bread, rye	28.6	6.5	23.2
Rolls	9.7	8.2	35.5
Bread, whole wheat	4.0	17.3	54.5
Bread, corn	4.0	7.5	22.0
Fruit cake	31.0	6.9	13.5
Oatmeal	5.6	11.3	56.1
Corn meal	4.0	7.5	22.0
Rice	16.4	15.4	28.8
Corn	21.3	14.2	14.2
Spaghetti	29.3	3.8	13.2
Sweet rolls	16.2	8.1	21.3
Flour, enriched	21.6	17.9	21.3
Group 4			
Potatoes, baked	32.9	10.0	14.1
Potatoes, boiled	55.9	10.0	14.1
Potatoes, fried	14.2	10.0	20.0
Potatoes, powdered	42.3	4.4	9.0
Potatoes, canned	19.9	10.0	14.1
Potato chips	13.5	10.0	42.0
Group 5			
Cabbage, raw	6.0	25.0	30.2
Cabbage, cooked	5.9	2.0	17.0
Celery, raw	10.1	5.9	11.5
Lettuce	11.1	24.0	24.0
Asparagus	5.7	58.0	64.0
Group 6			
Peas, cooked	12.3	6.0	22.4
Beans, cooked	10.0	10.0	40.0
Lima beans, frozen	9.4	8.8	31.3

TABLE 6-4   (Continued)

Food	Intake,[a] g	Folacin,[b] μg/100 g	
		Free	Total
Group 7			
Carrots, raw	8.8	13.8	18.3
Carrots, cooked	8.3	7.9	10.0
Onion, raw	6.8	14.8	16.3
Onion, cooked	6.8	7.1	8.0
Turnips, cooked	7.7	10.0	15.0
Group 8			
Tomatoes, fresh	24.5	4.1	5.6
Tomatoes, juice	13.3	4.7	10.7
Tomatoes, canned	11.2	2.0	3.0
Tomatoes, catsup	12.1	9.8	14.8
Tomatoes, soup	13.1	2.0	3.0
Cucumber	5.4	16.4	24.0
Group 9			
Oranges	12.0	13.4	24.0
Grapefruit, juice	8.7	3.5	5.0
Apples, fresh	27.7	3.3	5.8
Apple, sauce	5.1	3.3	3.5
Apple, juice	12.8	1.0	2.0
Bananas	14.3	11.6	20.4
Peaches	10.8	1.5	3.3
Pineapple, canned	6.5	5.1	6.0
Grapes	11.8	3.3	5.0
Apricots	11.0	3.0	4.0
Strawberries, frozen	19.5	15.0	15.0
Orange, juice	9.9	30.0	30.0
Raspberries, frozen	10.3	2.8	5.1
Group 10			
Peanut butter	5.8	19.8	79.0
Shortening	14.0	–	–
Salad dressing	6.8	0.5	1.0
Group 11			
Sugar, white	76.9	–	–
Sugar, brown	33.5	–	–
Jam	8.8	7.2	8.0
Pudding mix	4.4	2.9	2.9
Maple syrup	6.0	–	–
Honey	1.8	0.6	1.5
Candy	11.4	–	–
Salt	7.1	–	–
Pickles	8.4	–	–

[a]Quantity eaten per person per day.
[b]Data from Toepfer *et al.* (1951), Hoppner *et al.* (1972, 1973), Table 2, and unpublished data.

and provide approximately 2,780 kcal of energy and 88 g of protein per day (Thompson *et al.*, 1973).

The results of the "calculated" versus "analyzed" folacin contents of the composite diet are given in Table 6-5. Calculated total folacin (197 μg) compared favorably with analyzed total folacin (194 μg); calculated free folacin (117 μg) was slightly higher than analyzed free folacin (103 μg). This was generally true for all of the individual food groups, indicating that free folacin is more easily destroyed than total folate during preparation. The calculated values of folacin content also provided some insight to the origins of folacin in each food group. Similar analytical values for free (110 μg) and total folacin (240 μg) were obtained when the diet was prepared with foods collected in a different location. Both free and total folacin values compare favorably with average values reported by others (Hurdle and Path, 1968; Van de Mark and Wright, 1972; Moscovitch and Cooper, 1973), but they provide only 50–60 percent of the total folacin cited in the present RDA for total food folacin (Committees on Dietary Allowances and Interpretation of the Recommended Dietary Allowances, 1974).

Although an average diet such as this has the same limitations as any 'average' or 'normal' value in that it reveals little concerning individual variations, it does provide useful information on the basic per capita intake of folacin.

TABLE 6-5 Folacin Intake from Food Groups Estimated by Analysis and by Calculation

Food Group	Intake, g/person/day	Folacin by Analysis, μg		Folacin by Calculation, μg	
		Free	Total	Free	Total
1. Dairy products	493.4	19.2	33.6	23.3	23.7
2. Meat, poultry, fish	194.0	32.0	59.2	21.0	26.7
3. Cereal products	260.4	20.1	36.2	23.6	61.3
4. Potatoes	178.7	5.7	21.3	15.5	27.7
5. Leafy vegetables	38.8	4.9	5.6	8.2	14.1
6. Legumes	31.7	7.0	14.8	2.6	9.7
7. Root vegetables	38.4	0.9	1.5	4.1	5.3
8. Garden fruits	79.6	9.4	10.4	4.2	6.6
9. Fruits	160.4	1.9	3.4	12.2	16.5
10. Oils and fats	26.6	0.9	3.5	1.1	4.7
11. Sugar and adjuncts	158.3	1.1	4.1	0.8	0.8
TOTAL	1,660.3	103.1	193.6	116.6	197.1

LIMITATIONS OF CURRENT DATA

Table 6-1 reveals that current information on folacin content of foods is scarce and very basic. It refers to only a small part of the wide range of foodstuffs in existence today. This deficiency is compounded by the fact that for each individual food there is a wide range of folacin content, and the number of samples that were analyzed for most foods was limited. Few studies have been made of the folacin pattern in foods (Chan *et al.*, 1973) and diets (Butterworth *et al.*, 1963; Hoppner *et al.*, 1973).

Murphy *et al.* (1973) have pointed out many of the problems associated in evaluating original data. One of these problems is that insufficient attention has been given to the proper description and definition of samples.

From Table 6-1 it can be seen that variations of the method employed to measure the folacin content of foods in these studies varied widely. Earlier studies (Toepfer *et al.*, 1951; Teply *et al.*, 1953; Burger *et al.*, 1956; Hardinge and Crooks, 1961; Santini *et al.*, 1962) were carried out prior to the widespread use of ascorbate to protect against loss of labile folacin. Similarly, *Streptococcus faecalis* was used often rather than *Lactobacillus casei*. Other differences, such as the use of hog kidney or chicken pancreas conjugase, pH of incubation, ascorbate strength, conjugase concentration, etc., are prevalent today. In addition to those already mentioned, the limitations were also notable in the diet studies. Despite the diversity in sample definition and methodology with which current data on folacin content of foods and diets were evolved, many of the published data are comparable and do constitute a basic pool that must be improved by generating improved data.

CONCLUSIONS

A survey of the available data on folacin content of foodstuffs indicates that they do not meet present demands. It appears that there is a need for additional data on folacin activity in all types of foods, raw and processed.

To produce improved data and establish meaningful tables in the future, consideration should be given to evaluation and standardization of the current methodology for analyzing folacin in foods and providing an adequate description of the sample.

Furthermore, it would appear from present findings and other reports (Hurdle and Path, 1968; Van de Mark and Wright, 1972; Moscovitch and Cooper, 1973) that the current RDA (Committees on Dietary Allowances and Interpretation of the Recommended Dietary Allowances, 1974) for total food folacin for the adolescent, nonpregnant, and nonlactating adult is difficult to attain from an average composite diet.

DISCUSSION

HERBERT: When you talk about comparisons between calculated and analyzed values, were the calculations made from prior analysis in your laboratory of the same fresh foods?

HOPPNER: The data used to derive the "calculated" values came from earlier analysis of foodstuffs that we have reported.

BUTTERWORTH: Did you make any allowance for the fact that food might have been consumed raw by the individual, and yet cooked or autoclaved in your analysis?

HOPPNER: The diet composites were prepared according to general kitchen practice. Where foods are eaten either cooked or raw, they were added in equal proportion cooked and raw into the composite.

BUTTERWORTH: But, the individual might have consumed it raw, and yet when you took it into the lab to do the *L. casei* assay, you autoclaved it.

HOPPNER: Yes, the composites were treated like individual foods. They were autoclaved as stipulated in the method.

COOPER: Did you assay the diet mixed in the proportions normally taken by the person?

HOPPNER: The proportion of each food item was based on per capita disappearance statistics.

COOPER: But were foods analyzed in the form in which they are served? For example, consider cole slaw. Would you assay the cabbage mixed with the vinegar, which releases free folic acid, which in turn is broken down?

HOPPNER: The composites, or food groups, were a mixture of several individual foods. For instance, carrots were added raw and cooked together with other vegetables.

COOPER: Would they be added to meat, because people tend to have the carrots and meat on the same plate?

HOPPNER: Oh, yes. The composites in this study were analyzed individually. However, we have also analyzed total composites of all the foods used in this diet. The intake ranged between 197 to 250 μg/person/day. It depends on the proportion of each food in the diet and where the food is collected.

COOPER: The correlations between calculated and assay values, I think, are surprisingly good. The number may be different, but the rank order of the individual foods being studied is the same. We did a study in which the calculations for folate intakes were based on the values you gave here, giving a median intake of about 80 μg of free folate per day. Those diets were assayed, and the value was actually much more like the ones that you have given in your calculations, but the rank/order of the patients was very similar, suggesting that you just have to calculate to adjust the slope.

HOPPNER: I think the studies that have been made in the past comparing analyzed versus calculated values have shown reasonable agreement. I would like to make a few remarks about the analysis of free folate. It is very crude in the routine analysis of foods and probably gives rise to inflated values. As Dr. Scott mentioned earlier, autolysis can take place in several ways. I think that total folate is the value that we have to focus on when we talk about requirements. However, the amount of free folate as part of the total polyglutamyl folate structure in foods may be useful in assessing the efficiency of utilization. It may also be of interest to industry with respect to processing losses, since free folate is more readily destroyed.

HERBERT: In the final analysis, we are going to have to do what those concerned with iron have done. That is, we are going to have to use the term absorbability as a synonym for availability. Anything less is not going to be adequate for human nutrition studies.

LITERATURE CITED

Burger, M., Hein, L. W., Teply, L. J., Derse, P. H., and Krieger, C. H. 1956. Vitamin, mineral and proximate composition of frozen fruits, juices and vegetables. Agric. Food Chem. *4*:419–425.

Butterfield, S., and Calloway, D. H. 1972. Folacin in wheat and selected foods. J. Am. Diet. Assoc. *60*:310–314.

Butterworth, C. E., Jr., Santini, R., Jr., and Frommeyer, W. B., Jr. 1963. The pteroylglutamate components of American diets as determined by chromatographic fractionation. J. Clin. Invest. *42*:1929–1939.

Chan, C., Shin, Y. S., and Stockstad, E. L. R. 1973. Studies of folic acid compounds in nature. III. Folic acid compounds in cabbage. Can. J. Biochem. *51*:1617–1623.

Chanarin, I., Rothman, D., Perry, J., and Stratfull, D. 1968. Normal dietary folate, iron, and protein intake, with particular reference to pregnancy. Br. Med. J. *2*:394–397.

Chung, A. S. M., Pearson, W. N., Darby, W. J., Miller, O. N., and Goldsmith, G. A. 1961. Folic acid, vitamin B_6, pantothenic acid and vitamin B_{12} in human dietaries. Am. J. Clin. Nutr. *9*:573–582.

Committee on Dietary Allowances and Committee on Interpretation of the Recommended Dietary Allowances. 1974. Recommended dietary allowances, 8th rev. ed. National Academy of Sciences, Washington, D.C. 128 pp.

Dominion Bureau of Statistics. 1965. Publication No. 5502, Food balance sheet. Dominion Bureau of Statistics, Ottawa, Canada.

Dong, F. M., and Oace, S. M. 1973. Folate distribution in fruit juices. J. Am. Diet. Assoc. *62*:162–166.

Eichner, R. E., Buergel, Nancy & Hillman, R. S. 1971. Experience with an appetizing, high protein, low folate diet in man. Am. J. Clin. Nutr. *24*:1337–1345.

Food and Nutrition Board. 1968. Recommended dietary allowances, NAS Publication no. 1694. National Academy of Sciences, Washington, D.C. 101 pp.

Fung-Miller, C., Guadagni, D. G., and Kon, S. 1973. Vitamin retention in bean products: cooked, canned, and instant bean powders. J. Food. Sci. *38*:493–495.

Data on Folacin Activity in Food

Hardinge, M. G. and Crooks, H. 1961. Lesser known vitamins in foods. J. Am. Diet. Assoc. *38*:240–245.

Henderson, J. O. 1969. Folic acid—a review of current literature. Aust. J. Dairy Technol. *42*:143–144.

Herbert, V. 1963. A palatable diet for producing experimental folate deficiency in man. Am. J. Clin. Nutr. *12*:17–20.

Hoppner, K. 1971. Free and total folate activity in strained baby foods. Can. Inst. Food Sci. Technol. J. *4*:51–54.

Hoppner, K., Lampi, B., and Perrin, D. E. 1972. The free and total folate activity in foods available on the Canadian market. Can. Inst. Food Sci. Technol. J. *5*:60–66.

Hoppner, K., Lampi, B., and Perrin, D. E. 1973. Folacin activity of frozen convenience foods. J. Am. Diet. Assoc. *63*:536–539.

Hurdle, A. D. F., and Path, M. C. 1968. An assessment of the folate intake of elderly patients in hospital. Med. J. Aust. *55*:101–104.

Hurdle, A. D. F., Barton, D., and Searles, I. H. 1968. A method for measuring folate in food and its application to a hospital diet. Am. J. Clin. Nutr. *21*:1202–1207.

Lowenstein, L., Cantlie, G., Ramos, O., and Brunton, L. 1966. The incidence and prevention of folate deficiency in a pregnant clinic population. Can. Med. Assoc. J. *95*:799–806.

Moscovitch, L. F., and Cooper, B. A. 1973. Folate content of diets in pregnancy: comparison of diets collected at home and diets prepared from dietary records. Am. J. Clin. Nutr. *26*:707–714.

Murphy, E. W., Watt, B. K., and Rizek, R. L. 1973. Tables of food composition: availability, uses, and limitations. Food Technol. *27*:40–52.

Perry, Janet. 1971. Folate analogues in normal mixed diets. Br. J. Haematol. *21*:435–441.

Read, A. E., Gough, K. R., Pardoe, J. L. and Nicholas, A. 1965. Nutritional studies on the entrants to an old people's home with particular reference to folic—acid deficiency. Br. Med. J. *2*:843–848.

Santini, R., and Corcino, J. J. 1974. Analysis of some nutrients of the Puerto Rican diet. Am. J. Clin. Nutr. *27*:840–844.

Santini, R., Jr., Berger, F. M., Berdasco, G., Sheehy, T. W., Avileo, J., and Davila, I. 1962. Folic acid activity in Puerto Rican foods. J. Am. Diet. Assoc. *41*:562–567.

Santini, R., Brewster, C., and Butterworth, C. E., Jr. 1964. The distribution of folic acid active compounds in individual foods. Am. J. Clin. Nutr. *14*:205–210.

Smith, D. C. 1971. Pesticide residues in the total diet in Canada. Pestic. Sci. *2*:92–95.

Streiff, R. R. 1971. Folate levels in citrus and other juices. Am. J. Clin. Nutr. *24*:1390–1392.

Thompson, J. N., Beare-Rogers, J. L., Erdody, P., and Smith, D. C. 1973. Appraisal of human vitamin E requirement based on examination of individual meals and a composite Canadian diet. Am. J. Clin. Nutr. *26*:1349–1354.

Teply, L. J., Derse, P. H., Krieger, C. H., and Elvehjem, C. A. 1953. Vitamin B_6, folic acid, beta-carotene, ascorbic acid, thiamine, riboflavin, and niacin content and proximate composition. Agric. Food Chem. *1*:1204–1207.

Toepfer, E. W., Zook, E. G., Orr, M. L., and Richardson, L. R. 1951. Folic acid content of foods, microbiological assay by standardized methods and compilation of data from literature. Agriculture handbook No. 29. Human Nutrition and Home Economics Bureau, U.S. Department of Agriculture, U.S. Government Printing Office, Washington, D.C. 116 pp.

Van de Mark, M. S., and Wright, A. C. 1972. Hemoglobin and folate levels of pregnant teenagers. J. Am. Diet. Ass. *61*:511–516.

Watt, B. N., and Murphy, E. W. 1970. Tables of food composition: Scope and needed research. Food Technol. *24*:674–684.

7

Use and Significance
of Folate Binders

SHELDON P. ROTHENBERG, MARIA DA COSTA, *and*
CRAIG FISCHER

Although there has been a great deal of information accumulated in the past 10 years about the complexing of vitamin B_{12} with a number of specific binding proteins, until recently little was known about the binding of the functionally and clinically related vitamin folic acid (PGA) to specific macromolecules. Studies of folates have, for the most part, been directed at determining the state of oxidation, the form of the carbon unit carried, the number of glutamate residues, and the biochemical function of each coenzyme in a variety of biosynthetic reactions involving transfer of carbon molecules.

In order to discuss the use and significance of folate binders, the terminology, origin, properties, structure, and other characteristics of these binders should be precisely defined. Although some of this information on folate binders has become available in recent years, not all of these definitions are known at the present time; hence, some freedom for speculation will be necessary in this discussion.

The terminology used when describing these binders should be first defined. At this time the evidence suggests that there are two categories of folate binders—specific and nonspecific. A specific binder may be defined as a macromolecule with a binding site structured for complexing with a specific moiety of the folate molecule. The affinity constant for such binding should be high, usually greater than 10^5–10^6 L/M; and this type of binding should, in general, demonstrate saturation kinetics.

Binders of folate and/or bound forms of folate have been identified in milk (Ghitis, 1967; Metz *et al.*, 1968), liver (Zamieroski and Wagner, 1974; Corrocher *et al.*, 1974), kidney (Kamen and Caston, 175), intestinal epithelium (Garth and Rowe, 1972; Zamieroski and Wagner, 1974), leukemic granulocytes (Rothenberg, 1970; Rothenberg and da Costa, 1971), and granulocytes from women who are pregnant or taking oral contraceptives (da Costa and Rothenberg, 1974a). Where studied, the properties of these tissue binders suggest that some may fulfill these criteria for specific binders. A specific folate binder is also present in some human serums (Rothenberg *et al.*, 1972; Waxman and Schreiber, 1973), though it may not be detected when tested for the binding of exogenous folate because it is saturated with endogenous folate. In pig plasma (Mantzos *et al.*, 1974) and in human subjects who have folate deficiency (Waxman and Schreiber, 1973; Rothenberg, 1973), liver disease (Rothenberg, 1973) leukemia (da Costa and Rothenberg, 1974a), uremia (Hines *et al.*, 1973), and in women who are pregnant or taking oral contraceptives (da Costa and Rothenberg, 1974a) the serum binder may be present in the unsaturated state. Zettner and Duly claim from recent studies that virtually all serums from normal subjects and patients contain a specific folate binder (Zettner and Duly, 1974).

A nonspecific binder of folate may be defined as a macromolecule that does not require a specific conformational structure either on the macromolecule or folate and that has a low binding affinity, usually about 10^3 or 10^4 L/M or less. This type of binding reaction usually does not demonstrate saturation kinetics.

The major fraction of endogenous folate in serum appears to be nonspecifically bound. Studies by Markkanen (1968) and Markkanen and co-workers (Markkanen and Peltola, 1971; Markkanen *et al.*, 1972) using gel filtration have shown that a variable fraction of endogenous serum folate is associated with a protein fraction; however, this probably represents mostly nonspecific binding because it has been shown that folate activity in serum is freely diffusible (Condit and Grob, 1958; Retief and Huskisson, 1970) and is extractable by charcoal (Herbert *et al.*, 1962; Retief and Huskisson, 1970). PGA added to most serum(s) is also dialyzable (Hampers *et al.*, 1967; Retief and Huskisson, 1970) and is removed when sufficient charcoal is used (Metz *et al.*, 1968). Elsborg (1972), using PGA, and Spector *et al.* (1975), using N^5-methyltetrahydrofolate (methyl-FH_4), have demonstrated also that the binder(s) in serum for these folates is not saturable and can be duplicated by albumin. Additional evidence that the major fraction of endogenous folate in serum is nonspecifically bound is that it can be assayed in whole serum without extraction using either microbiological (Herbert, 1966) or radiometric methods (Waxman *et al.*, 1971; Rothenberg *et al.*, 1972). This indicates that the pteridine moiety of folate is sterically available to participate in other reactions.

There is evidence that red cell folate is coupled to macromolecules (Iwai *et al*, 1964), and this macromolecular–folate complex was termed folic acid precursor substance(s). Though this precursor activity precipitated with ammonium sulfate and filtered through G-50 Sephadex columns with the hemoglobin fraction of the hemolysate, it is probably nonspecifically bound folate because studies in our laboratory and that of Schreiber and Waxman (1974) have shown that red cell folate can be measured by radioassay without extraction, indicating that the pteridine moiety of the molecule is either free or very loosely bound.

Milk also contains a folate binder (Ghitis, 1967; Metz *et al.*, 1968), which has now been purified from cow (Salter *et al.*, 1972), goat (Rubinoff *et al.*, 1975), and human milk (Waxman, 1974) using affinity chromatography and which has properties that satisfy those of a specific binder. The specificity and high affinity of the milk-derived folate binder have been exploited in the recent development of radioassays for serum and red cell folate (Waxman *et al.*, 1971; Rothenberg *et al.*, 1972; Schreiber and Waxman, 1974).

The folate binder in chronic granulocytic leukemia cells (CML) was the first specific binder the properties of which have been defined (Rothenberg and da Costa, 1971; da Costa and Rothenberg, 1974a). It was first identified during the study of dihydrofolate reductase activity by CML cell lysates when it was observed that a tracer concentration of [^{3}H]PGA was not reduced to tetrahydrofolate unless unlabeled folate was added to the reaction mixture. The nature of this phenomenon became apparent when it was shown that the tracer [^{3}H]PGA was directly bound to a large molecule and, therefore, could not be enzymatically reduced. The addition of unlabeled folate to the reaction simply inhibited this binding of the [^{3}H]PGA, which then became available for reduction by dihydrofolate reductase.

PGA is coupled to the binder from CML cells by a noncovalent linkage since the binding decreases sharply below pH 5.0 and since bound PGA will also dissociate as the hydrogen ion concentration increases. The binder, as well as the binder–PGA complex, is resistant to heating at 56° C. The association reaction for the complex is very rapid at room temperature and there is also very little dissociation of bound folate in the crude lysate after the addition of a swamping concentration of unlabeled folic acid—even over a 24-h incubation period.

Recent studies during the purification of the folate binder from CML cells have indicated that there are two proteins with binding determinants for [³H]PGA (Fischer *et al.*, 1975). One elutes from DEAE–cellulose with dilute phosphate buffer, pH 6.0, and has a molecular weight of 34,000. A second more acidic protein elutes with 0.1 M phosphate buffer, pH 7.0, and has a molecular weight of 44,000. The affinity of both binding proteins was highest for PGA and dihydrofolate, and, with these more purified preparations, concentrations of methyl-FH₄ 10 times greater than PGA did inhibit the binding of the [³H]PGA, but no binding determinants were observed for formyl-FH₄ or methotrexate.

Recently, experiments have been conducted to study the intracellular properties and subcellular localization of the folate binder in these leukemic granulocytes (da Costa and Rothenberg, 1974b, 1975). Sonic extracts of the nuclear fraction and heavy mitochrondria of these cells demonstrated the most binder per fraction, while the least binding was observed with the microsomes. When these same CML cells were incubated with [³H]PGA, for 18 h and then subjected to subcellular separation, the most radioactivity accumulated in the cytosol and nuclear fractions. It was significant, however, that 92 percent of the radioactivity in the cytosol was dialyzable, whereas only 12 percent of the nuclear accumulation was lost by dialysis. These results indicate that a major compartment of intracellular folate binder is in the nuclei. Since the binder also has a high affinity for dihydrofolate, a coenzyme generated in the biosynthesis of thymine, these studies suggest that it may have some function in *de novo* DNA synthesis.

Antiserums to each of the binder–protein fractions separated by DEAE–cellulose chromatography have been obtained by immunization of rabbits and have been used to define the immunochemical specificity of each binder. These antiserums have also been used to develop a radioimmunoassay to detect and measure these binders in cells, tissue extracts, and serum, even when saturated by endogenous folate, since these saturated binders cannot be detected by the binding of exogenous tracer PGA.

The principle of this radioimmunoassay is diagrammatically illustrated in Figure 7-1 as applied to the more acidic binding fraction from the CML cells, abbreviated here as B binder. When the B-[³H]PGA complex reacts with the anti-B antiserum, the whole complex—(B-[³H]PGA,–AB)—precipitates at 25 percent ethanol. The (B-[³H]

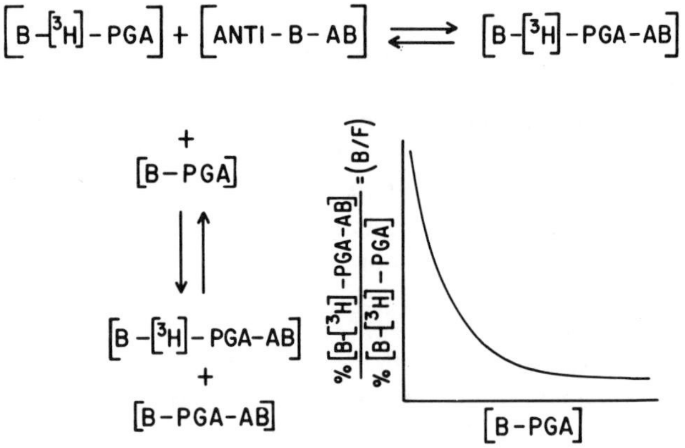

$$\left[\text{B--}[^{3}\text{H}]\text{--PGA}\right] + \left[\text{ANTI--B--AB}\right] \rightleftharpoons \left[\text{B--}[^{3}\text{H}]\text{--PGA--AB}\right]$$

FIGURE 7-1 The principle of the radioimmunoassay for the folate-binding protein(s) (see text for explanation).

PGA) complex not bound to antibody does not precipitate at this concentration of alcohol. When binder saturated with unlabeled PGA is added to the reaction system containing a limited binding capacity of the antiserum, less of the (B–[^{3}H]PGA) complex precipitates with the antibody. If the ratio of bound to free (B–[^{3}H]PGA) (B/F) is plotted as a function of the (B–unlabeled PGA) concentration, a dose–response curve, as shown diagrammatically in Figure 7-1, is obtained. Folate binder, immunochemically similar to this folate binder in the CML cells, if present in extracts of other tissues or biological fluids, can be measured by this radioimmunoassay. An example of the application is shown in Figure 7-2. The dose–response curve was obtained using concentrations of B-binder calculated from the quantity of PGA bound—assuming an equimolar binding ratio. Lysates of leukemic cells that did not bind exogenous [^{3}H] PGA nevertheless had experimental B/F values that fell on the dose–response curve. The lysate from granulocytes from a pregnant woman had a very low B/F value, indicating a high concentration of binder immunochemically similar to the CML binder.

This type of competitive inhibition radioimmunoassay can also be used to demonstrate that the folate binder in a number of sources may all be immunologically related and that tissue extracts and biological fluids that do not bind exogenous PGA may nevertheless contain the binding protein. To do this, an aliquot of the test material (e.g., serum, leukocyte lysates, tissue extract, etc.) is added to the tracer B–[^{3}H]PGA, and a concentration of the antiserum is diluted to bind about 50 percent of this

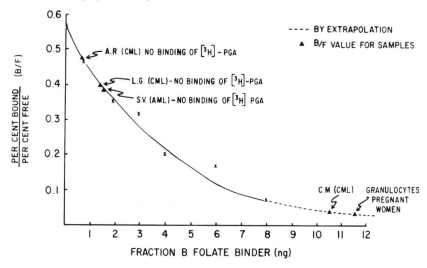

FIGURE 7-2   Radioimmunoassay dose–response curve obtained when the B-binder fraction saturated with PGA competed with the B-binder saturated with [³H]PGA for binding sites on the antibody to B-binder. The values on the ordinate are expressed as nanograms of protein, which were calculated from the quantity of PGA bound assuming a 1:1 binder–PGA ratio. The ratio of antibody bound (B-[³H]PGA) to free (B-[³H]PGA) (B/F) was plotted against concentrations of the same binder saturated with PGA. The B/F values for lysates prepared from other leukemia cells and granulocytes from a pregnant woman are indicated on the curve.

labeled complex. The results of this experiment are illustrated in Figure 7-3. The closed bar on the left side of the figure shows that 50 percent of the [³H] PGA,–binder complex was precipitated with the antiserum. This precipitation was decreased by competitive inhibition when CML binder saturated with cold PGA was added to the reaction mixture. The next series of lined bars shows the inhibition observed when different samples of biological material were added to the reaction mixture. All serums, including normals, inhibited the reaction of the [³H]PGA–binder complex with the antiserum. Thus, an antigenic protein similar to the folate binder in CML cells must be present in serum, as well as in normal granulocytes and leukemic cells other than CML.

It is significant that two lysates prepared from the ascitic form of L-1210 murine leukemia, a normal human liver homogenate, and some tumor homogenates also inhibited the reaction, indicating that immunologically similar determinants were present in these tissues or fluids, as shown in Figure 7-4. The results of these radioimmunoassay

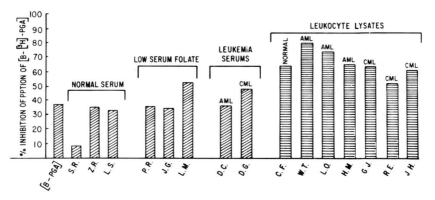

FIGURE 7-3 The competitive inhibition of the antibody binding of B-[³H]PGA by samples of different biological material (see text for explanation). Samples are identified by initials of patients.

experiments strongly suggest a structural relationship, which crosses, not only tissue but also species differences, between the folate binders.

Evidence is also available that indicates that the folate binder in serum may be derived from granulocytes. The first clue to this notion was the early observation that the unsaturated serum folate binder in a CML

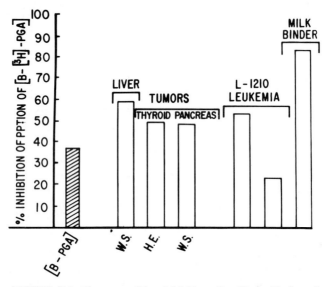

FIGURE 7-4 The competitive inhibition of antibody binding of (B-[³H]PGA) by samples of biological material (see text for explanation). Samples are identified by initials of patients where applicable.

patient disappeared as the peripheral granulocyte count decreased transiently to subnormal levels following treatment with busulfan (Rothenberg and da Costa, 1971).

The second piece of evidence suggesting that the granulocyte is the source of the serum folate binder were experiments with short-term cultures of CML granulocytes (da Costa and Rothenberg, 1974b, 1975). Over an incubation period of 5-h, the folate binding capacity of the culture medium increased. This apparent secretion of the binder from cells was not inhibited by puromycin, cycloheximide, or actinomycin D, indicating that this was a stored intracellular protein. Secretion was inhibited by incubation at 4° C or with N-ethylmaleimide, indicating that this process was mediated by an energy-dependent transport system. Recent studies by Colman and Herbert (1974a) that demonstrate that lithium added to whole blood results in an increase in PGA binding by plasma are additional support for the notion that granulocytes may release folate binder.

From the information so far accumulated about the folate binder(s) from all sources, no definitive function for them is apparent. Accordingly, at this time speculation about use and significance will be derived from the defined properties of these binders.

Serum Protein Binder

It is evident that methyl-FH_4 in serum is either free or loosely bound to albumin and represents the biologically important circulating folate. This nonspecific binding of methyl-FH_4 may, nevertheless, be physiologically important because it could prevent the loss of folate by excretion, particularly by the kidney.

There is a small compartment of bound folate that is in an oxidized form. Evidence for this was reported previously from our laboratory using a radioimmunoassay specific for oxidized folate (da Costa and Rothenberg, 1971). Additional evidence for this has been obtained from experiments where serum folate was measured in our laboratory using *Lactobacillus casei* and *Streptococcus faecalis* by the method of Cooperman (1967) before and after treatment with charcoal. The results are shown in Figure 7-5. As expected, the *L. casei* activity was significantly greater than the *S. faecalis* activity in the untreated serums. With the charcoal-treated serums, however, the *L. casei* activity decreased 79 percent, approaching the concentration of the *S. faecalis* activity in the untreated serums. There was some decrease in the *S. faecalis* activity in the charcoal-treated serums, but it was significantly less than that observed for the *L. casei* activity. These experiments support the notion

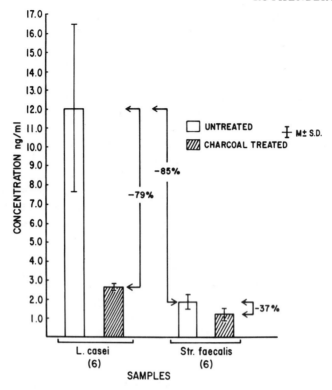

FIGURE 7-5   Microbiological assay of serums before and after
treatment with 5 mg/ml of Norit A charcoal. Values in parentheses
indicate number of samples.

that the oxidized folate in serum is, for the most part, protein bound and
not extractable with charcoal, while the reduced folate is free or weakly
bound and charcoal extractable.

Further support for this notion was obtained from experiments in
which serums were similarly assayed after extraction with and without
ascorbate in the extraction buffer. The results are shown in Figure 7-6.
L. Casei activity in serums extracted without ascorbate decreased to
levels virtually equivalent to *S. faecalis* activity. *S. faecalis* activity
was essentially unchanged by extraction without ascorbate. These
experiments demonstrate that there are two compartments of circulating serum folate—a free, nonspecifically bound compartment representing 5-methyltetrahydrofolate that is extractable with charcoal and
is heat labile in the absence of ascorbate and a bound compartment

comprised of oxidized folate that is not extractable with charcoal and that is stable to heat in the absence of ascorbate.

The compartment of free, reduced folate most likely represents the route for the transfer of biologically active folate from one tissue site to another. No such function can be derived for the compartment of bound, oxidized folate. If, as we now believe, most of the binding protein in serum is derived from granulocytes, oxidized folate coupled to this protein is very tightly bound at neutral pH. Waxman and Schreiber (1974) have also shown that folate bound to this serum binder is not taken up by a number of cell systems. Thus, at this time, it is not possible to assign either a use or a significance to this serum folate binder although its properties would satisfy the criteria of a specific binder. The low concentration of this binder in serum and the small fraction of serum folate in this compartment suggests that a function for this binder may be in intracellular folate metabolism.

Intracellular Protein Binder

One can speculate on a number of possible functions for the intracellular folate binder based on its subcellular location and properties. First, because the binder identified in CML cells has a high affinity

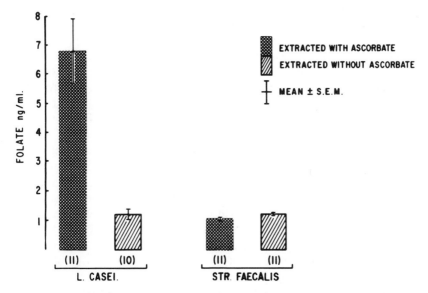

FIGURE 7-6 Microbiological assay of serums extracted with and without ascorbate in the extraction buffer. Values in parentheses indicate number of samples.

for dihydrofolate (FH$_2$), it may have a role in de novo thymine–DNA synthesis. Toward this notion, we studied the effect of exogenous PGA and FH$_2$ in cell cultures of CML cells containing a high and low concentration of unsaturated binder (da Costa et al., 1972). We observed that when PGA and FH$_2$ were added to CML cells with low unsaturated binder concentration there was a significant increase in the incorporation of [^{3}H]deoxyuridine (dU) into DNA. This incorporation was either not observed or markedly diminished when the PGA or FH$_2$ was added to the CML cells with a high concentration of unsaturated binder. Of particular interest was the observation that, after the CML patient with high binder was treated for a number of weeks with large doses of folic acid orally (60 mg per day), the unsaturated folate binding capacity of the cells decreased, and then, when cultured with PGA and FH$_2$, there was stimulation of [^{3}H]dU incorporation into DNA. The recent subcellular identification of saturated and unsaturated folate binder in the nuclear fraction of CML cells would also provide support for the hypothesis that it has some role in thymine–DNA synthesis. One notion would be that this binder may control the concentration of free dihydrofolate so that it would be a substrate rate-limiting biosynthetic process rather than an enzyme rate-limiting system.

Folate binder in the cytosol may also function to accumulate folate or prevent efflux of cellular folate when the extracellular folate concentration decreases below normal. It is unlikely that bound folate can function as a coenzyme, so some mechanism must also be operative to dissociate the folate–protein complex and shift the equilibrium toward a greater concentration of free folate when it is needed for metabolic processes or if it is to be secreted. The folate binder extracted from hog kidney is more likely to have such a "storage" function than the binder in CML cells because it appears to have greater affinity for N^5-methyltetrahydrofolate (Kamen and Caston, 1975).

Finally, another speculative function for the intracellular folate binder is antibacterial, as has been proposed for the intracellular activity of transcobalamin I. The folate binders from CML cells separated by DEAE–cellulose completely inhibited the growth of L. casei and S. faecalis. Ford (1974) has also demonstrated that folate bound to sow, cow, or goat milk is not available for uptake by enteric bacteria and has proposed that this binding of folate in the intestinal tract may "spare" the vitamin for absorption and regulate the ecology of the gut microflora in the neonatal period.

With the rapid progress being made into elucidating the nature and function of folate blinders from various biological sources, it is perhaps now appropriate to establish more precise terminology to describe these factors. The term folate binding protein, we believe, is too generic and fails to separate specific and nonspecific binding. This term, which is now being used to describe the folate binding protein concentration in serum, we also believe is incorrect. It is inaccurate to express the binder concentration by the amount of exogenous [³H]PGA bound because this reflects only the unsaturated folate binding capacity. The unsaturated folate binding capacity may or may not be related to the total concentration of the folate binding protein. Examples of the number of possible combinations of binder–protein concentration and unsaturated folate binding capacity are shown in Figure 7-7. In normal serum (bar A) the total binding protein expressed as 5 arbitrary units has little or no unsaturated binding capacity. In another serum (bar B), the total binding may still be 5 units, but the unsaturated binding capacity may be evaluated because there is less endogenous oxidized folate on this protein. This may represent the situation in folate deficiency. Bar C shows an increase in the total binding protein, which, nevertheless, remains abnormally unsaturated. This may occur with

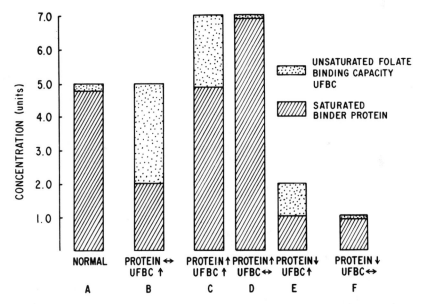

FIGURE 7-7 Examples of variations of total binder protein concentration with different levels of unsaturation. The total binder concentration is shown in arbitrary units and represents the sum of the saturated and unsaturated binder concentration (reproduced with permission: Clin. Haematol., East Sussex, England).

binder released from granulocytes in CML or in liver disease. In the serum shown in bar D, the protein may be similarly increased but saturated with endogenous folate like the normal and, therefore, would not be detected by the binding of exogenous [^{3}H]PGA. The latter situation may be observed in uremia (Hines et al., 1973). It is also possible to speculate on the occurrence of a low building protein concentration that is unsaturated (Bar E) or a low protein concentration that is saturated (bar F).

To identify these combinations of binding protein concentration and the unsaturated binding capacity will require more complex methodology than simply adding [^{3}H]PGA to serum and determining the amount bound. The total protein will have to be measured directly, as by radioimmunoassay, or by measuring the sum of the endogenous oxidized folate and unsaturated binding capacity. Colman and Herbert (1974b) have briefly described treating serum at an acid pH with charcoal to strip endogenous bound folate and then measuring the increase in the binding of [^{3}H]PGA. This finding is based on the previously reported methods of preparing unsaturated folate binding proteins in milk (Rothenberg *et al.*, 1972) and hog kidney (Kamen and Caston, 1975).

It might be worthwhile for this workshop to adopt a name for the folate binder that would not be as broad and nonspecific as the term "folate binding protein." Since the parent compound of folates is pteroic acid, which also appears to react with the milk, serum, and granulocyte binder, appropriate names might be transpteroyl or trans-folyl. This would also permit the addition of descriptive prefixes as information about specificity of these binders becomes available.

ACKNOWLEDGMENTS

This work has been supported by NIH grants CA 08976 and RO1 AM 16220. M. da Costa is supported by The National Leukemia Association, Inc., and Dr. C. Fischer is supported by The Kresevich Research Foundation.

We would like to thank Patricia Ferdinand and Zoltan Rosenberg for their technical assistance.

DISCUSSION

KRUMDIECK: Am I right in saying then that the *Streptococcus faecalis* assay of serum could be taken as a rough measure of the binding capacity in that sense?

ROTHENBERG: You would have to do two determinations. First, you would have to measure the amount of exogenous PGA bound by the serum. Second, you would have to take the same serum sample and either treat it with charcoal or extract it without ascorbate, and then assay it with either *L. casei* or *S. faecalis*. The methyltetrahydrofolate is nonspecifically bound, or free, and labile, so that it would be extracted by the charcoal or destroyed by the boiling. The oxidized folate remaining would then support the growth of either *L. casei* or *S. faecalis*. The total of those two folate measurements would represent the molar equivalents for the concentration of the binder in serum. Assuming a molecular weight of 40,000 for the binder, the amount of binder protein per milliliter of serum can be calculated.

HERBERT: We find that with stripping at pH 4.3, we get data that support the data you just presented in folate deficiency, normals, in pregnancy, and in certain tissues such as liver and renal.

ROTHENBERG: I offer a note of caution, because during the purification of the CML binder using a PGA-sepharose affinity column we have found that dissociating the complex at low pH may denature a fraction of the binder protein. But, of course, the binder is in a more purified state. In serum, the binder might very well be less labile, so your acid treatment may not denature it. This is the only caution I suggest. If your data support it, fine. We are planning to measure the binder in serum by acid stripping of endogenous folate and then measuring the amount of exogenous [^{3}H]PGA and comparing it to the direct measurement of the binder protein by radioimmunoassay.

WAXMAN: Does your peak A immunologically cross react with peak B?

ROTHENBERG: Yes, definitely, very definitely.

HOFFBRAND: Dr. Blair, I think, has shown that some N^{10}-formylfolic acid is in normal plasma. Do you think this is the oxidized folate that is bound to your binder?

ROTHENBERG: It certainly could be. We did not test N^{10}-formylfolate, but N^{10}-methylfolate reacts with the binder. I suspect that N^{10}-formylfolate will also react as long as that 5,6 area of the pteridine ring is not reduced and the 2-hydroxy position is intact.

HOFFBRAND: Dr. Blair says that N^{10}-formylfolate is less than 1 ng/ml of normal plasma and that it does nothing.

ROTHENBERG: It may serve no known function. If complexed to the binder in plasma, it is unlikely that it could be taken up by cells.

SCOTT: Blair *et al.* used an aseptic addition technique and found that the *S. faecalis* activity, which they ascribe to be N^{10}-formylfolic acid, did not have to be extracted. This is a discrepancy.

ROTHENBERG: If the assay is run at a low pH, the folate might dissociate slowly.

HERBERT: I think he ran it at 6.1, did he not?

ROTHENBERG: We did not study the equilibrium constants at pH 6.1. Now, it could be that at pH 6.1 there is slow release of folate. As the organism utilizes the free folate, more of the bound dissociates. After an 18- or 24-h growth period, all of the bound folate could dissociate because the affinity of the transport system of the microorganism may be greater than the affinity for folate by the binder at this pH.

LITERATURE CITED

Colman, N., and Herbert, V. 1974a. Release of folate binding protein FBP from granulocytes. Enhancement by lithium and elimination by fluoride. Studies with normal pregnant, cirrhotic and uremic persons. Proc. 17th Annu. Meet. Am. Soc. Hematol *155*. (Abstract)

Colman, N., and Herbert, V. 1974b. Measurement of total folate binding capacity (TFBC) of serum after removal of endogenous folate at acid pH. Clin. Res. *22*:700. (Abstract)

Condit, P. T., and Grob, D. 1958. Studies on the folic acid vitamins. I. Observations on the metabolism of folic acid in man and on the effect of aminopterin. Cancer *11*:525–536.

Cooperman, J. 1967. Microbiological assay of serum and whole blood folic acid activity. Am. J. Clin. Nutr. *20*:1015–1024.

Corrocher, R., De Sandre, G., Pacor, M. L. and Hoffbrand, A. V. 1974. Hepatic protein binding of folate. Clin. Sci. Mol. *46*:551–554.

da Costa, M., and Rothenberg, S. P. 1971. Identification of an immunoreactive folate in serum extracts by radioimmunoassay. Br. J. Haematol. *21*:121–130.

da Costa, M., and Rothenberg, S. P. 1974a. Appearance of a folate binder in leukocytes and serum of women who are pregnant or taking oral contraceptives. J. Lab. Clin. Med. *83*:207–214.

da Costa, M., and Rothenberg, S. P. 1974b. Studies of the folate binding factor in cultures and subcellular fractions of chronic myelogenous leukemia cells. Clin. Res. *22*:486. (Abstract)

da Costa, M., and Rothenberg, S.P. 1975. Subcellular localization and release of folate binding protein from chronic myelogenous leukemia cells in vitro. (Submitted for publication)

da Costa, M., Rothenberg, S. P., and Kamen, B. 1972. DNA synthesis in chronic myelogenous leukemia cells: Comparison of results in cells containing folate binding factor to replicating cells without binder. Blood *39*:621–627.

Elsborg, L. 1972. Binding of folic acid to human plasma proteins. Acta Haematol. *48*:207–212.

Fischer, C., da Costa, M., and Rothenberg, S. P. (In press). Heterogeneity and properties of folate binding protein from chronic myelogenous leukemia cells. Blood.

Ford, J. E. 1974. Some observations on the possible nutritional significance of vitamin B_{12}—and folate binding proteins in milk. Br. J. Nutr. *31*:243–257.

Garth, I. L., and Rowe, P. B. 1972. Folate binding by the brush border membrane proteins of small intestinal epithelial cells. Biochem. *9*:1696–1703.

Ghitis, J. 1967. The folate binding in milk. Am. J. Clin. Nutr. *20*:1–4.

Hampers, C. L., Streiff, R., Nathan, D. C., Snyder, D., and Merrill, J. P. 1967. Megaloblastic hematopoiesis in uremia and in patients on long term hemodialysis. N. Engl. J. Med. *276*:551–554.

Herbert, V. 1966. Aseptic addition method for lactobacillus casei assay of folate activity in human serum. J. Clin. Pathol. *19*:12–16.

Herbert, V., Larrabee, A. R., and Buchanan, J. N. 1962. Studies on the identification of a folate compound of human serum. J. Clin. Invest. *41*:1134–1138.

Hines, J. D., Kamen, B., and Caston, D. 1973. Abnormal folate binding proteins in azotemic patients. Blood. *42*:997. (Abstract)

Iwai, K., Luttner, P. M., and Toennies, G. 1964. Blood folic acid studies. VII. Purification and properties of the folic acid precursors of human erythrocytes. J. Biol. Chem. *239*:2365–2369.

Kamen, B. A., and Caston, J. D. 1975. Identification of a folate binder in hog kidney. J. Biol. Chem. *250*:2203–2205.

Mantzos, J. D., Terzaki, A., and Gyftaki, E. 1974. Folate binding in animal plasma. Acta Haematol. *51*:204–210.

Markkanen, T. 1968. Pteroylglutamic acid (PGA) activity of serum in gel filtration. Life Sci. *7*:887–895.

Markkanen, T., and Peltola, O. 1971. Carrier proteins of folic acid activity in human serum. Acta Haematol. *45*:176–179.

Markkanen, T., Pajula, R. L., Virtanin, S., and Himanen, P. 1972. New carrier protein(s) of folic acid in human serum. Acta Haematol. *48*:145–150.

Metz, J., Zalusky, R., and Herbert, V. 1968. Folic acid binding by serum and milk. Am. J. Clin. Nutr. *21*:289–297.

Retief, F. P., and Huskisson, Y. J. 1970. Folate binders in body fluids. J. Clin. Pathol. *23*:703–707.

Rothenberg, S. P. 1970. A macromolecular factor in some leukemic cells which binds folic acid. Proc. Soc. Exp. Biol. Med. *133*:428–432.

Rothenberg, S. P. 1973. Application of competitive ligand binding for the radioassay of vitamin B_{12} and folic acid. Metabolism *22*:1075–1082.

Rothenberg, S. P., and da Costa, M. 1971. Further observations on the folate-binding factor in some leukemic cells. J. Clin. Invest. *50*:719–726.

Rothenberg, S. P., da Costa, M., and Rosenberg, Z. 1972. Radioassay for serum folate: Use of a sequential-incubation, ligand-binding system. N. Engl. J. Med. *286*:1335–1339.

Rubinoff, M., Schreiber, C., and Waxman, S. 1975. Isolation and characterization of folate binding protein (FBP) from goat milk by affinity chromatography. Fed. Proc. *34*:904. (Abstract)

Salter, D. N., Ford, J. E., Scott, K. J., and Anderson, P. 1972. Isolation of the folate binding protein from cows milk by the use of affinity chromatography. Fed. Eur. Biochem. Soc. Lett. *20*:302–306.

Schreiber, C., and Waxman, S. 1974. Measurement of red cell folate levels by ^{3}H pteroylglutamic acid ([3]H PteGlu) radioassay. Br. J. Haematol. *27*:551–558.

Spector, R., Lorenzo, A. V., and Drum, D. E. 1975. Serum binding of methyltetrahydrofolic acid. Biochem. Pharmacol. *24*:542–544.

Waxman, S. 1974. Isolation and characterization of a folate binding protein(s) FABP from human milk by affinity chromatograhy. Blood *44*:911. (Abstract)

Waxman, S., and Schreiber, C. 1973. Characteristics of folic acid-binding protein in folate-deficient serum. Blood *42*:291–301.

Waxman, S., and Schreiber, C. 1974. The role of folic acid binding protein (FABP) in the cellular uptake of folates. Proc. Exp. Biol. Med. *147*:760–764.

Waxman, S., Schreiber, C., and Herbert, V. 1971. Radioisotopic assay for measurement of serum folate levels. Blood *38*:219–228.

Zamieroski, M., and Wagner, C. 1974. High molecular weight complexes of folic acid in mammalian tissues. Biochem. Biophys. Res. Commun. *60*:81–87.

Zettner, A., and Duly, P. E. 1974. New evidence for a binding principle specific for folates as a normal constituent of human serum. Clin. Chem. *20*:1313–1319.

8

Measurement of Serum Folate Levels: Current Status of the Radioassay Methodology

SAMUEL WAXMAN *and* CAROL SCHREIBER

In 1959, Baker *et al.* (1959) reported that the folate status in man could be measured using a microbiological assay of serum folate activity with *Lactobacillus casei*. This procedure, while adequate, is tedious and requires the maintenance of a special laboratory for this purpose. Furthermore, the assay cannot be used easily with turbid or bacterially contaminated serum and gives false low values if the serum contains high levels of certain antibiotics or antifols (Beard and Allen, 1967).

With the appearance of isotopically labeled folate, the theory of radioassay became increasingly more attractive, and Rothenberg (1965) developed a radioenzymatic assay for folic acid (PteGlu) whereby dihydrofolate reductase obtained from chicken liver was used to reduce the [^{3}H]PteGlu to tetrahydrofolic acid with reduced triphosphopyridine nucleotide as the cofactor. Addition of stable PteGlu to the incubation mixture competitively inhibited the reduction, and this inhibition was quantified and standardized. However, interference by amethopterin and the inability to measure the already reduced folates that predominate in the serum made this approach impractical.

The folate binding properties of milk have been known since the report of Ghitis (1967) and the confirmations by Ghitis *et al.* (1969) and Ford *et al.* (1969). The discovery of a natural binder for several folates, including 5-methyltetrahydrofolic acid ($5CH_3FH_4$), that was not inhibited by antibiotics, antifols, pharmacologic doses of 5-formyltetrahydrofolic acid, or vitamin B_{12} offered an attractive concept for measuring serum and red cell folate levels as an alternative to bioassay.

SURVEY OF APPROACHES FOR RADIOASSAY OF FOLATES

A radioligand competitive inhibition assay was first reported by Metz *et al.* (1968). It utilized commercially available skimmed milk as the source of binding protein but lacked sufficient sensitivity for clinical application. Waxman *et al.* (1971) described a sensitive, direct competitive assay using specially prepared [^{3}H]$5CH_3FH_4$ that was not commercially available with high enough specific activity to permit widespread use of the assay. As an alternative, these authors suggested that commercially available [^{3}H]PteGlu be substituted for the [^{3}H]$5CH_3FH_4$ in a sequential assay system, i.e., the milk binder is first incubated with the unknown sample, and unoccupied binding sites are then titrated with the labeled tracer. In these assays, Carnation Instant Powdered Milk was used as the folate binding source, and the incubations were carried out at 23° C in 0.1 M Na-K PO_4 buffer at the pH optimum of 7.4. The standard curve ranged between 0 and 10 ng of stable $5CH_3FH_4$ using 0.5 ng of [^{3}H]PteGlu as the tracer. Hemoglobin-coated charcoal was used as the adsorbant for unbound folate, and the results were equivalent to the *L. casei* diagnostic groups. These results were confirmed by Tajuddin and Gardyna (1973) who added a serum blank to correct for nonspecific binding of [^{3}H]PteGlu to the assay material, and in the same year Archibald *et al.* (1972) duplicated the procedure with the single additional notation that serum binding may result in artificially elevated values. Similar methodology was employed by Rothenberg *et al.* (1972) who used partially purified binder extracted from cow's milk. The reactions were run at pH 8 in a borate–Ringer's buffer, and [^{3}H]PteGlu was reduced to 0.2 ng per assay. The standard curve had a sensitivity of 0–3 ng of $5CH_3FH_4$, permitting microliter quantities of serum to be assayed. To promote a noncompetitive system, the incubation temperature was dropped to 4° C when the [^{3}H]PteGlu was added to minimize displacement of the bound, reduced folate. Ascorbate was added to the serum samples to preserve endogenous folate. They found results clinically compatible with, but numerically lower than, results given by assay with *L. casei*.

In March of 1973, Mincey *et al.* (1973) confirmed the above, with the only change being a return to Carnation milk as the source of folate binder.

Waxman and Schreiber (1973) first reported the use of crystalline bovine beta lactoglobulin as a source of folate binding protein. Although it was soon recognized that the folate binder was a contaminant of the commercial preparation (Waxman and Schreiber, in press), the nature of the methodology produced a uniform stable binder that was consistent from batch to batch and from producer to producer. Furthermore, the protein solutions were stable to freeze–thawing, and the nature of the binding was such that the need for a sequential assay was eliminated and the less-time-consuming simultaneous additions could be employed. The authors demonstrated that binding was uniform and maximal within 10 min and showed no displacement of reduced by oxidized folates during the 30-min, 23° C assay period. Endogenous folate binding protein (FABP) present in some test sera was saturated with stable PteGlu, and these saturated samples served as the serum blank. Values obtained by this method correlated with *L. casei* assays and the clinical picture. Antifols, antibiotics, vitamin B_{12}, and 5-formyltetrahydrofolic acid (Leucovorin, Lederle Laboratories, Pearl River, N.Y.) did not inhibit binding. No ascorbate or other reducing agents were necessary to preserve serum folate when the samples were centrifuged and stored at $-10°$ C within 1 h after clotting.

Leonard *et al.* (1973) at the Istanbul Symposium described studies of the technical aspects of the radioassay, adapting the methodology of Waxman and Schreiber (1973). They performed their studies with partially purified milk binder and used a sequential two-temperature assay system in borate–Ringer's buffer. Excellent correlation with *L. casei* assays were found.

Many workers have constructed assays utilizing binders other than bovine milk. Mantzos *et al.* (1971) used pig plasma binder in a simultaneous assay at 23° C using $[^{14}C]5CH_3FH_4$ as the tracer. Free folate was separated from bound folate by filtering through G-25 Sephadex columns. The serum binders were destroyed by autoclaving in the presence of ascorbate. Their results were numerically lower than those obtained with the *L. casei* assay but were equal when a correction factor was used. Gyftaki *et al.* (1973) modified the assay, using $[^3H]PteGlu$ with pig plasma in a sequential system. Kamen and Caston (1974) used purified binder from hog kidney and employed this in a simultaneous system. The $5CH_3FH_4$ and $[^3H]PteGlu$ were first incubated at 4° C followed by a 23° C incubation in the presence of binder. An extremely sensitive standard curve was produced, ranging from 0 to 1.6 ng of

$5CH_3FH_4$, and ascorbate was added to the system throughout. Values obtained by this method were lower than those given by the *L. casei* assay.

Shaw (1974), questioned the validity of PteGlu-saturated serum blanks and returned to the Carnation Instant Powdered Milk in a sequential assay system using 0.1 M PO_4 buffer, pH 7.4, and unsaturated serum blanks. He found generally good correlation with *L. casei* assays but recognizes the fact that certain sera range widely from the expected microbiologic value. However, no clinical correlations were cited and no conclusions were drawn.

To attempt to overcome the problem of serum binding of [³H]PteGlu, Dunn and Foster (1973) extracted their samples by boiling in a water bath for 15 min in 0.05 M lysine buffer, pH 10.5. This procedure destroyed the serum binder and produced a cloudy but coagulum-free sample. The pH was returned to 7.4, and a modification of the beta lactoglobulin binding assay of Waxman and Schreiber was employed in a simultaneous incubation at room temperature. Interestingly enough, no ascorbate was added to the serum extracts and excellent correlation with *L. casei* assays was obtained. In 1974 J. K. Givas (personal communication) reported that partially purified milk binder is unable to distinguish reduced from oxidized folates at pH 9.3. This finding was confirmed by Longo and Herbert (1974b) and also duplicated by Waxman and Schreiber (unpublished results). Givas and Gutchko (1975) constructed standard curves using PteGlu as the standard and assayed serum samples treated with ascorbate and boiled in lysine buffer.

The use of [¹²⁵I]PteGlu has been reported recently as a method of radioassay that would eliminate the use of a liquid scintillation system. Longo and Herbert (1974a) have reported on the viability of this technique, but to date no publication of methodology has been noted. Waxman and Schreiber have been unable to demonstrate successfully the efficacy of these assays since serum appears to nonspecifically bind [¹²⁵I]PteGlu, (unpublished results).

Since the inception of the folate radioassay, commercially available kits have been appearing, and Waddel et al. (1975) have confirmed the correlation between diagnostic kits employing [³H]PteGlu radioassay and bioassay. At this time, folate radioassay in its various modifications is being used in clinical facilities throughout the world.

Subsequent to the establishment of serum folate assays, methodology has been presented for the determination of red cell and whole blood folates. Mincey et al. (1973) assayed red cell folates by hemolyzing whole blood collected in EDTA with distilled water containing ascorbic acid. The hemolysates, after standing at room temperature for 30 min, were stored frozen. Folate levels were determined by reference to a standard curve prepared with $5CH_3FH_4$. Rothenberg *et al.* (1974) also measured incubated hemolysates against $5CH_3FH_4$. Schreiber and Waxman (1974) reported the assay of untreated whole blood stored at 4° C and lysed immediately prior to incubation with [³H]PteGlu. In this procedure, folates are calculated against a standard curve prepared with either the folyl polyglutamate PteGlu[3] or PteGlu. They were unable to obtain comparative whole blood levels if the standard curve was constructed with $5CH_3FH_4$ or with polyglutamates of $5CH_3FH_4$ (Glu_5 or Glu_7). (Waxman and Schreiber, unpublished results). All of the authors report correlations between *L. casei* assays and the clinical status.

PROBLEMS TO RESOLVE

As the development of folate radioassay progresses and modifications are made to increase accuracy, they should at the same time provide methodology that can be simply and rapidly used in any clinical laboratory. Modifications that create problems of technique or unnecessary refinements are best left to research studies where the volume of material to be assayed is markedly diminished.

Taking each aspect of the radioassay point by point, we have been able to propose the following:

1. Several investigators have proposed the addition of gelatin, albumin, or folate-free serum to the standard curve. When the assays are run in siliconized glass tubes or disposable borosilicate glass tubes, we have found no significant difference in the slopes of the curves obtained.

2. Except for the use of pH 9.3 buffers where PteGlu has been used to construct the standard curves, stable $5CH_3FH_4$ has been the usual standard. We have found that commercially available $5CH_3FH_4$ may contain a significant amount of oxidized products (probably $5CH_3FH_2$), which when present will significantly increase the sensitivity of the standard curve, resulting in observed serum folate levels markedly lower than the expected values. The addition of ascorbate or mercaptoethanol to the solutions may not renature the already formed degradation products. We have found the use of ϵ_{max} to be effective in calculating only the amount of $5CH_3FH_4$ present in the solution, but this technique does not measure the small amount of oxidation prod-

ucts that will be present in direct proportion to the deterioration of the compound. We therefore purify commercial $5CH_3FH_4$ on DEAE–cellulose according to the method of Blair and Saunders (1970), store the preparations in 0.1 M mercaptoethanol at $-67°$ C, and assay for purity by *L. casei* versus *Streptococcus faecalis.*These purified preparations, while time-consuming to prepare, have been unchanged for 2 years. Moreover, with the introduction of a uniform binder such as beta lactoglobulin, a single standard curve may be prepared and used as a master with only periodic checking, provided a binding control is run with each assay. We have found complete duplication of the standard curves, and perhaps more importantly, the single curve diminishes the problems with frequent deterioration of $5CH_3FH_4$, the most unstable reagent used. The use of a pH of 9.3 to eliminate using a reduced folate for the standard curve may prove feasible. However, we feel that the similar binding of both oxidized and reduced folates may represent slow alkaline oxidation of the reduced folate rather than a change in the affinity of the binder for the different analogues and must be further evaluated.

3. We prefer to use mercaptoethanol rather than ascorbate for storing our reagents because of the extreme sensitivity of the binder to pH changes in the acid region. Ascorbate causes slow lowering of the pH even when the sample is well buffered. When the pH of the reactions falls below 7, spurious results may be obtained.

4. We have noted that there has been some controversy over the use of preservatives in the serum samples. Some workers routinely add 5 mg of ascorbate to the samples to preserve the folates. Other workers have found this to be unnecessary, even when they take their sample through a boiling step. We have found that, when serum is separated from the clot within 1 or 2 h and immediately stored at $-10°$ C, the folate is stable for a period of at least 4 weeks. A longer delay may require the use of a reducing agent.

5. The variation in the buffer systems does not seem to be very significant. No investigator to date has used molarities greater than 0.1, and, with the exception of Rothenberg's method and the pH 9.3 methods, all buffers have a pH range of 7.2 to 7.6. This is in keeping with the established pH optima of the milk binder. The choice of buffer can be left to the convenience of the individual laboratory.

6. The next important question concerns both the temperature of the incubation and the use of sequential versus simultaneous systems. This in turn relates to the preparation of the folate binder used. Many sources of folate binder are available. Some investigators have stayed with Carnation Instant Powdered Milk, which involves a simple weigh-

ing process, possibly dialysis to rid the preparation of substances that might interfere with the scintillation cocktails, and storage at 4° C. The disadvantage is that the milk preparation has a tendency to turn sour after several days, rendering it unusable. A new binding curve must also be constructed with each new preparation because of variation in the product. Other investigators have looked into the possibility of other processed milks such as goat milk, which offers higher binding capacities but has the same preparation problems as cow milk. The possibility of partially purifying the binder from cow or human milk has been explored by some laboratories. They find that these preparations are stable when stored frozen. Binders from various sources such as swine kidney and plasma are prepared according to the particular laboratory situation. We have found that the commercially available bovine beta lactoglobulin is a uniform binder preparation protected from degradation by its protein contaminant and is extremely stable to freeze–thawing (Waxman and Schreiber, in press). Binding curves are duplicated after simple weighing out, and 0.1 mg has been found to bind 50–60 percent of 0.5 ng of [^{3}H]PteGlu from every batch of beta lactoglobulin tested. It has also been noted that, while a sequential incubation can produce a standard curve of exquisite sensitivity, a more efficient simultaneous incubation in which the reaction is started with the addition of the binder produces a standard curve of sufficient sensitivity to allow the use of less than 0.5 ml of serum. We find that binding is complete within 10 min and unchanged for at least 2 h at room temperature. The 30-min time interval for incubation was chosen for convenience. We have found insignificant changes in either the curves or the serum folate levels when the reactions are run at 4° C and we have found no displacement of reduced by oxidized folates at either temperature during the duration of the assay period.

7. The use of various charcoal preparations as the molecular sieve can be left to the discretion of the individual laboratory. We have found that Norit A neutral decolorizing carbon coated with hemoglobin (human) in a 1:20 ratio is most effective in our hands. We recognize that other coats are equally as efficacious and, provided that the principles of the molecular sieve are adhered to, should not create any controversy. It is to be noted that even the most carefully stored hemoglobin-coated charcoal preparations have a tendency to lose their effectiveness after approximately 1 to 2 months.

8. [^{3}H]PteGlu preparations with sufficiently high specific activity are available from several major suppliers. We have found that an occasional lot number of [^{3}H]PteGlu does not bind normally, and these have always been accepted for return by the supplier. We have found storage at −70° C in slightly alkaline phosphate buffer to be effective

for the duration of the preparation with only slight increases in the buffer control. Working solutions are kept at $-10°$ C and thawed prior to use. The suitability of [^{125}I]PteGlu presently available is still under consideration.

9. Scintillation cocktails are left to the individual laboratory to conform with their particular circumstances. Obviously the cocktail must be such as to prevent precipitation of the proteins and capable of taking up sufficient amounts of test solution for accurate quantitation.

10. The final and perhaps most controversial of the questions involves the serum folate binder, its effect on the measurement of folate levels, and the methods used to eliminate its interference or correct for its presence. The presence of folate binding protein in some sera has been observed by many investigators and appears to contribute to an artifactual lowering of serum folate levels unless it is corrected or eliminated (Rothenberg *et al.*, 1972; Waxman and Schreiber, 1973; Dunn and Foster, 1973; Eichner *et al.*, in press). This lower folate value obtained in some unextracted sera may be due to competition between endogenous unsaturated folate binder and milk binder for [^{3}H]PteGlu, or it may be due to a pool of endogenous-bound folate that is not available for measurement by radioassay unless released from the binder. Some workers, as previously discussed, go through a boiling step and others saturate the binder with excess stable PteGlu and use this saturated sample as a binding control. In both instances, the folate values become compatible with both *L. casei* assays and the clinical status. Waxman and Schreiber include a serum binder tube and PteGlu-saturated serum tube to search for patients who have elevations in folate binding protein. Many investigators have questioned the validity of PteGlu correction of the elevated serum folate binding protein because it results in "excess binder" for [^{3}H]PteGlu in the tubes where it occurs. When a standard curve is prepared with the folate binder (i.e., beta lactoglobulin) close to binding excess (at the point where binding of [^{3}H]PteGlu approaches a plateau), the small amount of endogenous folate binding protein present in 0.4 ml of serum, even in circumstances of extreme elevation (45–50 percent binding of 0.5 ng of [^{3}H]PteGlu), will not significantly affect the level of folate obtained. However, the question of whether there is a pool of non-radioassayable, bound endogenous folate can be answered only by doing both whole serum radioassay and heat-extracted radioassay.

CONCLUSIONS

In conclusion, we postulate that the ideal clinical radioassay for the measurement of serum folate levels should be accurate but at the same time simple enough to allow for large numbers of samples to be processed without the danger of either time running short or fatigue with meticulous technique causing unnecessary error.

Therefore, we propose the following:

1. A master standard curve be prepared with highly purified $5CH_3FH_4$ as a function of the reciprocal of the percent bound to produce a straight line. With each day's run, only a [^{3}H]PteGlu standard, buffer control, and 0 tube need be run. Alternatively, a pH 9.3 assay may be utilized, involving the standard curve to be constructed with PteGlu.

2. A buffer system close to normal serum pH to eliminate the need for corrections when larger amounts of serum are used.

3. Use of commercially prepared bovine beta lactoglobulin as the folate binder to eliminate elaborate purifications by laboratories whose main function is not research but clinical.

4. The use of a standard range where binder can always be in near excess to eliminate interference from the serum folate binding factor when present and allow a whole serum assay (unextracted).

5. A heat-extracted serum tube to determine if there is a pool of bound endogenous serum folate.

6. The use of a short-term (30 min) room temperature simultaneous addition procedure with untreated serum samples.

7. The use of a stable molecular sieve with short contact time that does not alter the bound–free ratio upon prolonged contact time.

8. A serum binder tube and PteGlu-saturated serum tube to measure folate binding protein.

However, there continue to be objections to this postulated format, and consequently an organized multi-laboratory comparative study is necessary. Thus far, only one group has compared and reported on the results obtained by the whole serum radioassay defined above, those obtained with a heat-extraction radioassay, and those obtained with a standard microbiologic assay (Eichner *et al.*, in press). There appears to be a close correlation between the whole serum radioassay and microbiologic assay in the normal folate range but a disparity when the serum contains folate binding protein. Further collaborative studies such as this are necessary to standardize methodology in this field. This type of study is all the more urgent since a variety of commercial kits for the radioassay of serum folates are already in extensive clinical use. These tests use different binders, standards, tracers, and incubation times. We recently surveyed 62 independent clinical facilities and found that almost half were using radioassay methods for the measurement of serum folate levels. Almost without exception each laboratory had modified a published procedure, and the result was 25 significantly different radioassay procedures. Most laboratories claimed good clinical correlations, but very few performed concomitant microbiologic assays for comparison. Thus, it appears that there may be a premature utilization of a variety of folate radioassays by clinical laboratories and producers of commercial kits who are not able to evaluate the most acceptable procedure.

The radioassays for folate and folate binding protein have allowed new observations and have opened several new research questions such as: (i) Is a certain portion of serum folate bound to specific endogenous folate binding proteins? (ii) Is this protein-bound folate handled differently from "free" folate and is it perhaps of pathophysiologic significance? (iii) Is a specific form of folate (i.e., oxidized) bound in the serum to specific folate binding proteins? (iv) Are folate binding proteins of clinical importance? (v) Does the microbiologic assay measure protein bound and free folates?

A multifaceted radioassay similar to that proposed could measure: (i) Whole serum folate (theoretically unbound folate); (ii) heat-extracted folate (theoretically bound + unbounded folate); (iii) endogenous bound folate (heat-extracted folate − whole serum folate); (iv) [^{3}H]PteGlu serum-binding capacity (unsaturated folate binding protein); (v) total folate binding capacity (endogenous-bound folate + unsaturated folate binding protein); (vi) levels of oxidized folates by means of anti-PteGlu antiserum.

The patterns obtained from these studies may result in a greater understanding of the complex folate nutritional status in man.

ACKNOWLEDGMENTS

This research was supported by NIH grants AM16690-02 and CA14491-02A2, the Chemotherapy Foundation, Inc., the United Leukemia Fund, and the Gar Reichman Memorial Fund.

DISCUSSION

HERBERT: Dan Longo in our laboratory has worked on a pH 9.0 radioassay and has found that he is unable to tell pteroylglutamic acid (PGA) apart from methyl folate. Therefore, one can use stable PGA, instead of unstable methyl folate, both as nonradioactive standard and as radioassay material. Also, we have found that iodinated folic acid can be used and that it works well with the assay. We can assay serum and red cell folate and get essentially identical results for serum folate using the [^{125}I]PGA pH 9.3 assay versus the [^{3}H]PGA pH 9.3 assay versus the *L. casei* assay. For red cell folate we get lesser correlation with *L. casei*.

We have also found that about half of the samples of milk, either fresh or powdered, contain a material that splits folate off from the endogenous serum folate binding protein. Therefore, if one uses such a milk, or such milk powders, one does not have to worry at all about whether the serum contains an endogenous folate binder, because this crude milk contains a substance, not yet isolated, that splits the serum folate that is bound off its binder. And that is probably another reason we get results highly similar to *L. casei* assay results.

We prefer working with liquid milk. Powdered milk has the asset that it can be stored for a longer period of time. It can be stored on the shelf in the laboratory for 6 months or longer, and not only is the folate binder intact, but the splitter that I mentioned is also intact after 6 months on the lab shelf.

LITERATURE CITED

Archibald, E. L., Mincey, E. K., and Morrison, R. T. 1972. Estimation of serum folate levels by competitive protein binding assay. Clin. Biochem. *5*:232–241.

Baker, H., Herbert, V., Frank, O., Pasher, I., Hutner, S. H., Wasserman, L. R., and Sobotka, H. 1959. A microbiologic method for detecting folic acid deficiency in man. Clin. Chem. *5*:275–280.

Beard, M. E. J., and Allen, D. M. 1967. The effect of antimicrobial agents on the *Lactobacillus casei* folate assay. Am. J. Clin. Pathol. *48*:401–404.

Blair, J. A., and Saunders, K. J. 1970. A convenient method for the preparation of dl-5-methyltetrahydrofolic acid (dl-5-5,6,7,8-tetrahydropteroyl-L-monoglutamic acid). Anal. Biochem. *34*:376–381.

Dunn, R. T., and Foster, L. B. 1973. Radioassay of serum folate. Clin. Chem. *19*:1101–1105.

Eichner, E. R., Paine, C. J., Dickson, V. L., and Hargrove, M. D., Jr. (In press). Clinical and laboratory observations on serum folate binding protein. Blood.

Ford, J. E., Salter, D. N., and Scott, K. J. 1969. The folate binding protein in milk. J. Dairy Res. *36*:436–446.

Ghitis, J. 1967. The folate binding in milk. Am. J. Clin. Nutr. *20*:1015–1024.

Ghitis, J., Mandelbaum-Shavit, F., and Grossowicz, N. 1969. Binding of folic acid and derivatives by milk. Am. J. Clin. Nutr. *22*:156–162.

Givas, J. K., and Gutcho, S. 1975. pH dependence of the binding of folates to milk binder in radioassay of folates. Clin. Chem. *21*:427–428.

Gyftaki, E., Loukopoulos, D., Kesse-Elias, M., and Alevizou-Terzaki, V. 1973. Estimation of serum folic acid with competitive protein binding method in beta thalassaemia. International Atomic Energy Agency Symposium on Radioimmunoassay and Related Procedures in Clinical Medicine and Research, Istanbul, Turkey.

Kamen, B., and Caston, D. 1974. Direct radiochemical assay for serum folate: Competition between ^{3}H-folic acid and 5-methyltetrahydrofolic acid for a folate binder. J. Lab. Clin. Med. *83*:164–174.

Leonard, J. P., Taymans, F., and Beckers, C. 1973. A radioassay for serum folate using milk protein as ligand-binding system, pp. 221–231. International Atomic Energy Agency Symposium on Radioimmunoassay and Related Procedures in Clinical Medicine and Research, Istanbul, Turkey.

Longo, D. L., and Herbert, V. 1974a. Simple radioassay for serum and red cell folate based on three new findings. Am. Soc. Hematol., Atlanta, Ga., no. 163.

Longo, D. L. and Herbert, V. 1974b. Simplifying serum folate radioassays: Equal binding of methyltetrahydrofolate (MTHF) and pteroylglutamic acid (PGA) by milk binder at pH 9.3; discovery of a serum folate releasing factor in crude milk binder. Clin. Res. *22*:701. (Abstract)

Mantzos, J., Gyftaki, E., Alevizou-Terzaki, V., Manesis, E., and Malamos, B. 1971. Determination of serum folates by the use of competitive protein binding: Preliminary studies. Jahrestag. Ges. Nuclearmed. Antwerpen.

Metz, J., Zalusky, R., and Herbert, V. 1968. Folic acid binding by serum and milk. Am. J. Clin. Nutr. *21*:289–297.

Mincey, E. K., Wilcox, E., and Morrison, R. T. 1973. Estimation of serum and red cell folate by a simple radiometric technique. Clin. Biochem. *6*:274–284.

Rothenberg, S. P. 1965. A radioenzymatic assay for folic acid. Nature *206*:1154–1156.

Rothenberg, S. P., da Costa, M., and Rosenberg, Z. 1972. A radioassay for serum folate: Use of a two-phase sequential incubation, ligand-binding system. N. Engl. J. Med. *286*:1335–1139.

Rothenberg, S. P., da Costa, M., Lawson, J., and Rosenberg, Z. 1974. The determination of erythrocyte folate concentration using a two-phase ligand-binding radioassay. Blood *43*:437–443.

Schreiber, C., and Waxman, S. 1974. Measurement of red cell folate levels by ^{3}H-pteroylglutamic acid (^{3}H-PteGlu) radioassay. Br. J. Haematol. *27*: 551–558.

Shaw, W., Slade, B. A., Harrison, J. W., and Nino, H. V. 1974. Assay of serum folate: Difference in serum folate values obtained by *L. casei* bioassay and competitive protein binding assay. Clin. Biochem. *7*:165–178.

Tajuddin, M., and Gardyna, H. A. 1973. Radioassay of serum folate with use of a serum blank and nondialyzed milk as folate binder. Clin. Chem. *19*:125–126.

Waxman, S., and Schreiber, C. 1973. Measurement of serum folate levels and serum folic acid binding protein by ^{3}H-PGA radioassay. Blood *42*:281–290.

Waxman, S., and Schreiber, C. 1975. The isolation of the folate binding protein from commercially purified bovine beta lactoglobulin. FEBS Lett. *55*:128–130.

Waxman, S., Schreiber, C., and Herbert, V. 1971. Radioisotopic assay for measurement of serum folate levels. Blood *38*:219–228.

Waddell, C. C., Domstad, P. A., Brown, J. A., and Lawhorn, B. K. 1975. Serum folate levels; comparison of microbiologic assay and radioisotopic method. Clin. Res. *23*:284. (Abstract)

9

Folate Polyglutamate Synthesis and Breakdown in Human Cells

A. V. HOFFBRAND, E. TRIPP, *and* A. LAVOIÉ

Recent evidence strongly suggests that folate polyglutamates are, in general, the naturally occurring folate coenzymes for the folate-mediated reactions in amino acid metabolism and purine and pyrimidine synthesis in mammalian cells (Baugh and Krumdieck, 1969; Hoffbrand, 1975). The alternative concept, that these compounds are only storage forms of the vitamin, is no longer acceptable. Folate polyglutamates are the major form of folate in mammalian (and other) cells, accounting for up to 90 percent or more of cell folate, and biochemical studies *in vitro* have shown that the reduced folate polyglutamates are more active than the corresponding folate monogluta-mates as coenzymes in folate-mediated reactions, such as serine–glycine interconversion (Blakley, 1957) and homocysteine methylation to methionine (F. W. Cheng and E. L. R. Stokstad, submitted for publication), and are more active substrates for the reducing enzymes, dihydrofolate reductase and 5,10-methylenetetrahydrofolate reductase (F. W. Cheng and E. L. R. Stokstad, submitted for publication; Coward et al., 1974).

Moreover, mammalian cells with a genetic inability to synthesize folate polyglutamates require extra thymidine, adenosine, and glycine, compounds whose *de novo* synthesis is known to require folate coenzymes in their culture medium for growth. (McBurney and Whitmore, 1974). In bacteria, the enzyme thymidylate synthetase has also been shown to be more effective with a folate polyglutamate coenzyme (Kislieuk *et al.*, 1974), but, as yet, similar studies of the mammalian enzyme have not been reported.

Since the circulating form of folate in plasma is a monoglutamate compound, 5-methyltetrahydrofolate, mammalian cells must each build up all their own folate (polyglutamate) coenzymes from this substrate. The reactions involved in the synthesis of folate polyglutamate compounds are, therefore, of particular interest. A separate enzyme is concerned with hydrolysis of folate polyglutamates to the monoglutamate state, but the role of this enzyme in general folate metabolism is not completely defined. This paper concerns the recent advances in knowledge about the mechanisms of action and functions of these two important enzyme systems.

FOLATE CONJUGASE (PPH, γ-GLUTAMYLCARBOXYPEPTIDASE)

Pteroylpolyglutamate hydrolase (PPH) hydrolyzes the γ-peptide bonds of folate polyglutamates (pteroylpolyglutamates). It is not only specific for the glutamate–glutamate linkage but is also capable of hydrolyzing γ-peptide linkages of other derivatives of folic acid (PteGlu), e.g., PteGlu–glycine or PteGlu–aspartate, though at a lower rate. The pH optimum is low (4.6), and the enzyme is localized in lysosomes. The enzyme is an exopeptidase with a preference for the longer chain derivatives, splits off glutamate moieties singly, and hydrolyzes folate polyglutamates down to monoglutamate derivatives. The mechanisms by which folate monoglutamates are degraded in the body to nonfolate compounds are unknown, but PPH is probably not involved. The molecular weight of PPH is unknown, although in gel filtration studies the rat enzyme has an apparent molecular weight of 63,000 (Jagerstad *et al.*, 1973), and the human jejunal enzyme behaves as though its molecular weight is about 83,000, and the enzyme in human serum behaves as though its molecular weight is 110,000 (Lavoie *et al.*, 1975). Further evidence for differences between the enzymes from these two human tissues is that the serum enzyme is less stable to heat than the jejunal enzyme (Lavoie et al., 1975). Taken together, these studies suggest that human PPH may exist in isoenzyme forms.

The enzyme in the duodenal and jejunal mucosal cells is almost certainly involved in the absorption of dietary folate polyglutamates. The concentration of enzyme in the lumen of the small intestine is extremely low, and *in vitro* studies using everted sacs (Rosenberg *et al.*, 1969) and isolated mucosal cells (Halsted and Gotterer, 1974) show that, in the rat at least, direct hydrolysis in the mucosa is possible. This is also suggested by kinetic studies of folate polyglutamate transfer across segments of dog intestine (Baugh *et al.*, 1975). The folate polyglutamate presumably enters the mucosal cell intact, but, despite the lysosomal localization of PPH, there is no evidence that the uptake is via pinocytosis. Back diffusion of folate monoglutamates from the mucosa may partly account for the appearance of folate monogluta-mates in the lumen of the small intestine after infusion of polyglutamate derivatives (Baugh *et al.*, 1975). It has been suggested that certain diseases (e.g. tropical sprue, adult coeliac disease) and drugs such as oral contraceptives and anticonvulsants interfere specifically with ab-sorption of dietary folate by reducing the mucosal cell concentration of PPH or by inhibiting the enzyme. However, there is as yet no evidence that diseases of the small intestine affect absorption of dietary folate because of an enzyme deficiency rather than because of damage to the absorptive surface. Indeed, in untreated adult coeliac disease, the concentration of jejunal PPH, like that of other lysosomal enzymes, is increased above normal and falls to normal when a gluten-free diet is given (Hoffbrand *et al.*, 1970; Jägerstad *et al.*, 1974), and no drug has been conclusively shown to cause malabsorption of dietary folate by inhibiting mucosal PPH.

PPH is also involved in recycling of cell folate polyglutamates when cells die, though it has not been established whether the enzyme in serum, in the dying cell itself, or, in some cases, in the reticuloendothe-lial cell engulfing the dying cell is concerned. The more speculative suggestion has been made that the enzyme PPH is concerned in regulat-ing the size of intracellular folates according to the proliferative activity of cells by reducing the polyglutamate chain length in actively dividing and proliferating cells (Krumdieck *et al.*, 1975). This theory implies that lower polyglutamates of folates may be the more active coenzymes for reactions in DNA synthesis. As mentioned earlier, however, the balance of evidence suggests that folates of shorter glutamate chain length are, in general, less active as coenzymes than the longer-chain derivatives. Moreover, studies in human and rat tissues (Lavoie *et al.*, 1975) do not show any change in size of intracellular folate polygluta-mates according to the proliferative activity of the cells, and the same is true when fetal and adult mouse and chick liver are compared or when the intracellular folates in *Escherichia coli* or *Lactobacillus casei* at different stages of cell proliferation are compared (Scott *et al.*, 1975).

SYNTHESIS OF FOLATE POLYGLUTAMATES

Only a few studies have been performed so far on the size and formation of human folate polyglutamates, though a number of studies of folate polyglutamate synthesis have recently been performed in bacterial and animal tissues. We have studied the synthesis of folate polyglutamates from tritium labeled folic acid and folinic acid (5-formyltetrahydrofolate) and from ^{14}C-labeled 5-methyltetrahydrofolate in human lymphocytes transformed with phytohemagglutinin. The cells are incubated with the labeled folate compound for periods up to 72 h. After washing the cells three times in ice-cold phosphate-buffered saline, pH 7.0, the labeled folates were recovered by extraction either by heating to 115° C for 5 min in 0.1 M phosphate buffer, pH 8.5, containing 1.5 g of ascorbate per 100 ml and 0.1 M mercaptoethanol or using 5 M urea and trichloroacetic acid (Baugh *et al.*, 1974). The labelled folates were cleaved at the 9–10 bond either by potassium permanganate oxidation (Houlihan and Scott, 1972) or by zinc reduction (Baugh *et al.*, 1974), and the resulting paraaminobenzoateglutamate fractions were chromatographed on DEAE–cellulose using a KCl gradient (Figure 9-1).

A typical time course of conversion of [^{3}H]PteGlu into lymphocyte folate is shown in Figure 9-2. After 4 h of incubation, nearly all the labeled intracellular folate is still in the monoglutamate form, but small amounts of labeled polyglutamates are already present (the major forms are tri-, tetra-, and pentaglutamates). After 24 h, substantially less labeled monoglutamate is present, and the proportion of the label in tetra-, penta-, and hexaglutamates has risen. After 72 h of incubation, the proportion of monoglutamate has fallen still further, and the proportions of tetra-, penta-, and hexa-derivatives have risen with significant amounts of hepta- and, in some experiments, traces of octa-derivatives also present. These findings are similar to those obtained in studies of the time course of folate polyglutamate formation in mammalian liver from injected tritiated folic acid (Corrocher *et al.*, 1972).

The range and mean distribution of the labeled folate according to the glutamate chain length after 72 h of incubation in seven normal cultures is shown in Table 9-1. This shows that tetra- and penta-derivatives are almost equal in proportion, with hexa-, tri-, and hepta-

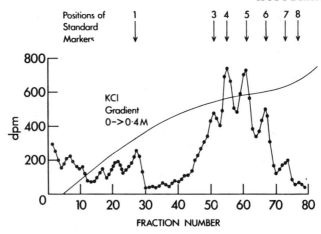

FIGURE 9-1 DEAE–cellulose chromatography of labelled human PHA-stimulated lymphocytes incubated for 72 h with [³H]PteGlu. A 2-μCi (28-ng) portion of 3′,5′,9-[³H]folic acid, 31 Ci/mmol (Radiochemical Centre, Amersham) was added to each 3-ml culture bottle containing 3×10^6 normal lymphocytes and PHA. In this experiment, a total of 21×10^6 lymphocytes were cultured. After 72 h of incubation at 37° C, the cells were harvested, and folates were extracted, cleaved by KMnO₄, and chromatographed (see text). Vertical scale = dpm from 2.5 ml of each 3.8-ml fraction (reproduced from A. V. Hoffbrand, E. Tripp, and A. Lavoie. Clin. Sci. Mol. Med. *50*:63, 1976, with kind permission of the authors, editor, and publisher).

derivatives being the next most frequent. It is likely that the proportion of labeled monoglutamate in these experiments is considerably higher than the proportion of folate monoglutamates in the endogenous lymphocyte folates because the cells are incubated (until analysis) in a medium containing a high concentration of the labeled monoglutamate PteGlu and it is likely that the ability of the cells to take up [³H]PteGlu from these high external concentrations in most experiments exceeds the ability of the cells to convert this to polyglutamate derivatives. Microbiological studies of endogenous lymphocyte folate confirm that the proportion that is monoglutamate is very much lower than these incorporation studies would suggest in view of the substantial proportion of lymphocyte folate that is microbiologically active folate triglutamate (Krumdieck *et al.*, 1975).

The enzyme that synthesizes folate polyglutamates (pteroylpolyglutamate synthetase [PPS] or pteroylpolyglutamate ligase) has been studied in extracts of *E. coli* (Griffin and Brown, 1964), *Neurospora*

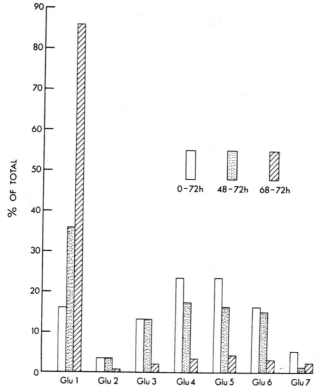

FIGURE 9-2 A typical experiment to illustrate the time course of formation of labelled pteroylpolyglutamates from [³H]PteGlu. The experimental conditions were similar to those described for Figure 1 except zinc cleavage was used to hydrolyze the C_9–N_{10} bond before chromatography. 18×10^6 lymphocytes were used for each time point.

crassa (Sakami *et al.,* 1973), rat liver (Spronk, 1973), and sheep liver (Gawthorne and Smith, 1973). The enzyme requires ATP, Mg^{++}, K^+, and a pH around neutral. Coenzyme A stimulates the reaction but apparently is not essential. In *N. crassa,* two enzymes are concerned; one adds the first glutamate and the second adds subsequent glutamate moieties (Sakami *et al.,* 1973).

Methotrexate (10^{-5} M) reduces but does not completely abolish the conversion of [³H]PteGlu to polyglutamate derivatives in human lymphocytes. Traces of di- and tetraglutamates are formed, as well as a larger proportion of triglutamate. Total cell uptake of [³H]PteGlu is

TABLE 9-1   Composition of Labeled Cell
Folate after Incubation of PHA-Stimulated
Lymphocytes with [^{3}H] PteGlu (0–72 h)[a]

Glutamate Chain Length	Percent of Total	
	Range of 7 Experiments	Mean
1	4–42	22.4
2	1–3	2.0
3	4–17	12.7
4	7–26	20.5
5	15–25	20.1
6	8–22	15.6
7	0–13	5.7
8	0–4	1.1

[a]Reproduced from A. V. Hoffbrand, E. Tripp, and
A. Lavoie, Clin. Sci. Mol. Med. *50:*63, 1976, with kind
permission of the authors, editor, and publishers.

reduced by methotrexate (10^{-5} M) by a third over the 48–72 h of culture
(Table 9-2). On the other hand, methotrexate has no effect on the
formation of labeled folate polyglutamates when labeled folinic acid is
the substrate (Table 9-2). These results show that a reduced folate is
the preferred form of folate monoglutamate from which polyglutamate
synthesis takes place in human cells. Some, but not all, workers have
found that unreduced pteroylpolyglutamates are formed from injected
^{3}H-labeled-folic acid ([^{3}H]PteGlu) in the livers of guinea pigs and rats
pretreated with methotrexate. However, the hepatic uptake of the
labeled[^{3}H]PteGlu was substantially reduced by the presence of
methotrexate, and the proportion of polyglutamate derivatives formed
was low in all studies (Corrocher and Hoffbrand, 1972; Brown *et al.*,
1974; Shin *et al.*, 1974).

The exact nature of the reduced folate monoglutamate compound (or
compounds) used by PPS in human tissues as the starting point for
polyglutamate synthesis is not established. Results in *E. coli, N.
crassa,* and rat liver show that tetrahydrofolate and not methyltetrahydrofolate is preferred (Griffin and Brown, 1964; Sakami *et al.*,
1973; Spronk, 1973). This may also be so in human tissues since when
folate polyglutamates are synthesized from methyltetrahydrofolate
labeled in the methyl group, the radioactive label cannot be detected in
the polyglutamates (Lavoie *et al.*, 1974). These results suggest that the
methyl group is completely removed before glutamate addition takes

TABLE 9-2   Composition of Labeled Cell Folate after Incubation of
PHA-Stimulated Lymphocytes with [^{3}H] PteGlu or [^{3}H] CHO-H$_4$ PteGlu
(24–72 h) with or without Methotrexate (10^{-5} M)

Glutamate Chain Length	Percentage of Total			
	[^{3}H]PteGlu		[^{3}H]CHO-H$_4$ PteGlu	
	Control	+ Methotrexate	Control	+ Methotrexate
1	4	71.5	10	17
2	1	0.5	9	10
3	11	24	16	13
4	24	4.0	20	18
5	21	0	35	36
6	22	0	8	5
7	13	0	2	1
8	4	0		

place. An alternative explanation for this indirect evidence that methyl-tetrahydrofolate is not used as such for polyglutamate synthesis in human cells but is first "demethylated" is that the labeled methyl group is removed from folate polyglutamates after, rather than before, they have been synthesized. This is less likely, however, since a substantial proportion of cell pteroylpolyglutamates are methylated.

The question of the nature of the exact folate substrate for PPS *in vivo* is important since all cells are presented with folate from plasma as methyltetrahydrofolate to which all dietary folates are converted by the small intestine. If indeed tetrahydrofolate, not methyltetrahydrofolate, serves as substrate for pteroylpolyglutamate synthesis, the biochemical reaction in which the methyl group is removed from methyltetrahydrofolate is placed in a key position in folate metabolism between plasma folate on the one hand and intracellular folate polyglutamate coenzymes on the other hand (Figure 9-3). The reaction concerned with the removal of the methyl group is the methylation of homocysteine to methionine, and this reaction also requires vitamin B$_{12}$ in the form of methylcobalamin as coenzyme. Studies with vitamin B$_{12}$-deficient human lymphocytes and bone marrow show that transfer of the methyl group from methyltetrahydrofolate *in vitro* is defective in these cells and can be corrected by adding vitamin B$_{12}$ (Lavoie *et al.*, 1974; Taylor *et al.*, 1974). Thus, the original "methylfolate" trap hypothesis (Noronha and Silverman, 1961; Herbert and Zalusky, 1962) can now be expanded to explain why plasma folate accumulates and intracellular folate content is reduced in vitamin B$_{12}$ deficiency and exactly how

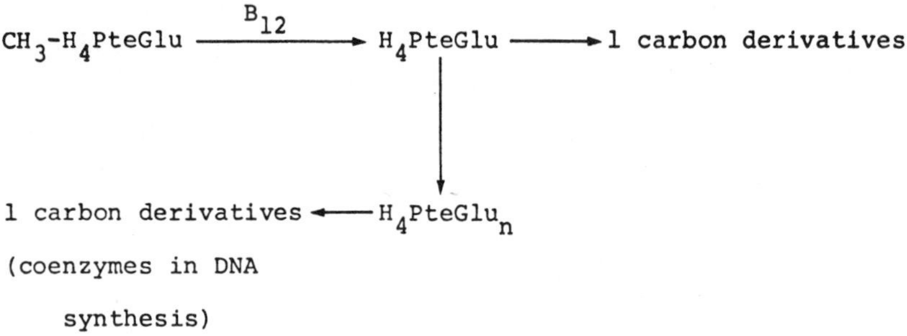

$$CH_3\text{-}H_4PteGlu \xrightarrow{\quad B_{12}\quad} H_4PteGlu \longrightarrow 1 \text{ carbon derivatives}$$

$$1 \text{ carbon derivatives} \longleftarrow H_4PteGlu_n$$

(coenzymes in DNA

   synthesis)

FIGURE 9-3   Proposed role of vitamin B_{12} in formation of intracellular folate poly-glutamate coenzymes from plasma folate (5-methyltetrahydrofolate).

synthesis of folate coenzymes from plasma folate may be reduced (Figure 9-3). Lack of a "pileup" of intracellular methyltetrahydrofolate in vitamin B_{12}-deficient cells that we (Hoffbrand and Tripp, unpublished observations) and others (Chanarin *et al.*, 1974) have observed may be due to failure of cells to retain this monoglutamate derivative as effectively as they retain the folate polyglutamates to which it is normally converted after "demethylation."

SUMMARY

Human intracellular folates, studied in phytohaemagglutinin-transformed lymphocytes, consist mainly of pteroyltetra-, penta-, and hexaglutamate derivatives. These polyglutamate compounds are likely to be the natural folate coenzymes in reactions in purine and pyrimidine synthesis and in amino acid metabolism. Cells contain an enzyme, pteroylpolyglutamate synthetase (PPS), capable of building up these polyglutamate derivatives from pteroylmonoglutamates and a second enzyme, pteroylpolyglutamate hydrolase (PPH, folate conjugase, γ-glutamylcarboxypeptidase), which splits the polyglutamate derivatives to the pteroylmonoglutamate state.

Previous biochemical studies with the rat liver enzyme have shown that PPS requires a reduced folate as substrate and that tetrahydrofolate rather than methyltetrahydrofolate is the preferred substrate. *In vitro* studies of the synthesis of pteroylpolyglutamate compounds in human lymphocytes using radioactively labeled folic acid, folinic acid, or 5-methyltetrahydrofolate as precursors have now been carried out. Results suggest that tetrahydrofolate rather than methyltetrahydrofolate is also the preferred substrate in human tissues. This observation implies that vitamin B_{12} may have a key role in the synthesis of folate coenzymes since it is needed in the homocysteine–methionine reaction by which methyltetrahydrofolate (which is the form of folate which cells take up from plasma) is converted to tetrahydrofolate. Lack of vitamin B_{12} may, therefore, deprive cells of tetrahydrofolate from which all the folate polyglutamate derivatives, the folate coenzymes, are built.

The enzyme that hydrolyzes polyglutamate forms of folate, PPH (folate conjugase), is localized in lysosomes and has a pH optimum of about 4.6. It is concerned with the hydrolysis of dietary folates during their absorption and with the recycling of folates after cell death, but the theory that the enzyme is also involved in changing the length of the glutamate side chain of folates in viable cells according to their proliferative state is not supported by most recent data. Recent heat stability and gel filtration studies suggest that the enzyme PPH may exist in different forms (possibly isoenzymes) in human tissues.

ACKNOWLEDGMENT

We wish to thank E. Buehring, E. L. R. Stokstad, and J. Perry for the standard folate polyglutamate markers. A. V. H. is supported by the Leukaemia Research Fund and Medical Research Council, and A. L. was a recipient of a Research Fellowship from the Medical Research Council of Canada.

LITERATURE CITED

Baugh, C. M., and Krumdieck, C. L. 1969. Naturally occurring folates. Ann. N.Y. Acad. Sci. *186*:7–28.

Baugh, C. M., Braverman, E., and Nair, M. G. 1974. The identification of polyglutamyl chain lengths in bacterial folates. Biochemistry *13*:3952–3957.

Baugh, C. M., Krumdieck, C. L., Baker, H. J. and Butterworth, C. E., Jr. 1975. Absorption of folic acid poly-γ-glutamates in dogs. J. Nutr. *105*:80–89.

Blakley, R. L. 1957. The interconversion of serine and glycine: Some further properties of the enzyme system. Biochem. J. *65*:342–348.

Brown, J. P., Davidson, G. E., Weir, D. G., and Scott, J. M. 1974. Specificity of folate-γ-L-glutamate ligase in rat liver and kidney biosynthesis of poly-L-glutamates of unreduced methotrexate and the effect of methotrexate on folate polyglutamate biosynthesis. Int. J. Biochem. *5*:727–733.

Chanarin, I., Perry, J., and Lumb, M. 1974. The biochemical lesion in vitamin B_{12} deficiency in man. Lancet *i*:1251–1252.

Corrocher, R., and Hoffbrand, A. V. 1972. Subcellular localisation and effect of methotrexate on the incorporation of radioactive folic acid into liver folate. Clin. Sci. *43*:815–822.

Corrocher, R., Bhuyan, B. K., and Hoffbrand, A. V. 1972. Composition of pteroylpoly-glutamates (conjugated folates) in guinea-pig liver and their formation from folic acid. Clin. Sci. *43*:799–813.

Coward, J. K., Parameswaran, K. N., Cashmore, A. R., and Bertino, J. R. 1974. 7,8-Dihydropteroyl oligo-γ-L-glutamates: Synthesis and kinetic studies with purified dihydrofolate reductase from mammalian sources. Biochemistry *13*:3899–3903.

Gawthorne, J. M., and Smith, R. M. 1973. The synthesis of pteroylpolyglutamates by sheep liver enzymes *in vitro*. Biochem. J. *136*:295–301.

Griffin, M. J., and Brown, G. M. 1964. The biosynthesis of folic acid. III. Enzymatic formation of dihydrofolic acid from dihydropteroic acid and of tetrahydropteroylpoly-glutamic acid compounds from tetrahydrofolic acid. J. Biol. Chem. *239*:310–316.

Halsted, C. H., and Gotterer, G. S. 1974. Correlation of folate conjugase and mucosal uptake of pteroylpolyglutamate. Clin. Res. *22*:359A.

Herbert, V., and Zalusky, R. 1962. Interrelationships of vitamin B_{12} and folic acid metabolism: Folic acid clearance studies. J. Clin. Invest. *41*:1263–1276.

Hoffbrand, A. V. (In press). Synthesis and breakdown of natural folates (pteroylpoly-glutamates). *In* Progress in ahematology, E. Brown, ed.

Hoffbrand, A. V., Douglas, A. P., Fry. L., and Stewart, J. S. 1970. Malabsorption of dietary folate (pteroylpolyglutamates) in adult coeliac disease and dermatitis her-petiformis. Br. Med. J. *4*:85–89.

Houlihan, C. M., and Scott, J. M. 1972. The identification of pteroylpentaglutamate as the major folate derivative in rat liver and the demonstration of its biosynthesis from exogenous (^{3}H) pteroylglutamate. Biochem. Biophys. Res. Commun. *48*:1675–1681.

Jägerstad, M., Lindstrand, K., and Westesson, A.-K. 1973. Hydrolysis of conjugated folic acid by pancreatic 'conjugase'. Scand. J. Gastroenterol. *7*:593–597.

Jägerstad, M., Lindstrand, K., Norden, A., Westesson, A.-K., and Lindberg, T. 1974. The folate conjugase activity of the intestinal mucosa in celiac disease. Scand. J. Gastroenterol. *9*:255-259.

Kislieuk, R. L., Gaumont, Y., and Baugh, C. M. 1974. Polyglutamyl derivatives of folate as substrates and inhibitors of thymidylate synthetase. J. Biol. Chem. *249*:4100–4103.

Krumdieck, C. L., Boots, L. R., Cornwell, P. E., and Butterworth, C. E., Jr. (In press). Estrogen stimulation of conjugase activity in the uterus of ovariectomized rats. Amer. J. Clin. Nutr., Vol. 28.

McBurney, M. W., and Whitmore, G. F. 1974. Isolation and biochemical characteristics of folate deficient mutants of Chinese hamster cells. Cell *2*: 173–182.

Noronha, J. M., and Silverman, M. 1961. On folic acid, vitamin B_{12}, methionine and formiminoglutamic acid metabolism. *In* Vitamin B_{12} and intrinsic factor, H. C. Hein-rich, ed. Enke Verlag, Stuttgart. pp. 728–736.

Lavoie, A., Tripp, E., and Hoffbrand, A. V. 1974. The effect of vitamin B_{12} deficiency on methylfolate metabolism and pteroylpolyglutamate synthesis in human cells. Clin. Sci. Mol. Med. *47*:617–630.

Lavoie, A., Tripp, E., and Hoffbrand, A. V. (In press). Sephadex-gel filtration and heat stability of human jejunal and serum pteroylpolyglutamate hydrolase (folate con-jugase). Evidence for two different forms. Biochem. Med.

Lavoie, A., Tripp, E. Parsa, K., and Hoffbrand, A. V. 1975. Polyglutamate forms of folate in resting and proliferating mammalian tissues. Clin. Sci. Mol. Med. *48*:67–73.

Rosenberg, I. H., Streiff, R. R., Godwin, H. A., and Castle, W. B. 1969. Absorption of polyglutamic folate: Participation of deconjugating enzymes of the intestinal mucosa. N. Engl. J. Med. *280*:985–988.

Sakami, W., Ritari, S. J., Black, C. W., and Rzepka, J. 1973. Polyglutamate synthesis by *Neurospora crassa*. Fed. Proc. *32*:471A.

Scott, J. M., Houlihan, C. M., Bassett, R., and Weir, D. G. 1975. Folate polyglutamates during development in mammalian cells and during growth cycle in micro-organisms. Eur. Afr. Soc. Haematol., London. (Abstract)

Shin, Y. S., Buehring, K. U., and Stokstad, E. L. R. 1974. The metabolism of methotrexate in *Lactobacillus casei* and rat liver and the influence of methotrexate on metabolism of folic acid. J. Biol. Chem. *249*:5722–5777.

Spronk, A. M. 1973. Tetrahydrofolate polyglutamate synthesis in rat liver. Fed. Proc. *32*:471A.

Taylor, R. T., Hanna, M. L., and Hutton, J. J. 1974. 5-Methyltetrahydrofolate homocysteine cobalamin methyltransferase in human bone marrow and its relationship to pernicious anemia. Arch. Biochem. Biophys. *165*:787–795.

10

Regulation of Folate Metabolism by Vitamin B_{12}

E. L. R. STOKSTAD

A direct metabolic link between vitamin B_{12} and folic acid was first established with the observation that the excretion of formimino-glutamic acid (FiGlu) was increased in vitamin B_{12} deficiency (Silverman and Pitney, 1958; Rabinowitz and Tabor, 1958). The addition of methionine to the vitamin B_{12}-deficient diet decreased the FiGlu excretion to normal (Silverman and Pitney, 1958; Rabinowitz and Tabor, 1958; Brown et al., 1960). Similarly, it was reported that the excretion of formate (Freidman et al., 1954; Stokstad et al., 1966) and im-idazolecarboxamide (McGeer et al., 1965; Oace et al., 1968) was increased in cobalamin deficiency and restored to normal by the addition of dietary methionine. Each of these metabolites is further metabolized by a folate-dependent reaction, and there is no evidence that cobalamin is directly involved. In clinical deficiencies of both folic acid and vitamin B_{12}, there is an increased excretion of FiGlu (Luhby et al., 1959; Zalusky and Herbert, 1961; Chanarin, 1963) and aminoimidazolecarboxamide (Luhby and Cooperman, 1962; Middletown et al., 1964). In all these cases, the effect of vitamin B_{12} deficiency is less marked than that of folic acid deficiency.

122

Two theories have been advanced to explain the effect of vitamin B_{12}:

1. Methyl trap theory. This was advanced by Noronha and Silverman (1962) and by Herbert and Zalusky (1962).
2. Membrane transport theory. This theory, advanced by Gawthorne and Smith (1973), proposes that vitamin B_{12} is involved in membrane transport of folic acid into the liver and thus accounts for the marked drop in hepatic folate levels in cobalamin deficiency.

METHYL TRAP THEORY

This theory holds that the 5-methyltetrahydrofolates accumulate in vitamin B_{12} deficiency. The metabolic scheme in which this would function is shown in Figure 10-1. This theory is also based on the premise that the equilibrium of the reduction of 5,10-methylenetetrahydrofolate to 5-methyltetrahydrofolate is very high and may be considered essentially irreversible under physiological conditions (Katzen and Buchanan, 1965; Kutzbach and Stokstad, 1971). Methyl folates can be converted to non-methyl forms only by reacting with homocysteine to give methionine in the cobalamin-dependent methyltransferase.

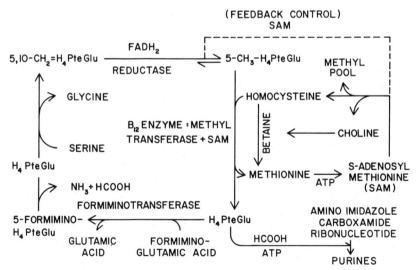

FIGURE 10-1   Interrelationship between folic acid, vitamin B_{12}, and methionine.

The effect of cobalamin deficiency on folate metabolism may be readily explained by the reduced reaction of methyltetrahydrofolate with homocysteine. It does not readily account for the action of methionine, which would be expected to reduce the reaction of methyltetrahydrofolates with homocysteine to give methionine on the basis of end product inhibition. Methionine repression of methylenetetrahydrofolate reductase has been observed in *Escherichia coli* (Katzen and Buchanan, 1965) and *Saccharomyces cerevisiae* (Combepine *et al.,* 1971), but no such repression has been found in mammalian tissue (Kutzbach *et al.,* 1967). Kutzbach and co-workers observed that hepatic methylenetetrahydrofolate reductase was unaffected by vitamin B_{12} deficiency and methionine (Kutzback *et al.,* 1967). They did find that the enzyme was inhibited by S-adenosylmethionine (SAM) but not by methionine. The effect of SAM was reversed by S-adenosylhomocysteine (Kutzbach and Stokstad, 1967, 1971). The 50 percent inhibition levels varied between 2.8 μM to 58 μM. The sensitivity of the enzyme to SAM inhibition was affected by aging of the enzyme preparation and degree of purity (Kutzbach and Stokstad, 1967, 1971). These 50 percent inhibition concentrations are similar to SAM levels of 33 to 110 nmol/g levels that have been found in rat liver (Vidal and Stokstad, 1974).

However, Gawthorne and Smith (1974), in studies with sheep, found that the 50 percent inhibition levels for SAM were much higher (approximately 500 nmol/ml) and that the levels of SAM in sheep liver (10–35 nmol/g) are too low to account for any regulatory effect.

Attempts were made to study the effect of methionine on folate metabolism using either tissue homogenates or liver slices. However, neither of these tissues resembled the whole animal in their response toward methionine. Batra *et al.* (1974) reported that liver homogenates from cobalamin-deficient rats degraded FiGlu slower than those from supplemented animals. However, the addition of methionine *in vitro* slightly decreased FiGlu degradation and therefore had an effect opposite to that which it had in the whole animal. The perfused liver was employed by Buehring *et al.* (1972) and was found to simulate the whole animal in its response to methionine. The metabolism of l-[2-^{14}C]histidine, when added to perfused livers from different dietary groups, was studied by measuring its conversion to respiratory $^{14}CO_2$ and to FIGLU. These results, presented in Table 10-1, show that the addition of methionine to the perfusion medium increases by 10-fold the respired $^{14}CO_2$ derived from histidine and decreases the amount of FiGlu found in the liver. Homocysteine had no effect. The $^{14}CO_2$ formation by the liver of an animal that had received dietary methionine ($-B_{12}$ + Met) was the

TABLE 10-1   Effect of Methionine on the Metabolism of [2-^{14}C] Histidine in the Perfused Rat Liver[a]

Group No.	Diet	Supplement in the Perfusion Medium	Respired $^{14}CO_2$, μmol	FiGlu in Liver, μmol	FiGlu in Perfusate, μmol
1	$-B_{12}-$Met	Hist	7.5 (2)	220 (2)	65 (2)
2	$-B_{12}-$Met	Hist + Met	80.0 (2)	90 (2)	55 (2)
3	$-B_{12}-$Met	Hist + Homo	10.0 (1)	215 (1)	–
4	$-B_{12}+$Met	Hist	10.0 (1)	170 (1)	60 (1)
5	$-B_{12}+$Met	Hist + Met	110.0 (1)	25 (1)	10 (1)

[a]The perfusion time was 2 h. The basal perfusion medium (100 ml) contained 500 μmol of L-histidine and 1.7 μCi of L-[2-^{14}C] histidine (specific activity, 58.3 mCi/mmol). When indicated, 200 μmol of L-methionine or 400 μmol of D,L-homocysteine thiolactone-HCl was added in the beginning of the perfusion and 100 μmol of methionine or 200 μmol of homocysteine was added at 30, 60, and 90 min. The values are expressed as the average of the number of animals shown in the parentheses. Abbreviations: Hist, histidine; Met, methionine; and Homo, homocysteine.

same as that from an animal on the $-B_{12}-$Met diet. Methionine added to the perfusate of a $-B_{12}+$Met animal markedly increased $^{14}CO_2$ production, which shows that the level of free methionine in the liver was rapidly exhausted. The effect of methionine added to the perfusate thus was similar to the effect of methionine in the whole animal in promoting the oxidation of [2−^{14}C] histidine to respiratory $^{14}CO_2$.

The effect of methionine on the metabolism of tritiated folic acid (500 μg) added to the perfusate was also investigated by Buehring *et al.* (1972). The distribution of folate derivatives in the liver and perfusate was determined by chromatography. The results which appear in Table 10-2 show that in the absence of methionine 70 percent of the tritiated folic acid was present as methyltetrahydrofolic acid. When methionine was added to the perfusate this was decreased to 3 percent, and the proportion of non-methyl derivatives such as tetrahydrofolate and 10-formyltetrahydrofolate increased. Methionine addition also increased the proportion of polyglutamate forms. These were 3 and 4 percent in the two livers without methionine and 8 and 25 percent in the two livers with added methionine. Methionine, however, did not influence the uptake of folic acid by the liver. The small amount of unchanged folic acid in the liver (6–13 percent) indicates that folic acid is rapidly reduced to tetrahydrofolic acid, and large amounts of reduced folates are excreted back into the perfusion media. Homocysteine plus betaine was as effective as methionine, while either one alone was inactive. Ethionine has the same effect as methionine in the perfused

TABLE 10-2 Effect of Various Components on the Metabolism of Folic Acid in Perfused Rat Liver[a]

Diet	Supplement to the Perfusion Medium	FiGlu in Liver	Folate in Liver (Perfusate), % of total	Distribution of Liver (Perfusate) Folates, %				
				F[b]	CH_3-FH_4[c]	FH_4[d]	CHO-FH_4[e]	Poly[f]
$-B_{12}$-Met	None	124	34 (66)	6 (33)	70 (55)	10	9	3
$-B_{12}$-Met	Methionine	6	48 (52)	9 (55)	3 (5)	46	27	8
$-B_{12}$+Met	None	140	32 (68)	13 (53)	65 (36)	6	6	4
$-B_{12}$+Met	Methionine	20	50 (50)	8 (44)	4 (3)	36	21	25
$-B_{12}$+Met	Ethionine	8	34 (66)		23	40	19	–
$-B_{12}$+Met	Homocysteine	115	34 (64)		78	6	4	–
$-B_{12}$+Met	Choline	125	29 (71)		78	4	4	–
$-B_{12}$+Met	Betaine	127	29 (71)		74	6	4	–
$-B_{12}$+Met	Homocysteine + Betaine	12	33 (67)		19	27	32	–

[a] The livers were perfused for 2 h with 6 μCi of [3H]folic acid (specific activity, 28 Ci/mmol), 500 μg of folic acid, and, when indicated, 200 μmol of L-methionine, 200 μmol of betaine, 400 μmol of D,L-homocysteine-thiolactone-HCl, and 400 μmol of D,L-ethionine. – indicates values not determined.
[b] PteGlu.
[c] 5-methyl-H4PteGlu.
[d] Sum of H4PteGlu and 5,10-methylene-H4PteGlu.
[e] Sum of 5,10-methenyl-H4PteGlu, 10-formyl-H4PteGlu, and 5-formyl-H4PteGlu.
[f] Pteroylpolyglutamates.

liver, which is consistent with its effect in decreasing FiGlu excretion in the vitamin B$_{12}$-deficient rat (Brown *et al.*, 1960) and the effect of *S*-adenosylethionine in inhibiting methylenetetrahydrofolate reductase (Kutzbach and Stokstad, 1967).

These data from studies with perfused liver support the view that methionine functions in regulating the proportion of methyl to non-methyl forms of tetrahydrofolic acid by its conversion to SAM, which in turn inhibits the reduction of methylenetetrahydrofolate to methyltetra-hydrofolate.

This mechanism of regulation provides a method of control of *de novo* synthesis of methyl groups. As SAM is the active methylating agent in most reactions, an increased need for methyl groups decreases the level of SAM. This then removes the inhibition of methylene reductase and permits increased formation of methyltetrahydrofolate for the methylation of homocysteine. This is in agreement with observations of du Vigneaud *et al.* (1953) that the *de novo* incorporation of deuterium into methyl groups is increased fourfold by the feeding of a labile methyl-free diet.

EFFECT OF VITAMIN B$_{12}$ ON HEPATIC FOLATE LEVELS

Another mechanism of vitamin B$_{12}$ action lies in its effect in increasing liver folate levels. Vitamin B$_{12}$ deficiency decreases liver folate levels by 50 percent in the rat (Kutzbach *et al.*, 1967; Gawthorne and Stokstad, 1971) and by 90 percent in sheep (Smith *et al.*, 1974). The hepatic uptake of an intravenous pulse dose of [^{3}H]folate is decreased in vitamin B$_{12}$ deficiency by 75 percent of the normal level in rats (Gawthorne and Stokstad, 1971) (Table 10-3). When methionine is administered either by feeding or by injection at the same time the folate is given, the folate uptake by the liver is increased to normal, as shown in Table 10-4 (Gawthorne and Stokstad, 1971). It can be seen that injection of vitamin B$_{12}$ (given concurrently with the [^{3}H]folate) had no effect on folate uptake in a 10-h period. A large dose of methionine (225 mg) I.P. promoted a higher [^{3}H] folate uptake than the control diet, while a smaller dose of methionine (40 mg) had little effect. Subsequent work (Vidal and Stokstad, 1974) showed that 12.5 mg of ethionine gave maximum hepatic uptake of [^{3}H]folate. This is in agreement with the fact that ethionine is rapidly converted to *S*-adenosylethionine, which is much more stable than SAM (Stekol, 1965) and gives about 10 times higher tissue levels of the *S*-adenosyl derivative than the same amount of methionine.

TABLE 10-3 Effect of Dietary Supplements of Vitamin B_{12} and Methionine on Liver and Plasma Folate Levels, Excretion of Formiminoglutamic Acid (FiGlu) and Methylmalonic Acid (MMA), and Uptake of Tritiated Folic Acid[a]

| Diet[b] | Folate Levels | | Urinary Excretion, μmol/100 g body wt/day | | Uptake of Tritiated Folate by Liver,[c] % |
	Liver, μg/g	Plasma, ng/ml	FiGlu	MMA	
$-B_{12}-$Met	3.1 ± 1.1[d]	74 ± 10	$33\ \ \pm 22$	$105\ \ \pm\ \ 80$	7.9 ± 1.7
$-B_{12}+$Met[e]	6.6 ± 2.4	55 ± 29	$3.9\ \ \pm\ \ 3.8$	$172\ \ \pm 116$	31.0 ± 7.7
$+B_{12}-$Met	9.5 ± 2.8	49 ± 6	$0.08 \pm\ \ 0.02$	$7.5 \pm\ \ 1.1$	25.5 ± 5.7
$+B_{12}+$Met	9.2 ± 0.7	52 ± 15	$0.05 \pm\ \ 0.01$	$7.4 \pm\ \ 1.1$	25.4 ± 3.8

[a]Data courtesy of S. Thenen (Ph.D. Thesis, University of California, Berkeley, 1970).
[b]Diets fed for 18 weeks; six animals per group.
[c]Uptake by liver in 24 h following I.V. dose of 5 μCi or 0.06 μg tritiated folate per 100 g body weight.
[d]± Standard deviation.
[e]Methionine given 24 h before injection.

TABLE 10-4   Effect of Intraperitoneal Supplements of Vitamin B_{12} and Methionine on Uptake of Intravenously Administered [^{3}H] Folic Acid by Rat Liver[a]

Diet Fed 15 Weeks	Supplement, I.P., for 10 h	[^{3}H] Folate Uptake, % in 10 h	Relative Uptake, %
Control[b]	–	11.4 ± 0.8	100
Basal[c]	–	4.1 ± 0.3	36
	B_{12}[d]	5.1 ± 0.4	45
	Met (40 mg)	5.5 ± 0.5	48
	B_{12}+Met (40 mg)	13.1 ± 1.1	115
	Met (225 mg)	17.8 ± 1.8	156
	B_{12}+Met (225 mg)	18.0 ± 0.7	158

[a]Data: Gawthorne and Smith (1974).
[b]+B_{12}+Met diet: basal diet with 100 μg of vitamin B_{12}/kg and 0.7 percent methionine added.
[c]–B_{12}–Met diet: deficient in vitamin B_{12}, only 0.2 percent methionine.
[d]Intraperitoneal injection of 2.5 μg of vitamin B_{12}.

Urinary excretion of folate following an I.P. dose of [^{3}H]folate is also increased in vitamin B_{12} deficiency (Vidal and Stokstad, 1974) (Table 10-5). The increase is due mainly to a large increase in the proportion of methyltetrahydrofolate. Administration of methionine or ethionine decreases the excretion and reduces the proportion of methyltetrahydrofolate in the urine. It should be noted that, with or

TABLE 10-5   Effect of Vitamin B_{12}, Methionine, and Ethionine on Hepatic Folic Acid Uptake and on Urinary Excretion of Folic Acid Derivatives[a]

Diet[b]	Liver Uptake	Radioactivity in Urine, % of original dose	Folate Distribution in Urine, % of original dose		
			PteGlu	Methyl[c] Folate	Non-Methyl[d] Folate
–B_{12}–Met	4.9	61	1.2	40	12
+B_{12}–Met	11.3	26	–	13	10
–B_{12}+Met	15.3	45	2.6	18	14
+B_{12}+Met	14.7	30	1.2	12	11
–B_{12}+Eth[e]	16.0	27	0.8	11	10

[a]Data courtesy of Vidal and Stokstad (1974).
[b]Diets, B_{12}, and methionine supplements given for 8 weeks.
[c]CH_3-H_4PteGlu.
[d]5-CHO-H_4PteGlu and 10-CHO-H_4PteGlu.
[e]Ethionine (0.4 percent) given in diet for 24 h plus 12.5 mg of ethionine given I.P. just before tritiated folate injection.

without vitamin B_{12}, only a small amount (about 4 percent) of the urinary folate consists of nonreduced PteGlu following an I.P. dose of [^{3}H]folate. This shows that when the [^{3}H]folate is administered I.P. it is very rapidly taken up by the liver, if we assume that formation of methyltetrahydrofolic acid occurs in the liver following I.V. or I.P. administration. In the vitamin B_{12}-deficient animal, only 4 percent of the I.P. dose of folate was retained by the liver 24 h following injection, but 61 percent had been excreted, practically all of which had been converted to reduced methyl- and formyltetrahydro- forms. Thus the decreased hepatic absorption of folate in the vitamin B_{12}-deficient animals would not appear to be reduced uptake but rather the failure of the liver to retain absorbed folate.

One theory to account for the effect of vitamin B_{12} deficiency in decreasing liver folate levels is based on the premise that polygluta-mates are formed more rapidly from tetrahydrofolate than from methyltetrahydrofolate. This is the case in the bacterial systems of *E. coli* (Griffin and Brown, 1964) and *Neurospora* (Sakami et al., 1973) where only tetrahydrofolate can serve as the substrate. However, the evidence in mammalian systems is conflicting. Spronk (1973), using a partially purified rat liver enzyme, obtained polyglutamate synthesis with tetrahydrofolic acid but not with methyltetrahydrofolic acid. Gawthorne and co-workers (Gawthorne and Smith, 1973, 1974), using a variety of subcellular fractions of sheep liver, found approximately equal activity with tetrahydrofolate, 5-formyltetrahydrofolate, and methyltetrahydrofolate as substrates for polyglutamate synthetase.

A second theory, proposed by Gawthorne and Smith (1973) to account for the decreased liver folate levels in vitamin B_{12} deficiency, is based on an impairment of membrane transport of folate. This is supported by the observation that the uptake of methotrexate by sheep liver slices is reduced 60 percent in a combined vitamin B_{12} and methionine deficiency (Gawthorne and Smith, 1973). However, the observation that injection of methionine prior to sacrifice only partially restores the absorption of methotrexate while restoring liver folate levels to normal (Gawthorne and Smith, 1974) suggests that the mecha-nism being measured by methotrexate uptake is not the same as that involved in folate uptake *in vivo*. Data relative to this question are also provided by the liver perfusion experiments presented in Table 10-2. The total uptake of added [^{3}H]folate by the perfused liver may be considered to be the difference between the total folate added and the amount of nonreduced folates in the perfusate. On this basis, the folate uptake by the two livers in the absence of methionine were 64 and 78 percent, while in the two livers with added methionine they were 72 and 78 percent. It would thus appear that there is little difference in folate absorption when measured in this way.

EFFECT OF VITAMIN B$_{12}$ DEFICIENCY ON ERYTHROCYTE AND SERUM FOLATE LEVELS

In clinical vitamin B$_{12}$ deficiency there is a decrease in erythrocyte folate levels (Cooper and Lowenstein, 1964) that is due primarily to a reduction of folyl polyglutamates with little change in monoglutamate levels (Jeejeebhoy *et al.*, 1965; Chanarin *et al.*, 1974). Serum folate levels are also increased in clinical vitamin B$_{12}$ deficiency (Herbert and Zalusky, 1962). We have found that rats on a low vitamin B$_{12}$ and methionine diet have elevated plasma folate levels (Gawthorne and Stokstad, 1971). These data, shown in Table 10-3, show that in combined vitamin B$_{12}$ and methionine deficiency in rats there is a reduction in liver folates and an increase in plasma folates. Refeeding of methionine with or without vitamin B$_{12}$ produces a rapid drop in plasma folate and a slower rise in liver folates (Gawthorne and Stokstad, 1971). In clinical vitamin B$_{12}$ deficiency, serum folate levels are elevated in 15 to 25 percent of the cases (Herbert and Zalusky, 1962), and there is a rapid drop of about 50 percent of cases to normal or subnormal levels when large amounts of cobalamin (100 to 1000 μg) are given. This may be compared with the rapid drop in plasma folates produced by vitamin B$_{12}$ and methionine feeding in rats.

EFFECT OF VITAMIN B$_{12}$ DEFICIENCY ON FOLATE METABOLISM IN BONE MARROW

In bone marrow from pernicious anemia patients, a decreased incorporation of deoxyuridine into DNA has been reported (Metz *et al.*, 1968; Waxman *et al.*, 1969). This has been shown by measuring the effect of preincubation with deoxyuridine on the incorporation of [³H]thymidine into DNA. This impaired conversion of deoxyuridine into thymidine can be restored by adding either folic acid (Metz *et al.*, 1968) or vitamin B$_{12}$ (Metz *et al.*, 1968; Waxman *et al.*, 1969). In folic acid-deficient marrow, the reduced *de novo* synthesis of thymine DNA can also be restored by adding methyltetrahydrofolate. In cobalamin-deficient marrow, methyltetrahydrofolate is ineffective (Metz *et al.*, 1968), demonstrating an impairment in the utilization of methyl folate. The addition of methionine decreased the *de novo* synthesis of thymine, while homocysteine promotes it. Thus, in bone marrow, methionine has a so-called "anti-folic-acid-like" effect. This is in contrast to that in perfused liver and the whole animal where methionine has a "pro-folic-acid-like" effect in facilitating folate dependent reactions (Buehr-ing *et al.*, 1972). This effect of methionine suggests that it functions in the bone marrow by end product inhibition in suppressing the conver-sion of methyltetrahydrofolate to tetrahydrofolate.

In view of these results with human bone marrow, we studied the regulatory effect of vitamin B_{12} and methionine on folic acid metabolism in rat bone marrow (Cheng *et al.*, in press). It was found that cobalamin deficiency in the rat did not decrease bone marrow folate levels although it does decrease liver folate levels (Kutzbach *et al.*, 1967; Gawthorne and Stokstad, 1971). The addition of methionine to cobalamin-deficient rat bone marrow culture increased the propor-tion of methyl folates and decreased the proportion of non-methyl forms, following a dose of [^{3}H]folic acid. This is consistent with its effect in inhibiting *de novo* thymine formation. It is also in contrast to the perfused liver, where addition of methionine decreases the propor-tion of methyl forms of folate. Thus, the regulatory mechanism of methionine on folate metabolism is quite different in the bone marrow than it is in the liver. Methylenetetrahydrofolate reductase is present in rat bone marrow and it is inhibited by SAM (Cheng *et al.*, in press) in a manner similar to that for the liver enzyme (Katzen and Buchanan, 1965; Kutzbach and Stokstad, 1967). However, it appears that end product inhibition by methionine is the predominant regulatory mecha-nism rather than the effect of SAM on methylenetetrahydrofolate reduc-tase.

This effect of methionine in inhibiting *de novo* thymine formation in cobalamin-deficient marrow is consistent with the failure of methionine to produce a reticulocyte response in pernicious anemia (Rundles and Brewer, 1958). This difference in the regulatory effect of vitamin B_{12} and methionine on liver and bone marrow helps to explain why methionine can have a "pro-folic-acid-like" effect in pernicious anemia in reducing FiGlu excretion (Zalusky and Herbert, 1962) and be ineffec-tive in producing a hematological response (Rundles and Brewer, 1958).

DISCUSSION

CHANARIN: I wonder to what extent Dr. Stokstad thinks that the data in one species can be related to another species? After all, man is the only animal that gets a megaloblastic anemia. To what extent would all these experiments differ if a more physiological form of folic acid than pteroylglutamic acid were used?

STOKSTAD: The only conclusion I would draw is that methionine regulates the methyl and non-methyl forms of folic acid in the rat and likely in man.

WAXMAN: We always talk about species differences; but how about tissue differences in the organism itself? (For example, the liver is interested in making protein; the bone marrow in proliferation, the intestinal mucosa in proliferation, the latter tissues having a requirement for the duplication of DNA. So, there has to be some mechanism whereby one-carbon moieties are directed for protein synthesis or DNA synthesis. One would guess, and I think there is some evidence, that SAM may be important in this regard and may determine folate metabolism. Increased tissue SAM may favor DNA synthesis by diverting 5,10-methylene THFA to methylation of deoxyuridylate. If there is a need for protein synthesis, decreased SAM may divert 5,10-methylene THFA to 5-methyl-THFA to provide additional SAM to initiate protein synthesis in these situations. Thus, folate biochemistry may differ from tissue to tissue depending on the tissue characteristics. For example, it appears that the central nervous system has a different folate system in which there is absence of dihydrofolate reductase. So, I think we have to think about the biochemistry of each particular organ that we are dealing with, not only of the total organism.

LITERATURE CITED

Batra, K. K., Buehring, K. U., and Stokstad, E. L. R. 1974. The effect of DL-methionine, vitamin B_{12} and thyroid powder on metabolism of formiminoglutamic acid in rats. Proc. Soc. Exp. Biol. Med. *147*:72.

Brown, D. D., Silva, O. L., Gardiner, R. C., and Silverman, M. 1960. Metabolism of formiminoglutamic acid by vitamin B_{12} and folic acid-deficient rats fed excess methionine. J. Biol. Chem. *235*:2058.

Buehring, K. U., Batra, K. K., and Stokstad, E. L. R. 1972. The effect of methionine on folic acid and histidine metabolism perfused rat liver. Biochim. Biophys. Acta *279*:498.

Chanarin, I. 1963. Urocanic acid and formimino-glutamic acid excretion in megaloblastic anaemia and other conditions: The effect of specific therapy. Br. J. Haematol. *9*:141.

Chanarin, I., Perry, J., and Lumb, M. 1974. The biochemical lesion in vitamin B_{12} deficiency in man. Lancet *i*:1251.

Cheng, F. W., Shane, B., and Stokstad, E. L. R. (In press). The anti-folate effect of methionine on bone marrow of normal and vitamin B_{12} deficient rats. Br. J. Haematol.

Combepine, G., Cossins, E. H., and Lor, K. L. 1971. Regulation of pteroylglutamate pool size by methionine in *Saccharomyces cerevisiae*. FEBS Lett. *14*:49.

Cooper, B. A., and Lowenstein, L. 1964. Relative folate deficiency of erythrocytes in pernicious anemia and its correction with cyanocobalamin. Blood *24*:502.

du Vigneaud, V., Kinney, J. M., Wilson, J. E., and Rachele, J. R. 1953. Effect of the presence of labile methyl groups in the diet on labile methyl neogenesis. Biochim. Biophys. Acta *12*:88.

Friedmann, B., Nakada, H. I., and Weinhouse, S. 1954. A study of the oxidation of formic acid in the folic acid-deficient rat. J. Biol. Chem. *210*:413.

Gawthorne, J. M., and Smith, R. M. 1973. The synthesis of pteroylpolyglutamates by sheep liver enzymes *in vitro*. Biochem. J. *136*:295.

Gawthorne, J. M., and Smith, R. M. 1974. Folic acid metabolism in vitamin B$_{12}$ deficient sheep. Effects of injected methionine on methotrexate transport and the activity of enzymes associated with folate metabolism in liver. Biochem. J. *142*:119.

Gawthorne, J. M., Stokstad, E. L. R. 1971. The effect of vitamin B$_{12}$ and methionine on folic acid uptake by rat liver. Proc. Soc. Exp. Biol. Med. *136*:42.

Griffin, M. J., and Brown, G. M. 1964. The biosynthesis of folic acid. III. Enzymatic formation of dihydrofolic acid from dihydropteroic acid and of tetrahydropteroylpoly-glutamic acid compounds from tetrahydrofolic acid. J. Biol. Chem. *239*:310.

Herbert, V., and Zalusky, R. 1962. Interrelations of vitamin B$_{12}$ and folic acid metabolism: Folic acid clearance studies. J. Clin. Invest. *41*:1263.

Jeejeebhoy, K. N., Pathare, S. M., and Noronha, J. M. 1965. Observations on conju-gated and unconjugated blood folate levels in megaloblastic anemia and the effects of vitamin B$_{12}$. Blood *26*:354.

Katzen, H. M., and Buchanan, J. M. 1965. Enzymatic synthesis of the methyl group of methionine. VIII. Repression-derepression, purification and properties of 5,10-methylenetetrahydrofolate reductase from Escherichia coli. J. Biol. Chem. *240*:825.

Kutzbach, C., and Stokstad, E. L. R. 1967. Feedback inhibition of methylenetetrahy-drofolate reductase in rat liver by S-adenosyl methionine. Biochim. Biophys. Acta *139*:217.

Kutzbach, C., and Stokstad, E. L. R. 1971. Mammalian methylenetetrahydrofolate reductase. Partial purification, properties, and inhibition by S-adenosylmethionine. Biochem. Biophys. Acta *250*:459.

Kutzbach, C., Gallow, E., and Stokstad, E. L. R. 1967. Influence of vitamin B$_{12}$ and methionine on levels of folic acid compounds and folate enzymes in rat liver. Proc. Soc. Exp. Biol. Med. *124*:801.

Luhby, A. L., and Cooperman, J. M. 1962. Aminoimidazolecarboxamide excretion in vitamin B$_{12}$ and folic deficiencies. Lancet *ii*:1381.

Luhby, A. L., Cooperman, J. C., and Teller, D. N. 1959. Histidine metabolic loading test to distinguish folic acid deficiency from vitamin B$_{12}$ in megaloblastic anemias. Proc. Soc. Exp. Biol. Med. *101*:350.

McGeer, P. L., Sen, N. P., and Grant, D. A. 1965. Excretion of 4(5)-amino-5(4)-imidazolecarboxamide and formimino-L-glutamic acid in folic acid and vitamin B$_{12}$ deficient rats. Can. J. Biochem. *43*:1367.

Metz, J., Kelly, A., Swett, V. C., Waxman, S., and Herbert, V. 1968. Deranged DNA synthesis by bone marrow from vitamin B$_{12}$-deficient humans. Br. J. Haematol. *14*:575.

Middletown, J. E., Coward, R. F., and Smith, P. 1964. Urinary excretion of AIC in vitamin B$_{12}$ and folic acid deficiencies. Lancet *ii*:258.

Noronha, J. M., and Silverman, M. 1962. On folic acid, vitamin B$_{12}$, methionine and formiminoglutamic acid metabolism, p. 728. *In* Vitamin B$_{12}$ and intrinsic factor, Second European Symposium, H. C. Heinrich, ed. F. Enke Verlag, Stuttgart.

Oace, S. M., Tarczy-Hornoch, K., and Stokstad, E. L. R. 1968. Urinary aminoimidazolecarboxamide in the rat as influenced by dietary vitamin B$_{12}$, methionine and thyroid powder. J. Nutr. *95*:445.

Rabinowitz, J. C., and Tabor, H. 1958. The urinary excretion of formic acid and formiminoglutamic acid in folic acid deficiency. J. Biol. Chem. *233*:252.

Rundles, W. R., and Brewer, S. S. Jr. 1958. Hematologic responses in pernicious anemia to orotic acid. Blood *13*:99.

Sakami, W., Ritari, S. J., Black, C. W., and Rzepka, J. 1973. Polyglutamate synthesis by *Neurospora crassa*. Fed. Proc. *32*:471.

Silverman, M., and Pitney, A. J. 1958. Dietary methionine and the excretion of formiminoglutamic acid by the rat. J. Biol. Chem. *233*:1179.

Smith, R. M., Osborne-White, W. S., and Gawthorne, J. M. 1974. Folic acid metabolism in vitamin B_{12}-deficient sheep. Effects of injected methionine on liver constituents associated with folate metabolism. Biochem. J. *142*:105.

Spronk, A. M. 1973. Tetrahydrofolate polyglutamate synthesis in rat liver. Fed. Proc. *32*:471.

Stekol, J. A. 1965. Formation and metabolism of S-adenosyl derivatives of S-alkylhomocysteines in the rat and mouse, p. 231. *In* Transmethylation and methionine biosynthesis, S. K. Shapiro and F. Schlenk, eds. University of Chicago Press, Chicago.

Stokstad, E. L. R., Webb, R. E., and Shah, E. 1966. Effect of vitamin B_{12} and folic acid on the metabolism of formiminoglutamate, formate, and propionate in the rat. J. Nutr. *88*:225.

Vidal, A. J., and Stokstad, E. L. R. 1974. Urinary excretion of 5-methyltetrahydrofolate and liver S-adenosylmethionine levels of rats fed a vitamin B_{12}-deficient diet. Biochim. Biophys. Acta *362*:245.

Waxman, S., Metz, J. and Herbert, V. 1969. Defective DNA synthesis in human megaloblastic bone marrow: Effects of homocysteine and methionine. J. Clin. Invest. *48*:284.

Zalusky, R., and Herbert, V. 1961. Failure of formiminoglutamic acid (FiGlu) excretion to distinguish vitamin B_{12} deficiency from nutritional folic acid deficiency. Am. Soc. Clin. Invest. *40*:1091.

Zalusky, R., and Herbert, V. 1962. Urinary formiminoglutamic acid as a test of folic acid deficiency. Lancet *i*:108.

11

Role of Intestinal Conjugase in the Control of the Absorption of Polyglutamyl Folates

IRWIN H. ROSENBERG

In 1970, Herbert Godwin and I proposed a scheme of the various possibilities by which polyglutamyl folate might be absorbed by the intestine (Rosenberg and Godwin, 1971). Figure 11-1 presents this scheme. There is a good deal of agreement because of observation by several investigators (Perry and Chanarin, 1968; Rosenberg et al., 1969; Butterworth et al., 1969) that folate from its heptaglutamate appears in the mesenteric circulation in the form of folyl monoglutamate. Much of the evidence indicates that hydrolysis occurs within or in intimate relation to the intestinal cell.

If there is conversion of the heptaglutamate to monoglutamate during transport across the epithelial cell, what controls the entire process? Is this a process the rate of which is controlled by the hydrolysis step? Or is this a process that is controlled by the ultimate transport and release of the monoglutamate? If this is a process in which there is the participation of intestinal enzymes, "conjugases," or polyglutamate hydrolases, does hydrolysis occur in a single step or in multiple stages?

To address the second question first, I will present a very rapid review of our experience with the chicken intestinal enzyme, the

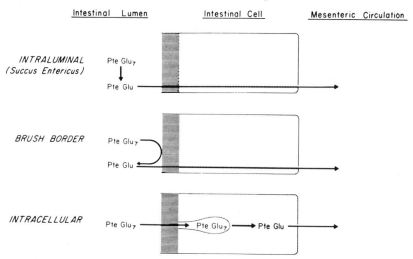

FIGURE 11-1   Scheme of three alternative possibilities for sequential hydrolysis and absorption of polyglutamyl folate (shown here as PteGlu$_7$) by intestine (Rosenberg and Godwin, 1971; permission to reprint Figure 7 from N. Engl. J. Med. *293*:1303–1308, 1971).

chicken intestinal conjugase. Much that was known and that we have learned indicates that the avian enzyme is different from the mammalian enzyme in some of its basic characteristics, but these studies give us an idea of how this complicated process can be dissected.

One of the ways that conjugated folate was first demonstrated was to show that there were forms of folate that would act as the vitamin for deficient chicks but would not support the growth of *Lactobacillus casei* (Hogan and Parrott, 1940). Thus the chick is known to be an organism that possesses conjugases and that can utilize conjugated folate. To study conjugase, we needed pure substrate, and in collaboration with J. Meienhofer we settled on a technique in which we used a solution phase for synthesis of the gammaglutamyl peptide (Meienhofer *et al.*, 1970) and condensed with pteroic acid (Figure 11-2). We put our tritium label in the pteroyl portion (Godwin *et al.*, 1972), and this provided a tool for study of the enzyme and for absorption studies. Hava Neumann, working in our lab, showed that, if one incubates pteroylheptaglutamate with crude chicken intestine and follows the sequence of events (Rosenberg and Neumann, 1974), at 1 h the disappearance of the heptaglutamate and the appearance of a peak that migrates as a diglutamate is seen. With increasing incubation time,

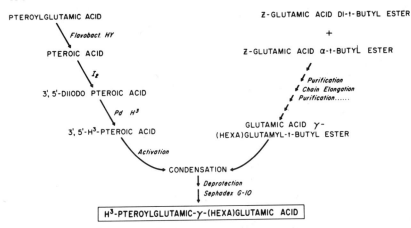

FIGURE 11-2   Scheme for chemical synthesis of pteroylpolyglutamates. For detail see Godwin *et al.* (1972) (reprinted by permission from Gastroenterology *60*:445, 1972).

we observed a progressive decrease in this pteroyldiglutamate intermediate and the appearance of final product, monoglutamate.

This indicates that there is a stepwise hydrolysis, and, the question is, is this a process that is being generated by a single enzyme or by multiple enzymes? For that purpose, Parmesh Saini, in our laboratory, used affinity chromatography to purify the enzyme from the chick intestine (Saini and Rosenberg, 1974). Figure 11-3 presents a polyacrilamide gel of the original homogenate of chick intestine after butanol extraction and after one purification step with ammonium sulfate. We obtained two protein bands after the affinity chromatography step, and after a gel filtration step we obtained a single band of protein that had activity against pteroylheptaglutamate.

As shown in the schematic high-voltage electrophoretogram in Figure 11-4, when the pteroylheptaglutamate is incubated with the crude intestine, a whole series of products is produced, including the monoglutamate as the major product, the diglutamate as another product, and several of the free gamma-glutamylpeptides, including glutamic acid. In incubations with the purified single protein, only the diglutamate (which has been known for some time to be the product of hydrolysis of heptaglutamate with chick *pancreas* enzyme) and a free pentagammaglutamylpeptide were seen. This indicated to us that the enzyme that we had purified was not carrying the process to completion and that instead there appeared to be a group of enzymes involved.

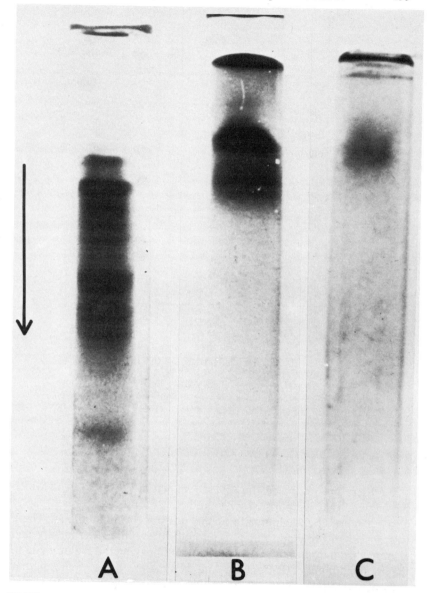

FIGURE 11-3   Polyacrilamide gel electrophoresis of chicken intestine during purification of "conjugase" using affinity chromatography. (A) Crude homogenate after butanol extraction and $(NH_4)_2SO_4$ fractionation; (B) two bands after affinity chromatography; (C) simple band of pure endopeptidase after gel filtration (Saini and Rosenberg, 1974; reprinted by permission from J. Biol. Chem. *249*:5131, 1974).

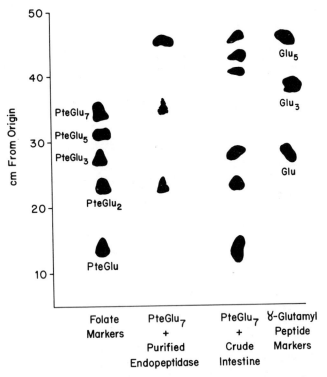

FIGURE 11-4 Drawing of a high-voltage electrophoregram showing the effect of crude chick intestine and purified endopeptidase on
PteGlu$_7$ (reprinted by permission from J. Biol. Chem. *249*:5126,
1974).

We therefore proposed the scheme shown in Figure 11-5, in which
the enzyme that we purified with the help of affinity chromatography
cleaved pteroylheptaglutamate at the position of diglutamate. There
was a second enzyme, which we could differentiate chemically and
also by chromatography, that is capable of cleaving the diglutamate to
the monoglutamate (Rosenberg and Neumann, 1974). Still another
enzyme, which we have subsequently had more opportunity to study,
is capable of hydrolyzing the free gamma-glutamylpeptide and has
many of the characteristics of gamma-glutamyl transpeptidases from
liver and intestine.

Evidence from our laboratory and from others seems to indicate that
in mammalian systems there may be a hydrolytic process that is more

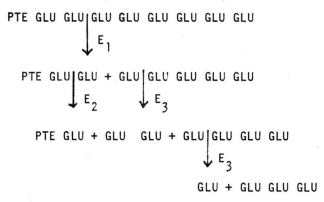

FIGURE 11-5   Scheme of multistep hydrolysis of pteroylglutamate by chick intestine.

characteristic of a gamma-glutamylcarboxypeptidase (Bird *et al.*, 1945; Baugh *et al.*, 1970) with stepwise hydrolysis of glutamic acid residues from the carboxyl end of the molecule. However, when we perform similar experiments in mammalian systems, we see monoglutamate as a very early product in the hydrolytic process. It is possible that in addition to gamma-glutamylcarboxypeptidase in mammalian systems there is also an enzyme analogous to the chick enzyme that acts as an endopeptidase. Parenthetically, this emphasizes a problem that needs to be solved before we can settle the issue of nomenclature for these enzymes.

Pratt and Cooper (1971), Perry and Chanarin (1970), and recently Olinger *et al.* have emphasized the importance of the conversion of monoglutamate to methyl folate during transport across the intestine. One of the ways that one could look at the question of whether the heptaglutamate and the monoglutamate enter by similar or parallel pathways is to determine whether folates derived from both substrates enter the same monoglutamate pool before release from the cell. So, we have designed experiments to compare kinetics of absorption of tritium-labeled monoglutamate and tritium-labeled heptaglutamate across rat intestine. My colleagues and I have recently reported *in vitro* studies showing that rates of hydrolysis of pteroylheptaglutamate by intestine greatly exceed folate transport rates even when hydrolysis is partly inhibited and the folate derived from heptaglutamate is meth-ylated as is the monoglutamate (Wagonfeld *et al.*, 1975).

If these *in vitro* studies are relevant to some aspects of folate and nutrition requirements in man, then we should see some documentation in our clinical investigations. Celiac sprue or gluten-induced enteropathy is a serious disease of the small intestine with marked aberration of intestinal mucosal cell structure and function. One would expect, therefore, to observe serious defects in intestinal absorption of folate, and folate deficiency is very common in this condition. One might also have expected that with the distortion of the intestinal epithelial cells there might be serious problems in mucosal digestive function as well as absorptive function. Hoffbrand *et al.* (1970) studied celiac patients using yeast polyglutamates and found a similar defective absorption of yeast folate and crystalline PGA (1970). We have confirmed these observations using the tritium-labeled synthetic pteroylheptaglutamate. We have measured folate absorption by urinary excretion after a flushing dose (Godwin and Rosenberg, 1975) in a number of untreated patients with celiac sprue (Santiago-Borrero *et al.*, 1973). The defect in absorption of the monoglutamate and the heptaglutamate is really quite similar in most of these patients. In only one patient was there substantially better absorption of the monoglutamate than the heptaglutamate. This suggested that inhibition of monoglutamate absorption in some way controlled heptaglutamate absorption also. There does not appear to be evidence for independent control of heptaglutamate absorption from these studies.

In confirmation of previous work presented by Hoffbrand *et al.* (1970) using the yeast polyglutamate assay, and similar to work recently reported by Halsted and his co-workers in tropical sprue (1973), we did not find a decrease in intestinal biopsy conjugase in untreated celiac disease. In fact, there is an increase in biopsy conjugase on a per weight or per milligram protein basis.

Another clinical observation that helps exclude the possibility that folyl heptaglutamate and monoglutamate are traversing the intestine by separately controlled mechanisms was made in a patient with a specific genetic defect in folate absorption (Santiago-Borrero *et al.*, 1973). If folyl polyglutamate were able to cross the intestine by a separate process from the monoglutamate, as is the case with some di- or tripeptides in patients with genetic amino acid transport defects, then one would predict that the individual who lacks the monoglutamate transport system might absorb folate from the polyglutamate. This was not the case in the patients studied; neither polyglutamate nor monoglutamate feeding caused an elevation in serum folate. Thus there appears to be a genetically determined mechanism that controls the absorption of the monoglutamyl folate and thereby controls absorption of its polyglutamate precursor.

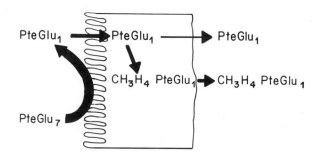

INTESTINAL   INTESTINAL   MESENTERIC
LUMEN   EPITHELIAL   CIRCULATION

FIGURE 11-6   Proposed scheme of the digestion and absorption of polyglutamyl folate by the intestine. Hydrolysis of the $PteGlu_7$ to $PteGlu_1$ by intestinal enzymes is rapid, while the overall rate of transport into the mesenteric circulation is controlled by the movement of the monoglutamyl folate, $PteGlu_1$. Under appropriate conditions a significant portion of $PteGlu_1$ is reduced and methylated in the intestinal cell and appears in the circulation as 5-methyltetrahydrofolate ($CH_3H_4PteGlu_1$).

Figure 11-6 illustrates our current conception of folate absorption and malabsorption. The site at which the polyglutamyl folate is hydrolyzed has not been determined, but after hydrolysis the product enters a common pathway of absorption with monoglutamyl folate and to some degree is converted to methyl folate. The rate of hydrolysis substantially exceeds the overall rate of transport. Thus, only a severe effect of hydrolysis would result in a slowing of transport, whereas any direct effect on the transport process would cause malabsorption of any dietary folate.

Certainly, we still need to determine the precise location of the hydrolysis. In both our *in vitro* flux studies and in perfusion studies, folyl monoglutamate accumulates on the mucosal side when one starts with heptaglutamate. This suggests that the hydrolytic process is occurring at the mucosal border of the cell, perhaps by a form of contact digestion (Ugolev, 1972). With the current momentum and technology in this field, we may hope that this question will be soon answered.

DISCUSSION

COOPER: Dr. Max Katz and I have attempted to utilize the perfusion system he has been using for B_{12} transport to determine if, in the rat, polyglutamate and monoglutamate biological folates are absorbed similarly. In this procedure, the arterial and venous blood supply to the small intestine are canulated and perfused with oxygenated perfusate solution. In this system, glucose is transported much more rapidly than xylose, and Dr. Katz has reported that vitamin B_{12} is found to be transported across the intestine into the portal perfusate. We have prepared a polyglutamyl folate cocktail by feeding [^{3}H]folate acid to *Lactobacillus casei* for 18 h and extracting folates as described by Buehring, Shin, and Stokstad. We treated half of both ^{14}C- and ^{3}H-labeled polyglutamylfolate with serum and autoclaved to produce a primarily monoglutamyl mixture of biological folates. This deconjugated mixture was mixed with the polyglutamyl material labeled with the other isotope and injected into the rat intestine, following which radioactivity was collected from the portal venous perfusate. Both polyglutamyl and mono-glutamyl labels appeared simultaneously in the perfusate and increased at the same rate. (Figure 11-7). Chromatography of the perfusate revealed that both

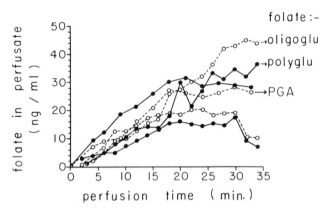

FIGURE 11-7   Radioactivity in portal venous perfusate after inject-ing a mixture of poly- and monoglutamyl folates into the intestinal lumen. Equal molar quantities of a mixture of polyglutamyl and monoglutamyl folates were injected into the intestinal lumen; each species was labeled with either ^{14}C or ^{3}H. – – – –, Radioactivity from polyglutamyl folate; ———, radioactivity from monoglutamyl folates. The line labeled PGA represents [^{14}C]folic acid mixed with [^{3}H]polyglutamyl folate; other solid lines represent polyglutamyl folates deconjugated by human serum conjugase (reprinted by per-mission from Br. J. Haematol. *16*:241, 1969).

labels were on monoglutamyl folate, but the material collected was insufficient quantitatively to allow us to identify which monoglutamyl folate appeared in the portal vein. We suspect, based on previous studies, that this was primarily methyltetrahydrofolate.

LITERATURE CITED

Baugh, C. M., Stevens, J. C., and Krumdieck, C. L. 1970. Studies of γ-glutamyl carboxy peptidase I. Biochim. Biophys. Acta *212*:116.

Bird, O. D., Robbins, M., Vanderbelt, J. M., and Pfiffner, J. J. 1945. Observations on vitamin B_c conjugase from hog kidney. J. Biol. Chem. *163*:649–659.

Butterworth, C. E., Jr., Baug, C. M., and Krumdieck, C. 1969. A study of folate absorption and metabolism in man utilizing carbon-14 labeled polyglutamates synthesized by the solid phase method. J. Clin. Invest. *48*:1131–1142.

Godwin, H. A., and Rosenberg, I. H. 1975. Comparative studies of the intestinal absorption of (^{3}H) pteroylheptaglutamate in man. Gastroenterology *69*:364–373.

Godwin, H. A., Rosenberg, I. H., Ferenz, C. R., Jacobs, P. M., and Meienhofer, Jr. 1972. The synthesis of biologically active pteroyloligo-γ-L-glutamates (folic acid conjugates). Evaluation of (^{3}H)-pteroylheptaglutamate for metabolic studies. J. Biol. Chem. *247*:2266–2271.

Halsted, O. H., Reisenauer,, and Corcino, J. J. 1975. Jejunal hydrolysis and uptake of conjugated folate in tropical sprue. Clin. Res. *23*:457A. (Abstract)

Hoffbrand, A. V., Douglas, A. P., and Fry, L. 1970. Malabsorption of dietary folate (pteroylpolyglutamates) in adult coeliac disease and dermatitis herpetiforms. Br. Med. J. *4*:85.

Hogan, A. G., and Parrott, E. M. 1940. Anemia in chicks caused by a vitamin deficiency. J. Biol. Chem. *132*:507–517.

Meienhofer, J., Jacobs, P. M., Godwin, H. A., and Rosenberg, I. H. 1970. Synthesis of hepta-L-glutamic acid by conventional and solid-phase techniques. J. Org. Chem. *35*:4137–4140.

Olinger, J., Bertino, J. R., and Binder, H. J. 1973. Intestinal folate absorption II. Conversion and retention of pteroylmonoglutamate by jejunum. J. Clin. Invest. *52*:2138–2144.

Perry, J., and Chanarin, I. 1968. Absorption and utilization of polyglutamyl forms of folate in man. Br. Med. J. *4*:546–549.

Perry, J., and Chanarin, I. 1970. Intestinal absorption of reduced folate compounds in man. Br. J. Haematol. *18*:329–339.

Pratt, R. D., and Cooper, B. A. 1971. Folates in plasma and bile of man after feeding ^{3}H folic acid and 5-formyl tetrahydrofolate (folinic acid). J. Clin. Invest. *50*:445.

Rosenberg, I. H., and Godwin, H. A. 1971. The digestion and absorption of dietary folate. Gastroenterology *60*:445–463.

Rosenberg, I. H., and Neumann, H. 1974. Evidence for a multi-step mechanism in the enzymatic hydrolysis of polyglutamyl folate by chicken intestine. J. Biol. Chem. *249*:5126–5130.

Rosenberg, I. H., Streiff, R. R., Godwin, H. A., and Castle, W. B. 1969. Absorption or polyglutamic folate: Participation of deconjugating enzymes of the intestinal mucosa. N. Engl. J. Med. *280*:985–988.

Saini, P. K., and Rosenberg, I. H. 1974. Isolation of pteroyl-*v*-oligoglutamyl endopeptidase from chicken intestine with the aid of affinity chromatography. J. Biol. Chem. *249*:5131–5134.

Santiago-Borrero, B. J., Santini, R., Jr., Perez-Santiago, E., and Maldonado, N. 1973. Congential isolated defect in folic acid absorption. J. Pediatr. *3*:450.

Ugolev, A. M. 1972. Membrane digestion. Gut *13*:735.

Wagonfeld, J. B., Dudzinsky, D., and Rosenberg, I. H. 1975. Analysis of rate-controlling processes in polyglutamyl folate. Clin. Res. *23*:259. (Abstract)

12

Plasma Conjugase Activity in Health and Disease

ERIK M. MAGNUS

Although it has been known for many years that conjugase (pteroyl-polyglutamyl hydrolase) exists in circulating human plasma (Wolff *et al.*, 1949), its functional role and clinical significance remain largely unknown. Many animal tissues, including brain, pancreas, liver, kidney, intestine, and bone marrow, have also been reported to contain conjugase (Laskowski et al., 1945) Erythrocytes, however, are notably devoid of the enzyme. Studies of conjugase were facilitated by the recent development of a simple *in vitro* assay by Krumdieck and Baugh (1970). This method is based on the amount of radioactivity liberated under standard conditions from pteroyl-triglutamate synthesized with a molecule of uniformly-labeled [^{14}C]glutamate in the terminal unit of the gamma peptide chain.

In an effort to discover if abnormally high or low levels of plasma conjugase activity are associated with specific disease entities, assays were performed routinely on 2,332 patients admitted to our medical department from June 1, 1974, through the end of May 1975. Pending analysis of the entire series, this report describes preliminary observations that indicate the occurrence of elevated values in metastatic

147

cancer, active liver disease, and in patients receiving phenytoin. Normal values were observed in pernicious anemia. Low values were observed in patients with widespread malignancy, hepatic coma, aplastic anemia, diabetes mellitus, and severe malnutrition.

METHODS

Conjugase assay was carried out by the method of Krumdieck and Baugh (1970) modified for use with plasma as follows (Krumdieck, personal communication):

1. Heparinized plasma is employed since citrate appears to inhibit conjugase activity;

2. A 2-ml portion of plasma added to 2 ml of 2 M mercaptoethanol and incubated in a water bath at 37° C for 12 min, or until a gel is formed. The gel and precipitate are removed by centrifugation at 9,000 × g for 30 min.

3. The clear supernatant fluid is used preparing duplicate tubes containing: 0.1 ml of L-glutamic acid, 0.001 M; 0.5 ml of acetate buffer, pH 4.5, 0.1 M; 0.5 ml of deionized water; and 0.1 ml of plasma supernate (mercaptoethanol treated).

4. Tubes are placed in a 37° C water bath for 5 min for thermal equilibration, after which the reaction is initiated by the addition of 0.25 ml of pteroylglutamyl-γ-glutamyl-γ-[U-^{14}C]glutamate, and mixed in a Vortex mixer. Substrate solution is standardized to contain 0.1 μmol/ml, with a specific activity of about 715,000 cpm/μmol.

5. The reaction is stopped promptly after 10 min by the addition of 0.5 ml of 10% trichloroacetic acid.

6. A 1.0-ml portion of charcoal suspension (2.5 g of activated charcoal in 500 ml of L-glutamic acid buffer, 0.05 M, pH 3.0) is added, and the solution is mixed.

7. Charcoal is removed by filtration through a Millipore filter (pore size, 0.45 nm) for counting in a liquid scintillation counter.

RESULTS

The plasma conjugase activity, expressed as radioactivity (counts per minute), released from "end-labeled" pteroyltriglutamate by 0.1 ml of plasma in 186 normal controls is presented in Table 12-1. The lowest and highest values were observed in males (140 and 465), and the range

TABLE 12-1   Plasma Conjugase Activity in
186 Controls[a]

Control	No.	Mean cpm	SD	Range
F	100	273	67	182–406
M	86	282	69	140–465

[a]379 cpm corresponds to 1 nm of glutamic liberated/10 min
by enzyme action. SD, standard deviation.

in females was 182 to 406. However, mean values were similar in males
and females (282 and 273, respectively).

Table 12-2 summarizes the results in 18 subjects receiving phenytoin
(diphenylhydantoin) for control of epilepsy. Conjugase activity was
significantly higher among 10 patients receiving 300 mg of the medication daily than among 5 patients receiving 200 mg daily. Conjugase
activity remained high in two patients even after supplementation with
oral folic acid in doses of 200 μg and 15,000 μg per day, respectively.

Table 12-3 presents results of conjugase activity in four patients with
vitamin B_{12} deficiency before and after therapy. It may be seen that,
although the activity is normal initially, it increases by approximately
50 percent after 10 days of treatment.

Figure 12-1 illustrates the sequential changes in plasma conjugase
activity following the daily oral administration of 1,000 μg of vitamin
B_{12}. This figure also illustrates the increase in red cell folate as
previously described (Butterworth *et al.*, 1966) and now explained by
vitamin B_{12}-facilitated synthesis of folic acid polyglutamates (Chanarin
et al., 1974).

TABLE 12-2   Plasma Conjugase Activity in Patients Receiving
Anticonvulsant Therapy (Diphenylhydantoin)

Diphenylhydantoin, mg/day	No.	Mean Conjugase, cpm
200	5	391
300	10	506
400	3	444
Those with low PF and low WBF	7	403
Those with low PF and normal WBF	5	472
Those with normal PF and low WBF	2	424
Those with normal PF and normal WBF	4	496
Anticonvulsant plus folate, 100 μg/day	1	444
Anticonvulsant plus folate, 200 μg/day	1	501
Anticonvulsant plus folate, 15,000 μg/day	1	531

TABLE 12-3   Conjugase Activity in B_{12}-Deficient
Patients[a]

Case No.	Conjugase Activity,[b] cpm	
	Before Therapy	10 Days after B_{12}
1	250	420
2	268	341
3	328	512
4	165	230

[a]Mean increase: 50 percent.
[b]Normal: 150–450.

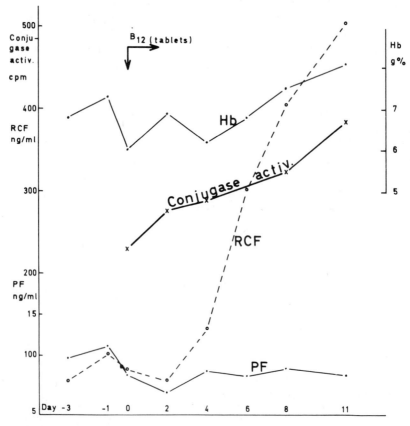

FIGURE 12-1   Chart showing sequential changes in hemoglobin, conjugase, red cell
folate, and plasma folate in response to oral administration of vitamin B_{12}, 1,000 mg daily,
in a 60-year-old man with pernicious anemia.

High values have been noted in patients with metastatic cancer of various types. In several patients followed at weekly or monthly intervals, there seemed to be a steady increase in plasma conjugase activity during the development of the disease in untreated subjects. Highest values were observed in a group of patients with pancreatic cancer, in whom the mean value was significantly greater than corresponding mean values in patients with cancer of the breast, prostate, respiratory tract, or gastrointestinal tract. Those with liver metastases at autopsy tended to have very high levels of plasma conjugase, but in some instances high values were observed in cancer patients with no involvement of liver or the biliary tract. High values were found in patients with biliary tract obstruction due to pancreatic tumor where there was no evidence of liver metastasis. High values were also observed in active liver disease.

Subnormal values of plasma conjugase were observed in subjects with advanced liver disease, such as cirrhosis with hepatic coma. Low values were also observed in chronic malnutrition, in some individuals with diabetes mellitus, and in debilitated individuals with terminal cancer. One patient with aplastic anemia had low plasma conjugase activity.

These preliminary observations suggest that assays of plasma conjugase activity may be of value in the diagnosis or monitoring of certain disease states. More experience is needed to delineate clear associations. However, the observation of elevated values in pancreatic cancer, biliary tract obstruction, active liver disease, and metastatic cancer involving the liver suggests that the pancreas and liver may contribute to the circulating pool of conjugase. It is hoped that further study of plasma conjugase will result in better understanding of disease processes related to folate metabolism in a wide variety of tissues.

LITERATURE CITED

Butterworth, C. E., Jr., Scott, C. W., Magnus, E., Santini, R., and Dempsey, H. 1966. Metabolic changes associated with recovery from vitamin B_{12} deficiency. Med. Clin. North Am. *50*:1627–1641.

Chanarin, I., Perry, J., and Lumb, M., 1974. The biochemical lesion in vitamin B_{12} deficiency in man. Lancet *2*:1251–1252.

Krumdieck, C. L., and Baugh, C. M. 1970. Radioactive assay of folic acid polyglutamate conjugase(s). Anal. Biochem. *35*:123–129.

Laskowski, M., Mims, V., and Day, P. 1945. Studies on the enzyme which produces the *Streptococcus lactis*-R stimulating factor from inactive precursor substance in yeast. J. Biol. Chem. *157*:731–739.

Wolff, R., Drouet, L., and Karlin, R. 1949. Occurrence of vitamin B_c conjugase in human plasma. Science *109*:612.

13

Automated Microbiological
Assay for Folic Acid

ERIK M. MAGNUS

The microbiological assay of folic acid in plasma and whole blood is time consuming. It involves, however, some steps in which automation may be useful. At Krohgstotten Hospital in Oslo, Norway, we have for the last 4 to 5 years utilized an automated method involving an "Auto-Lab" that is available commercially from a Swedish company. It consists of three main parts: a sampler, a water bath, and an analyzing unit.

The folate assay is, with some modifications, performed in plasma as reported by Waters and Mollin (1961) and in red cells as reported by Grossowicz et al. (1962). Plasma folate and whole blood folate are assayed in the same batch.

The first two steps are identical for the manual and the Auto-Lab procedure. It has been found practical to assay 60 samples in one batch when utilizing the Auto-Lab, usually 40 plasma samples and 20 whole blood samples. The dilution of samples and incubation of whole blood samples requires approximately 120 min. Deproteinizing by autoclaving takes about 60 min. The next step is to pipette exact amounts of standards and supernatants from plasma and whole blood samples into tubes and to add exact amounts of buffer and medium solutions. By the manual method, this requires about 80 min. To place empty plastic tubes in a conveyor belt in the Auto-Lab and to fill standards and supernatants from samples in plastic tubes and place them in a parallel running conveyor belt takes about 30 min. The Auto-Lab pipettes 0.5 ml from the samples and delivers it to the parallel tube on the other belt. Through the same pipette, 2 ml of buffer solution is flushed out into the same tube. The pipette is also rinsed on the outside while moving up and down through a ring-shaped device. Sterilized water flows on the inside of the ring and is sucked back by a vacuum pump. The next pipette delivers 2.5 ml of medium solution. The samples are brought directly to a water bath, and the used plastic tubes in the other belt are discarded. While the "Auto-Lab" is running, one can perform other tasks, such as preparing the records, while keeping an eye on the machine.

It is not necessary to sterilize the samples when they have been through the Auto-Lab. Half an hour before starting, the machine is continuously rinsed with sterilized water, and in the last 5 min buffer and medium solutions, respectively, are flushed through the syringes, the connections, and the pipettes.

Inoculation of the samples takes about 5 min. The water bath is covered by a drip-safe lid, so there is no need to cover the individual tubes.

Reading of the samples and calculating the results takes about 2 h when read in an ordinary densitometer. The Auto-Lab photometer reads the samples in 90 min and at the same time prints out the results. A stirrer stirs the samples before they enter the photometer. It is important that there is a lag time of at least 15 s from the time the sample is brought into the photometer until it is read. The technician can start to calculate the results as soon as the analyzing unit has given the first figures and will be finished almost as soon as the machine has printed out the last figures (Table 13-1 summarizes these time comparisons).

The cost for a 60-sample batch when utilizing Auto-Lab is 2.77 dollars per sample. The cost of using the manual assay is slightly less: 2.61 dollars per sample. On the other hand, this method is more time consuming, requiring 2 h and 20 min more than the automatic method for a 60-sample batch. It was found practical not to have more than 40 samples in one batch when we utilized the manual method. The expenses would thus be practically the same by both methods, but 20 more samples could be analyzed daily by using the automated analysis.

Pooled plasma from blood donors has repeatedly been assayed as a

TABLE 13-1   Time Comparisons of Manual and Auto-Lab Methods

Step	Time Required, min	
	Manual	Auto-Lab
1. Preparation of standard and samples, incubation	120	120
2. Deproteinizing by autoclaving	60	60
3. Pipetting of samples; adding buffer and medium	80	30
4. Sterilizing by autoclaving	60	–
5. Placing in water bath and inoculation	15	15
6. Reading of samples and calculating the results	120	90
Total time (60 samples/bath)	455	315

continuous check on the accuracy of the assay. It should be noted that the reproducibility seems to be better using the manual assay. Our experience is that the Auto-Lab sampler is reliable, and technical errors are easily detected. Theoretically the Auto-Lab method should yield more reliable results than a manual method. We have not yet been able to verify this.

It has not been necessary for me to ask the laboratory staff which method they prefer. They have been quick to point out the disadvantages of the old method and all the advantages of the automated procedure.

In conclusion, I recommend that the automated method for assaying folic acid be employed, but one should be very careful when selecting the machine.

DISCUSSION

KRUMDIECK: We put together a machine with an old fraction collector that cost us only about 1,600 dollars. The main innovation is a fiberoptic probe that dips into each tube when it is read after the incubation period. A swinging arm on the fraction collector aspirates a precise amount of sample and squirts it into a tube together with preinoculated medium. We use two carriers—one for the sample and one for the preinoculated medium. When the spool is full, we just take it out and put it in an incubator for 18 h. Then the following day, we put it back in the machine, and switch to 'read'. The fiberoptic probe goes in, and then it oscillates up and down, while the reading is being taken to keep the bacteria evenly suspended. We can run three samples per minute and read two samples per minute.

WAGNER: What is the relative cost of the microbiological assay compared to the radioimmunoassay?

HERBERT: The cost of the radioimmunoassay is largely the cost of the isotope. The cost of the microbiological assay is largely the cost of the technician.

SCOTT: Could we get a comment on the use of the chloramphenicol-resistant organism? We have been using it for a few years now, and have found it quite successful. It cuts a tremendous number of the problems associated with the conventional assay.

STOKSTAD: We have been using the chloramphenicol-resistant *L. casei* assay for a year or more and find that it works very well.

HERBERT: When John Scott was with us for a year, we compared the two methods, as we have done before, and really found no difference. One can do the aseptic addition method and eliminate the autoclaving step *with* or *without* the chloramphenicol-resistant strain, without any problem and without any sepsis.

LITERATURE CITED

Grossowicz, N., Mandelbaum-Shavit, F., Davidoff, R., and Aronovitch, J. 1962. Microbiological determination of folic acid derivatives in blood. Blood *20*:609–616.

Waters, A. H., and Mollin, D. L. 1961. Studies on the folic acid activity of human serum. J. Clin. Pathol. *14*:335–344.

14

Mechanisms in the Production of Megaloblastic Anemia

I. CHANARIN *and* JANET PERRY

The end point in the production of a megaloblastic anemia is the lack of a normally functioning folate coenzyme(s). We will try to review some of the current ideas about how lack of a folate coenzyme arises in the various disorders that lead to a megaloblastic anemia.

NATURE OF THE FOLATE COENZYME

There is increasing evidence that the coenzyme is folate polyglutamate and the monoglutamate is the transport form between different compartments of the body. In bacterial systems such as in clostridia, the apoprotein, e.g., formyl tetrahydrofolate synthetase, has a much greater affinity for polyglutamates than for monoglutamates (Curthoys and Rabinowitz, 1972). In thymidine synthesis in *Lactobacillus casei*, the polyglutamate is several times more active than the monoglutamate (Kisliuk *et al.*, 1973).

In mammalian cells, serine hydroxymethylase from rabbit liver shows a higher affinity for the triglutamate than for monoglutamate.

Dihydrofolate reductase from a human cell line was more active with polyglutamate than with monoglutamate folates (Morales and Greenberg, 1964; Greenberg *et al.*, 1966; Plante *et al.*, 1967; Coward *et al.*, 1974). McBurney and Whitmore (1974) described a mutant mammalian cell line from hamster ovary in which there was a failure to synthesize polyglutamate, all the cellular folates being monoglutamates. These cells required preformed thymidine, adenosine, and glycine. This is most persuasive evidence that the polyglutamate form was involved in the synthesis of these essential compounds—a function the monoglutamate was unable to perform.

PERNICIOUS ANEMIA

In pernicious anemia (PA), there is a fall in red cell folate polyglutamate (Table 14-1) with relatively little change in folate monoglutamate levels (Chanarin *et al.*, 1974a). Because of the relatively long survival of red cells, the red cell folate levels underestimate the extent of depletion of folate elsewhere in the body. The decline in the level of active folate coenzyme explains the known events in megaloblastic anemia in man. With treatment there is a striking increase in red cell methyltetrahydropteroylpolyglutamates without any change in the monoglutamates and shorter-chain polyglutamates (Figure 14-1).

There also appear to be significant differences between the pattern of folate in red cells in B_{12} and in folate deficiency (Table 14-2). Treated

TABLE 14-1 Red Cell Folate in the Absence of Conjugase Treatment (1–3 Glutamate Residues) and after Conjugase Treatment (Total Folate) Assayed with *L. casei*[a]

Folate Form	Vitamin B_{12} Deficiency (11)	Controls (31)	P
Free (1–3 glutamate residues)	85.4	86.3	NS[b]
Polyglutamate (4 or more residues)	103.4	202.8	>0.0025
TOTAL	193.9 (69–443)	289.2 (135–569)	>0.005

SOURCE: Chanarin *et al.*, The biochemical lesion in vitamin-B12 deficiency in man, Lancet *i*:1251–1252, 1974.
[a]The difference between these values represents longer chain folate polyglutamates.
[b]Not significant.

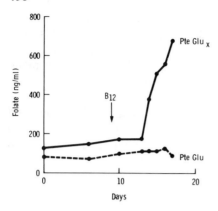

FIGURE 14-1 Effect of vitamin B_{12} therapy on short chain (PteGlu) and longer chain polyglutamates ($PteGlu_x$) in pernicious anemia (SOURCE: A. Wu, I. Chanarin, and A. J. Levi. Lancet *i*:829, Figure 1, 1974).

epileptic patients under the care of E. H. Reynolds had normal hemoglobin levels, but half were macrocytic. Their free folate levels were significantly lower than in the PA group. The polyglutamate levels were also reduced. In the few patients with severe folate deficiency, both parameters were very low.

There are various possible explanations for the low folate polyglutamate levels in PA.

1. There is a failure to transport methyltetrahydrofolate into B_{12}-deficient cells. This was demonstrated by the failure of lymphocytes in untreated PA to take up labeled methylfolate (Das and Hoffbrand, 1970; Tisman and Herbert, 1973). If folate cannot get into cells, it cannot be converted into the coenzyme. Evidence against this being the primary and the only lesion lies in the difference in free and polyglutamate forms in B_{12}- and folate-deficient red cells. The difference in short-chain folates indicates that in PA there is a block in converting monogluta-

TABLE 14-2 Short-Chain and Longer-Chain Folate Polyglutamates in Red Blood Cells in Controls, Pernicious Anemia, and Treated Epileptics Assayed with *L. casei*[a]

	Red Cell Folate, ng/ml	
Group	$5CH_3H_4PteGlu_{1-3}$	$5CH_3H_4PteGlu_{4-6}$
Controls (31)	86.3	202.8
B_{12} deficient (11)	85.4	108.4
Treated epileptics (42)	20.2	159.2

[a]Data published by permission of E. H. Reynolds.

mates to polyglutamates that does not appear to exist in primary folate deficiency. It is possible that the failure of methylfolate uptake by lymphocytes is secondary to the failure to shift monoglutamate to polyglutamate within the cell.

2. Is there a direct B_{12} requirement for folate polyglutamate synthesis? There is no direct evidence that this is the case. J. Perry has examined the polyglutamates present in normal, PA, and folate-deficient red cells. In all three there are penta- and hexafolate polyglutamates and no unusual forms except transiently after B_{12} treatment, when we found a peak that we think has four glutamic acid residues (Figure 14-2).

3. Spronk (1974) showed that rat liver synthesized polyglutamate from tetrahydrofolate but not from methyltetrahydrofolate. Lavoie *et al.* (1974) showed that human lymphocytes also failed to accumulate labeled polyglutamate after administration of methylfolate labeled in the methyl group.

Assuming that methyltetrahydrofolate cannot be used as a substrate for polyglutamate synthesis, the third hypothesis is that in pernicious anemia there is failure within the cell to convert methyltetrahydrofolate to tetrahydrofolate and so provide the proper substrate for polyglutamate synthesis. This is the methyl trap hypothesis put forward by Noronha and Silverman (1961) and Herbert and Zalusky (1962). This hypothesis indicates that conversion of homocysteine to methionine is accompanied by the coincident conversion of methyltetrahydrofolate to tetrahydrofolate and this, of course, is said to fail in B_{12} deficiency. There are various difficulties that must be explained before that hypothesis is accepted.

In attempting to test this hypothesis, we observed that intravenous methylfolate is cleared from plasma in patients with pernicious anemia in either a normal manner (Chanarin and Perry, 1968) or more rapidly than normal when there is a low red cell folate level (Figure 14-3). If methylfolate was not used, one might anticipate that it would accumulate in plasma as suggested by the elevated methyl folate level sometimes seen in untreated pernicious anemia. That this does not happen is perhaps surprising, but it is a fact. More important is that patients with congenital methyl-malonylaciduria, in which there is a lack of vitamin B_{12} coenzyme, a demonstrable failure of homocysteine–methionine conversion, and raised plasma levels of homocysteine and homocysteinuria, there is no effect on hemopoiesis, which is normoblastic. These children do not trap folate as methylfolate despite failure of the vitamin B_{12}-mediated homocysteine–methionine pathway (Levy *et al.*,

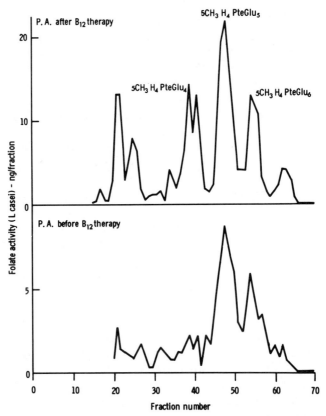

FIGURE 14-2 Chromatography of red cell folate before and 4 weeks after B_{12} therapy in pernicious anemia. Before treatment the usual 5- and 6-glutamic acid chains are present. A presumably transient peak of a 4-glutamic acid polyglutamate appeared after treatment (SOURCE: Perry *et al.*, Br. J. Haematol. *32*:243, Figure 3, 1976).

1970). For these reasons I think that the methylfolate trap remains unproven at present, although it provides the most attractive explanation for the changes in red cell folate in PA.

LESION IN MEGALOBLASTIC ANEMIA DUE TO ANTICONVULSANT DRUGS

The nature of the lesion produced by drugs such as diphenylhydantoin and barbiturates remains uncertain. Our studies were stimulated by the

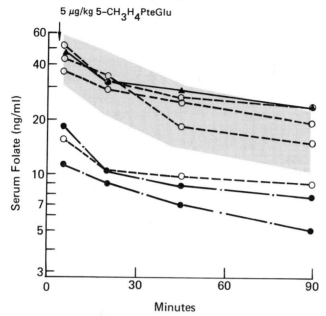

FIGURE 14-3   Serum folate levels after the I.V. injection of 5 μg/k of 5-methyltetrahydrofolate in controls (shaded area) and patients with untreated pernicious anemia (SOURCE: Chanarin and Perry, Br. J. Haematol. *14*:297, Figure 1, 1968).

evidence that in pernicious anemia vitamin B_{12} was concerned directly or indirectly with methylfolate transport. Could the anticonvulsant drugs likewise interfere with methylfolate transport? It has been shown many times that folate levels in cerebrospinal fluid (CSF) are abnormally low in treated epileptics. Further, about 50 percent of treated epileptics are macrocytic, and minor megaloblastic marrow changes are common.

To study transport of folate into CSF, we prepared methylfolate generally labeled with tritium of high specific activity. This was done by tritium exchange with folinic acid. 5-Formyltetrahydrofolate is easily converted into 5-methyltetrahydrofolate (Chanarin and Perry, 1967).

Following I.V. injection of labeled 5-methyltetrahydrofolate, a label appeared in the CSF in high concentration within 4 h, and after that the level declined. About one-quarter of the total dose was present in CSF, indicating considerable circulation of methylfolate between plasma and cerebrospinal fluid compartments (Chanarin *et al.*, 1974b).

The uptake of methylfolate in the choroid plexus of the pig was studied by Chen and Wagner (in press). Phenobarbitone caused significant inhibition in the transport of methylfolate by the choroid plexus and, if confirmed in man, would go a long way in explaining the mode of action of anticonvulsants since some, like primidone or mysoline, are converted in the body to phenobarbitone. On this basis one can anticipate that these drugs may interfere with transport of methylfolate into hemopoietic cells, and, if so, this could account for the megaloblastic process. Failure of transport into intestinal cells may account for the observations of impaired folate absorption recorded by some groups, although others, including ourselves, have failed to obtain similar results (Meynell, 1966; Dahlke and Mertens-Roesler, 1967; Gerson et al., 1970; Hoffbrand and Necheles, 1968; Rosenberg et al., 1968; Benn et al., 1971; Perry and Chanarin, 1972).

Another potentially important observation made by Chen and Wagner (in press) is that pteroylglutamic acid interfered with methylfolate transport into the CSF. Again, if confirmed in man, this could explain why folic acid can aggravate the neuropathy in patients with pernicious anemia. It could also explain the observation by Reynolds (1967) that folic acid in the long term aggravates epilepsy and increases fit frequency.

FOLATE AND ALCOHOLISM

The importance of folate deficiency in the development of megaloblastic anemia in alcoholics was shown by Sullivan and Herbert (1964), Eichner et al. (1972), Eichner and Hillman (1971), and others. It has led to the suggestion that alcohol exerts its effect directly on the folate pathways. We have had the opportunity of studying a different type of alcoholic in the United Kingdom (Wu et al., 1974, 1975). Studies in the United States have been done with so-called "skid row" alcoholics. In the United Kingdom we have studied a group of alcoholics who are still well integrated into the community, who do a normal day's work, and generally, but not always, consume an adequate diet. Under these circumstances we have been able to distinguish between the effects of dietary lack of folate on the one hand and the action of alcohol on the other. (see Tables 14-3 and 14-4). Each of the 84 patients we studied was taking more than 80 g of ethanol per day. Only one-third showed evidence of folate deficiency as judged by low serum, red cell, and liver folate concentrations. Liver for folate assay was obtained from a percutaneous biopsy. Two-thirds of our patients had no evidence of folate deficiency, but 85 percent were macrocytic; that

TABLE 14-3   Effect of Alcoholic Beverage Consumed on Serum, Red Cell, and Liver Folate in Alcoholics

Folate	Beer	Wine Spirits	Significance
Serum, ng/ml	5.0	2.8	<0.01
Red cell, ng/ml	404	292	<0.05
Liver, μg/g	4.8	3.1	<0.02

is, in the majority the macrocytosis was not associated with folate deficiency.

One-third of our patients showed megaloblastic marrow changes, although none were anemic. Nearly one-half of these megaloblastic patients had normal serum, red cell, and, in those in which it was assayed, normal liver folate levels. Thus macrocytosis and megaloblastosis can occur in alcoholism in the absence of folate deficiency, and we suggest that these are the result of the direct toxic action of alcohol on the erythroblast. Of course, they can also be produced by folate deficiency when it is present.

Folate deficiency was present in those on poor diets and those who drank spirits rather than beer, an aspect that has also been prominent in U.S. studies. I should add that macrocytosis disappeared in these patients who stopped consuming alcohol, but macrocytosis persisted, despite folate therapy over 6 months, in those who continued to drink alcohol.

FOLATE DEFICIENCY DUE TO INCREASED GROWTH REQUIREMENTS

Despite considerable uncertainty about man's folate intake, we can define a number of disorders in which folate deficiency arises because of either a temporary or long-standing increase in folate requirement.

TABLE 14-4   Effect of Diet on Serum, Red Cell, and Liver Folate in Alcoholics

Folate	Adequate	Inadequate	Significance
Serum, ng/ml	4.1	2.7	<0.05
Red cell, ng/ml	378	252	<0.02
Liver, μg/g	4.0	3.4	NS[a]

[a]Not significant.

The two most important situations are pregnancy and chronic hemolytic states. When megaloblastic anemia develops, there is often evidence that poor dietary folate intake was also a factor. Chronic
hemolysis is of little importance in Caucasians but of great importance
in non-Caucasians (for example, in West Africa, where one-third of the
population carries an abnormal hemoglobin—to which may be added
the hemolysis of chronic malaria).

Figure 14-4 presents a summary of data in pregnancy. The index of
folate status used in this study was the red cell folate level. The study
involved some 200 women, one half of whom were given a daily
supplement containing 200 μg of pteroylglutamic acid and the other
half a placebo (Chanarin *et al.*, 1968). Both preparations also contained
200 mg of iron. The 100-μg dose of folate was chosen as a result of
previous studies in which we had used inadequate folate supplements.
All the women had blood counts and red cell folates estimated regularly
throughout pregnancy, and all had a marrow aspiration performed in
the last few weeks of pregnancy.

The group not receiving folate showed a steady fall in red cell folate
levels throughout pregnancy. The group receiving 100 μg of folate
showed a rise in red cell folate in the earlier weeks of pregnancy, and
thereafter the red cell folate level was maintained. Thus the average

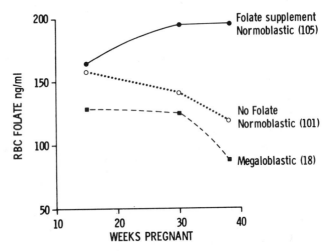

FIGURE 14-4   Effect of a folate supplement (100 μg daily) or a
placebo throughout pregnancy on red cell folate. Values in 18
women who had megaloblastic marrow changes in late pregnancy
are shown separately.

amount of additional folate required was 100 μg daily. Hansen and Rybo (1967) in Sweden showed that a supplement of 50 μg of folate daily failed to arrest the fall in red cell folate, 100 μg stabilized the level, and 200 μg daily was associated with a steady increase in RBC folate.

There were 18 patients whose marrows showed megaloblastic change at the end of pregnancy. These had significantly lower red cell folate levels when first seen in early pregnancy as compared to the rest of the women in this study. This reduced red cell folate level in early pregnancy can only be due to nutritional folate deficiency.

Pregnancy represents a standard folate stress. The way this stress is met depends on folate stores before pregnancy, and this in turn depends on dietary folate intake. Those whose diets supply inadequate amounts of folate both before and during pregnancy are unable to meet the folate stress in pregnancy and become megaloblastic. Temperley and his colleagues (1968) in Dublin, Ireland, have made similar observations using the serum folate level as criterion for deficiency.

INCREASED FOLATE REQUIREMENT DUE TO INEFFECTIVE HEMOPOIESIS

Folate deficiency develops in two-thirds of patients with pernicious anemia as assessed by the abnormally low red cell folate, and the considerable death of cells in the marrow may in part be the explanation of this. Chronic myelofibrosis is another disorder in which ineffective hemopoiesis is prominent. Folate deficiency is common in this group (Hoffbrand *et al.*, 1968).

NUTRITIONAL FOLATE DEFICIENCY

There remains considerable uncertainty about normal folate intake and requirement. We have previously published data suggesting a normal daily folate intake of 676 μg, of which 160 μg was short-chain folates (Chanarin *et al.*, 1968b). We now think that these values are too high. We have reassayed many individual food components as well as complete diets, and our estimate for folate content of mixed diets is 129 to 300 μg/day, a figure in keeping with that published by Cooper *et al.* (1970). We now believe that almost all the monoglutamates are absorbed, and we base this on observations we have made with tritium-labeled analogues using a fecal excretion method (Figure 14-5). Our results show that physiological folate analogues are almost completely

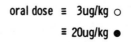

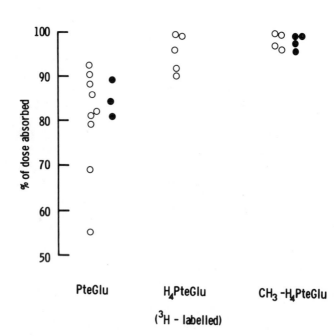

FIGURE 14-5   Absorption of folate analogues generally labelled with tritium by control subjects using a fecal excretion method (SOURCE: Hoffbrand *et al.*, Q. J. Med. N.S. *37*:493, Figure 3, 1968).

absorbed and better absorbed than pteroylglutamic acid. Free folate may constitute between 15 to 50 percent of dietary folate.

The availability of longer-chain folate polyglutamates for absorption in man remains uncertain, and the extent to which this absorption is influenced by conjugase inhibitors remains conjectural.

LITERATURE CITED

Benn, A., Swan, C. H. J., Cooke, W. T., Blair, J. A., Matty, A. J., and Smith, M. E. 1971. Effect of intraluminal pH on the absorption of pteroylmonoglutamic acid. Br. Med. J. *1*:148–150.
Chanarin, I., and Perry, J. 1967. A simple method for the preparation of 5-methyltetrahydropteroylglutamic acid. Biochem. J. *105*:633–634.

Chanarin, I., and Perry, J. 1968. Metabolism of 5-methyltetrahydrofolate in pernicious anemia. Br. J. Haematol. *14*:297–301.

Chanarin, I., Rothman, D., Ward, A., and Perry, J. 1968a. Folate status and requirement in pregnancy. Br. Med. J. *2*:390–394.

Chanarin, I., Rothman, D., Perry, J., and Stratfull, D. 1968b. Normal dietary folate, iron, and protein intake, with particular reference to pregnancy. Br. Med. J. *2*:394–397.

Chanarin, I., Perry, J., and Lumb, M. 1974a. The biochemical lesion in vitamin-B$_{12}$ deficiency in man. Lancet *i*:1251–1252.

Chanarin, I., Perry, J., and Reynolds, E. H. 1974b. Transport of 5-methyltetrahydrofolic acid into the cerebrospinal fluid in man. Clin. Sci. Mol. Med. *46*:369–373.

Chen, C. P., and Wagner, C. (In press). Life sciences.

Cooper, B. A., Cantlie, G. S. D., and Brunton, L. 1970. The case for folic acid supplements during pregnancy. Am. J. Clin. Nutr. *23*:848–854.

Coward, J. K., Parameswaran, K. N., Cashmore, A. R., and Bertino, J. R. 1974. 7,8-Dihydropteroyl oligo-gamma-L-glutamates: synthesis and kinetic studies with purified dihydrofolate reductase from mammalian sources. Biochemistry. *13*:3899–3903.

Curthoys, N. P., and Rabinowitz, J. C. 1972. Formyltetrahydrofolate synthetase; binding of folate substrates and kinetics of the reverse reaction. J. Biol. Chem. *247*:1965–1971.

Dahlke, M. B., and Mertens-Roesler, E. 1967. Malabsorption of folic acid due to diphenylhydantoin. Blood *30*:341–351.

Das, K. C., and Hoffbrand, A. V. 1970. Lymphocyte transformation in megaloblastic anemia: morphology and DNA synthesis. Br. J. Haematol. *19*:459–468.

Eichner, E. R., and Hillman, R. S. 1971. The evolution of anemia in alcoholic patients. Am. J. Med. *50*:218–232.

Eichner, E. R., Buchanan, B., Smith, J. W., and Hillman, R. S. 1972. Variations in the hematologic and medical status of alcoholics. Am. J. Med. Sci. *263*:35–42.

Gerson, C. D., Hepner, G. W., Brown, N., Cohen, N., Herbert, V., and Janowitz, H. D. 1970. Inhibition by diphenylhydantoin (dilantin) of folic acid absorption in man. J. Clin. Invest. *49*:33a. (Abstract)

Greenberg, D. M., Tam, B. D., Jenny, E., and Payes, B. 1966. Highly purified dihydrofolate reductase of calf thymus. Biochim. Biophys. Acta *122*:423–435.

Hansen, H., and Rybo, G. 1967. Folic acid dosage in prophylactic treatment during pregnancy. Acta Obstet. Gynecol. Scand. *46* Suppl. *7*:107–112.

Herbert, V., and Zalusky, R. 1962. Interrelations of vitamin B$_{12}$ and folic acid metabolism: folic acid clearance studies. J. Clin. Invest. *41*:1263–1276.

Hoffbrand, A. V., and Necheles, T. F. 1968. Mechanism of folate deficiency in patients receiving phenytoin. Lancet *ii*:528–530.

Hoffbrand, A. V., Chanarin, I., Kremenchuzky, S., Szur, L., Waters, A. H., and Mollin, D. L. 1968. Megaloblastic anaemia in myelosclerosis. Q. J. Med. N.S. *37*:493–516.

Kisliuk, R. L., Gaumont, Y., and Baugh, C. M. 1973. Polyglutamyl derivatives of folate as substrates and inhibitors of thymidylate synthetase. J. Biol. Chem. *249*:4100–4103.

Lavoie, A., Tripp, E., and Hoffbrand, A. V. 1974. The effect of vitamin B$_{12}$ deficiency on methylfolate metabolism and pteroylglutamate synthesis in human cells. Clin. Sci. Mol. Med. *47*:617–630.

Levy, H. L., Mudd, S. H., Schulman, J. D., Dreyfus, P. M., and Abeles, R. H. 1970. A derangement in B-12 metabolism associated with homocystinemia, cystathioninemia, hypomethioninemia and methylmalonic aciduria. Am. J. Med. *48*:390–397.

McBurney, M. W., and Whitmore, G. F. 1974. Isolation and biochemical characterization of folate deficient mutants of Chinese hamster cells. Cell. *2*:173–182.

168 CHANARIN AND PERRY

Meynell, M. J. 1966. Megaloblastic anemia in anticonvulsant therapy. Lancet *i*:487.

Morales, D. R., and Greenberg, D. M. 1964. Purification and properties of dihydrofolate reductase of sheep liver. Biochim. Biophys. Acta 85:360–376.

Noronha, J. M., and Silverman, M. 1961. *in* Vitamin B-12 and intrinsic factor 2, H. C. Heinrich, ed., p. 728. Stuttgart.

Perry, J., and Chanarin, I. 1972. Observations on folate absorption with particular reference to folate polyglutamate and possible inhibitors to its absorption. Gut 13:544–550.

Plante, L. T., Crawford, E. J., and Friedkin, M. 1967. Enzyme studies with new analogues of folic acid and homofolic acid. J. Biol. Chem. 242:1466–1476.

Reynolds, E. H. 1967. Effects of folic acid on the mental state and fit-frequency of drug-treated epileptic patients. Lancet *i*:1086–1088.

Rosenberg, I. H., Godwin, H. A., Streiff, R. R., and Castle, W. B. 1968. Impairment of intestinal deconjugation of dietary folate. A possible explanation of megaloblastic anemia associated with phenytoin therapy. Lancet *ii*:530–532.

Spronk, A. M. 1973. Tetrahydrofolate polyglutamate synthesis in rat liver. Fed. Proc. 32:471. (Abstract)

Sullivan, L. W., and Herbert, V. 1964. Suppression of hematopoiesis by ethanol. J. Clin. Invest. 43:2048–2062.

Temperley, I. J., Meehan, M. J. M., and Gatenby, P. B. B. 1968. Serum folic acid levels in pregnancy and their relationship to megaloblastic marrow change. Br. J. Haematol. 14:13–19.

Tisman, G. W., and Herbert, V. 1973. B-12 dependence of cell uptake of a serum folate: an explanation for high serum folate and cell folate depletion in B-12 deficiency. Blood 41:465–469.

Wu, A., Chanarin, I., and Levi, A. J. 1974. Folate deficiency in the alcoholic—its relationship to clinical and haematological abnormalities, liver disease and folate stores. Lancet *i*:829–830.

Wu, A., Chanarin, I., Slavin, G., and Levi, A. J. 1975. Macrocytosis of chronic alcoholism. Br. J. Haematol. 29:469–478.

15

Drug-Induced
Folate Deficiency

RONALD H. GIRDWOOD

First I must say how truly delighted I am to have been invited to participate in this Workshop. By chance I have recently been so overwhelmed with other medical matters that I have temporarily ceased to be actively involved in research in this field, but I am always delighted to return to discussions about folic acid and to learn of the new thoughts about the actions of the folates. My own interest was first aroused in 1938 when I saw women in pregnancy or the puerperium seriously ill with megaloblastic anemia. There was a certain mortality then, since folic acid was unknown and even our transfusion service was in a primitive state. Blood banks had not yet been introduced. We knew about Wills' factor and hoped that it would soon be isolated. My own next major encounter with megaloblastic anemia was when I saw it, almost on an epidemic scale, in the Far East in 1943. This was epidemic tropical sprue, but folic acid was not yet available as a therapeutic agent.

I feel sure that drug-induced folate deficiency is now a subject worth attention, and one about which we know little. It may be particularly important in those marginally deficient in folate.

169

DRUGS THAT REQUIRE CONSIDERATION

The drugs that have been claimed to cause megaloblastic anemia include:

(a) Those that interfere with the dihydrofolate reductase mechanism:

> Aminopterin
> Methotrexate
> Pyrimethamine
> Trimethoprim
> Triamterene (?)

(b) Drugs interfering with DNA synthesis:

> Cytosine arabinoside
> Mercaptopurine
> Thioguanine
> Cyclophosphamide
> Azathioprine
> 5-Fluouracil
> Hydroxyurea
> Arsenic (?)

(c) Antiepileptic drugs, acting by an unknown mechanism (e.g., interference with conjugases, displacement of folate from protein carriers, enzyme induction leading to folate destruction, coincidence of nutritional folate depletion):

> Phenytoin
> Primidone
> Phenobarbitone (?)

(d) Drugs interfering with vitamin B_{12} absorption:

> Metformin

(e) Uncertain or doubtful action:

> Oral contraceptives
> Ethyl alcohol
> Cycloserine
> Phenylbutazone

ORAL CONTRACEPTIVES

In considering any such list, there is little need to discuss further the drugs that may cause megaloblastic anemia by interference with DNA synthesis, and there is doubt about the mode of action of all the others, apart from the ones that interfere with the folate reductase mechanism. It is of considerable current interest to know whether contraceptive pills can by themselves cause megaloblastic anemia in a woman who has no other reason for the development of this complication. Shojania *et al.* (1968, 1969) reported that oral contraceptives led to a fall in serum and red cell folate levels, findings that were not confirmed by Spray (1968) or Paine *et al.* (1975). Reports of the occurrence of megaloblastic anemia have been given by Paton (1969), Streiff (1970), and others. Sometimes there are complicating factors. Thus, Wood *et al.* (1972) reported three patients who developed megaloblastic anemia when taking oral contraceptives, but one had gluten enteropathy, another had chronically poor nutrition, and a third had a diet that was rather low in folate content.

To obtain accurate data, we require a comprehensive reporting system. In the United Kingdom, the Committee on Safety of Medicines maintains an Adverse Reactions register. Doctors are asked to report adverse reactions to the Committee, and drug companies are obliged by law to do so if new preparations are marketed or unexpected reactions occur. One would imagine therefore that, if megaloblastic anemia commonly occurs from the taking of oral contraceptives, this would be reported reasonably often. I have obtained from the Committee permission to quote from the Register, and I can only say that helpful evidence is not available.

The relevant section in the Register is headed "Macrocytic Anemia." Megaloblastic anemia is not separately identified.

All the reports received between April 1964 and June 1973 in relation to drugs listed under (a) to (e) above are shown in Table 15-1. In this and the following tables, if an oral contraceptive contains both an oestrogen and a progestogen, the incident is recorded against each component, and hence there will be two reports of the same incident.

It can be seen that doctors probably do not trouble to report either anticonvulsant-induced megaloblastic anemia or that due to cytotoxic drugs or antimitotic agents. Hematologists, at least, have been anxious to trace incidents of co-trimoxazole-induced megaloblastic anemia, and eight reports have been made, but these may be subject to doubts about true cause and effect. It cannot really be said that there is any hard evidence from this Register to support the view that contraceptives are a causative agent.

It has been suggested that anticonvulsant drugs may cause abnormalities in the fetus, and indeed the companies marketing anticonvulsants in Britain have issued warnings about the possible danger of their use in pregnant epileptics. It is pointed out by the manufacturers that

TABLE 15-1   Macrocytic Anemia

Drug		Reports	Deaths
Phenytoin		11	7
Primidone		6	1
Phenobarbitone		7	3
Co-trimoxazole		8	0
Pyrimethamine		2	0
Azathioprine		1	0
Ethinyloestradiol	(Oestrogen)	3	0
Norethisterone	(Progestogen)	2	0
Ethynodiol	(Progestogen)	1	0

long-term anticonvulsant therapy can be associated with decreased serum folate levels, and there have, of course, been numerous reports to this effect. The statement is made that "the very slight risk of an abnormal fetus must be weighed against the risks of withholding treatment during pregnancy." Mention is made of the possibility that treatment with folic acid and vitamin B_{12}, "although controversial," should be considered. The subject of anticonvulsant drugs, epilepsy, and congenital malformations has been discussed by Mercier-Parot and Tuchmann-Duplessis (1974), Speidel and Meadow (1974), and Norris and Pratt (1974). The matter still requires elucidation.

A report of drugs that might be of interest in relation to folate deficiency or metabolic abnormalities and that have been reported to the Committee to have possibly caused multiple congenital abnormalities in the fetus is given in Table 15-2. This includes all the reports between April 1964 and June 1973 in relation to drugs suspected of

TABLE 15-2   Multiple Congenital Abnormalities

Drug		Reports	Deaths
Phenytoin		11	0
Primidone		6	0
Co-trimoxazole		1	0
Ethinyloestradiol	(Oestrogen)	5	0
Mestranol	(Oestrogen)	2	0
Norethisterone	(Progestogen)	5	0
Hydroxyprogesterone	(Progestogen)	3	0
Dydrogesterone	(Progestogen)	3	0
Ethynodiol	(Progestogen)	1	0
Megestrol	(Progestogen)	1	0

being able to cause folate abnormalities in any way. Some reports may relate to "hormonal" tests for pregnancy, involving the use of a mixture of an oestrogen and progestogen.

It does not follow in any instance that the congenital abnormalities were really due to the drugs. The *commonest* drug listed was, in fact, meclozine (12 reports), which is not included in the tables. It does not cause folate deficiency. This drug is given to control vomiting, and so it is probably often taken by pregnant women, including some who, even without taking it, no doubt, would have had infants with congenital abnormalities. Various *isolated* congenital abnormalities were also reported and are shown in Table 15-3 in relation to the drugs we are considering. Again, there were 12 reports of incidents after the taking of meclozine.

It will be seen that phenytoin and primidone, which are known to cause megaloblastic anemia by an unknown mechanism believed to involve folate metabolism, might be thought to demonstrate some evidence of being a cause of dysmorphogenesis in the fetus. To prove that there is a real danger requires a very large-scale investigation, possibly involving the administration of anticonvulsants to nonepileptics and also recording of the incidence of abnormalities in children of epileptics who have not received treatment. It should be noted that it is said that barbiturates impair the effectiveness of oral contraceptives (Garb, 1971) and that one manufacturer warns that some drugs, including barbiturates, hydantoin, or rifampicin, if given with oral contraceptives, may lead to occasional pregnancies. Presumably this drug interaction is by the induction of liver enzymes, but the problem of congenital abnormalities then requires even greater consideration, as

TABLE 15-3 Various Congenital Abnormalities

Drug		Reports	
Phenytoin		11	(+ 15 cleft palates)
Primidone		11	(+ 20 cleft palates)
Co-trimoxazole		1	
Ethinyloestradiol		12	
Mestranol		11	
Norethisterone		15	
Hydroxyprogesterone		6	
Dydrogesterone		8	
Ethynodiol		1	
Norethynodrel	(Progestogen)	3	
Ethisterone	(Progestogen)	3	

we have now come around to thoughts of unexpected pregnancies in patients receiving anticonvulsants and oral contraceptives together. Do we know what, if anything, oral contraceptives can do to folate metabolism? What happens if anticonvulsants are also taken? What if a dihydrofolate reductase inhibitor is added? Certainly there is nothing in Tables 15-2 or 15-3 to suggest any real problem with dihydrofolate reductase inhibitors, either alone or in conjunction with other drugs. However, I do feel that, in considering the possible effects of oral contraceptives, we are discussing a subject the importance of which is uncertain, and we do not know whether there is any disturbance of folate metabolism. It will perhaps be a suitable subject for a workshop in several years' time.

DIHYDROFOLATE REDUCTASE INHIBITORS

I feel that I should omit the earlier, more obvious, drugs, and refer to trimethoprim. The combination of sulphamethoxazole with trimethoprim has been freely used in the United Kingdom for several years and was introduced from the United States as a result of the fundamental work of Dr. Hitchings. We considered it to be a great advance in antibacterial therapy, but its use was not permitted in the United States until recently, and then only on a restricted basis. It is marketed in Britain as Bactrim and Septrin and in the United States as Bactrim and Septra.

I have referred elsewhere (Girdwood, 1973) to the small-scale investigation we did when one of my colleagues, Norman Horne, was doing a trial of ampicillin and Septra in two groups of bronchitic patients over a period of 1 yr. There is nothing to report about the patients receiving ampicillin, and in Table 15-4 I have updated the results relating to the patients receiving Septra.

The numbers would have been larger, but three patients did not attend for the full length of the trial, four withdrew because of upper-gastrointestinal discomfort, one developed a rash, one emigrated, and one was found to have gluten enteropathy and was therefore unsuitable.

It will, however, be seen that in this small trail there was no evidence that two tablets of Septra twice daily (320 mg of trimethoprim plus 1,600 mg of sulphamethoxazole) for 1 yr caused any abnormality of folate metabolism, and the lobes of the granulocyte nuceli were not altered. This lack of effect is not surprising when it is realized that

TABLE 15-4 Septra Trial

Test	Pre	6 Months	12 Months
Hb (g/100 ml)	15.6 ± 1.8[a]	14.6 ± 1.4	14.4 ± 0.94
Platelets	222 ± 68	209 ± 80	244 ± 80
Plasma folate	8.6 ± 4.7	8.1 ± 3.9	9.6 ± 4.97
Red cell folate	330 ± 109	298 ± 123	346 ± 182
Plasma B_{12}	408 ± 108	392 ± 195	392 ± 216
No.	18	18	15

[a] ± Standard deviation.

trimethoprim is 50,000 times more active against bacterial dihydrofolate reductase than against that of man.

There has been a relatively small number of reports of megaloblastic anemia occurring after the administration of tablets of co-trimoxazole, but I have referred to this elsewhere (Girdwood, 1973), pointing out that the cases have always been complex ones, as have any alleged examples that I have seen myself, numerous possible other factors being involved. However, Chanarin (Chanarin and England, 1972) has produced evidence to suggest that the drug might inhibit the normal reticulocyte response in the treatment of pernicious anemia with vitamin B_{12}. In Table 15-1 there are eight reports of macrocytic anemia after administration of co-trimoxazole, but without knowing details we cannot be sure whether or not other factors were involved. However, reporting of side effects of this drug is certainly being done, because, like any sulphonamide, the sulphamethoxazole part of co-trimoxazole may cause thrombocytopenia. The Committee on Safety of Medicines has 32 reports of thrombocytopenia from co-trimoxazole during the same period as the eight reports of macrocytic anemia.

It would obviously be unwise to use co-trimoxazole in the treatment of patients already folate deficient for some other reason, although I have seen nothing anywhere to suggest that there is any danger from giving this drug together with anticonvulsants, and in a few short-term experiments with this combination we found no change in serum folate levels. A larger experiment should be done in a hospital dealing with large numbers of epileptics. If a patient has sprue or primary folate deficiency, it is obviously necessary to give folic acid before using Septra. Fortunately, the folic acid, although available to the patient, cannot be utilized by bacteria, and so even combined therapy with Septra and folic acid is possible.

ETHYL ALCOHOL

In the United States it appears that folate deficiency and megaloblastic anemia are not uncommonly found in alcoholics (Herbert *et al.*, 1963; Klipstein and Lindenbaum, 1965). In Britain the problem of alcoholism is less severe, and there is little published evidence that folate depletion occurs. However, Wu *et al.* (1975) studied 84 English patients who regularly took more than 80 g of alcohol daily (see Chapter 14).

Is there really a considerable problem of folate deficiency in alcoholics, and is it greater in some countries than in others? I wonder, too, whether we are very ignorant not only about the incidence of drug-induced megaloblastic anemia, but, in many instances, about its mechanisms. I think, too, that much has to be learned about the extent to which the drugs we have been considering prove a hazard to the fetus. Perhaps the danger is slight, but so is our information.

LITERATURE CITED

Chanarin, I., and England, J. M. 1972. Toxicity of trimethoprim-sulphamethoxazole in patients with megaloblastic haemopoiesis. Br. Med. J. *1*:651–653.
Garb, S. 1971. Clinical guide to undesirable drug interactions and interferences. Harvey Miller & Medcalf, London.
Girdwood, R. H. 1973. Trimethoprim/sulphamethoxazole: Long-term therapy and folate levels. Med. J. Aust. (Special Suppl.) *1*:34–37.
Herbert, V., Zalusky, R., and Davidson, C. S. 1963. Correlation of folate deficiency with alcoholism and associated macrocytosis, anemia and liver disease. Ann. Intern. Med. *58*:977–988.
Klipstein, F. A., and Lindenbaum, J. 1965. Folate deficiency in chronic liver disease. Blood *25*:443–456.
Mercier-Parot, L., and Tuchmann-Duplessis, H. 1974. The dysmorphogenic potential of phenytoin: experimental observations. Drugs *8*:340–353.
Norris, J. W., and Pratt, R. F. 1974. Folic acid deficiency and epilepsy. Drugs *8*:366–385.
Paine, C. J., Grafton, W. D., Dickson, V. L., and Eichner, E. R. 1975. Oral contraceptives, serum folate, and hematologic status. J. Am. Med. Assoc. *231*:731–733.
Paton, A. 1969. Oral contraceptives and folate deficiency. Lancet *i*:418.
Shojania, A. M., Hornandy, G., and Barnes, P. H. 1968. Oral contraceptives and serum folate level. Lancet *i*:1376–1377.
Shojania, A. M., Hornandy, G., and Barnes, P. H. 1969. Oral contraceptives and folate metabolism. Lancet *i*:886.
Speidel, B. D., and Meadow, S. R. 1974. Epilepsy, anticonvulsants and congenital malformations. Drugs *8*:354–365.
Spray, G. H. 1968. Oral contraceptives and serum folate levels. Lancet *ii*:110–111.
Streiff, R. R. 1970. Folate deficiency and oral contraceptives. J. Am. Med. Assoc. *214*:105–108.

Wood, J. K., Goldstone, A. H., and Allan, N. C. 1972. Folic acid and the pill. Scand. J. Haematol. 9:539–544.

Wu, A., Chanarin, I., Slavin, G., and Levi, A. J. 1975. Folate deficiency in the alcoholic—its relationship to clinical and haematological abnormalities, liver disease and folate stores. Br. J. Haematol. 29:469–478.

16

Mechanism of Uptake of Folate Monoglutamates and Their Metabolism

JOSEPH R. BERTINO, P. F. NIXON, *and* A. NAHAS

INTRODUCTION

Although it is now clear that almost all mammalian cells examined have the folate coenzymes present in polyglutamate forms (Baugh and Krumdieck, 1971) and that these forms are probably the active coenzymes in cells (Coward *et al.*, 1974, 1975), folates are transported at the monoglutamate level, with the possible exception of intestinal transport. In man the predominant circulating folate in serum, and presumably the transport form, is 5-methyltetrahydrofolate (MeFH$_4$). It is of most relevance, therefore, to study the uptake of this compound by cells that require folate for DNA replication and growth. In addition, the transport of folic acid, the commercially available, stable, oxidized folate form, and 5-formyltetrahydrofolate (leucovorin, citrovorum factor, fFH$_4$) are also of importance since these compounds are used therapeutically. These compounds are converted to other folate coenzymes by cells, however, thus complicating analysis of the transport phenomena. For this reason and because of its importance in the treatment of neoplastic diseases, methotrexate (MTX), a nonmetabolizable folate analogue, has been used extensively for transport studies.

178

PREPARATION OF RADIOLABELED FOLATE COENZYMES

Measurement of intracellular metabolism of folate coenzymes has been facilitated by the use of doubly labeled folate coenzymes and the use of chromatographic procedures (Nixon and Bertino, 1970). The metabolism of the one carbon moiety with ^{14}C can thus be followed as well as the fate of the pteridine nucleus labeled with tritium (9,3′,5′). Furthermore, the folate coenzymes of interest, fFH_4 and $MeFH_4$, can be prepared as the physiologically active diasteriomers (Nixon and Bertino, 1971). The key reaction in the synthesis of these coenzymes from radiolabeled folate is the use of the enzyme dihydrofolate reductase to produce the physiologically active diasteriomer rather than the racemic mixture that would result from chemical reduction of folate or dihydrofolate to tetrahydrofolate. By utilizing commercially available folic acid of very high specific activity for these studies, labeled by tritium in the 9,3′,5′ position, labeled material can be prepared with high specific activity. However, because of the limitation of the specific activity possible with ^{14}C, the activity of the second label introduced into the one carbon moiety is limited (approximately 50 μCi/μmole). The doubly labeled material can be conveniently prepared by mixing the ^3H-labeled and ^{14}C-labeled compounds prepared as described (Bertino and Nixon, 1971).

Transport of Folates in Mouse Tumor Cells

MTX transport has been extensively studied in mouse tumor cells beginning with the early work of Fischer (1962) and Hakala (1965a, 1965b). MTX has been found to be transported across the membrane of mouse tumor cells, in particular the S-180 (Hakala, 1965a), the L1210 (Kessel and Hall, 1967; Goldman, 1971), and the L5178Y (Fischer, 1962) cell lines by a carrier-mediated process. The uptake is rapid and temperature dependent and is inhibited by ouabain and p-chloromercuribenzoate (PCMB). The reduced folates $MeFH_4$ and fFH_4 competitively inhibit methotrexate influx, whereas folic acid, only in very large doses, partially inhibits this process (Nahas et al., 1972). If cells are preloaded with MTX and then resuspended in MTX-free media, efflux of MTX occurs at 37° C to levels that are just sufficient to bind intracellular dihydrofolate reductase (DHFR). Efflux is stimulated by the addition of the reduced folates $MeFH_4$ and fFH_4 but not by folic acid. In recent years, our laboratory (Nahas et al., 1969, 1972) and that of Goldman (1971) have also studied the transport of fFH$_4$ in mouse leukemia cells. Folate transport has also been studied in erythrocytes (Izak et al., 1968; Bobzien and Goldman, 1972) and bone marrow cells (Corcino et al., 1971). In the L1210 mouse leukemia cell, both of these compounds are rapidly accumulated. fFH$_4$ uptake is inhibited by MeFH$_4$ and MTX in a competitive manner. MeFH$_4$ uptake is inhibited also by MTX and fFH$_4$ competively, but not by folic acid (Nahas et al., 1969). When efflux of fFH$_4$ was studied, it was found that radioactivity was displaced by MeFH$_4$ and MTX but not by folic acid in similar concentration. Chromatography of the cell supernatant after incubation of the cells with doubly labeled fFH$_4$ demonstrated that this coenzyme was metabolized rapidly to other folate coenzymes within the cell (Nahas et al., 1972).

MeFH$_4$ uptake and turnover was studied in L1210, L1210R (methotrexate resistant), and L5178Y leukemia cells (Nixon et al., 1973). Analysis of cell extracts showed that, for each cell line, 80 percent of the total cell ^{14}C-methyl group was transferred to macromolecular compounds within 5 min, and 82 to 91 percent was transferred at time intervals up to 60 min. Of the total cell ^{3}H, more than 87 percent remained identifiable as MeFH$_4$ at 60 min. Thus, although most of the ^{14}C-methyl group was transferred from MeFH$_4$, the major intracellular labeled folate remained as MeFH$_4$, indicating rapid resynthesis. The initial transfer of the ^{14}C appeared to be into [^{14}C]methionine, but trichloroacetic acid-insoluble materials, presumably RNA, DNA, and protein, were also progressively ^{14}C labeled. In L1210 cells, the rate of thymidylate biosynthesis was estimated by two different approaches. The first approach was to incubate L1210 cells with fFH$_4$ labeled in the 6 position with tritium and then measure transfer of the ^{3}H to thymidylate. At 1 hr, 28 percent of the cell folate had been used for thymidylate biosynthesis. This value was confirmed by a second approach in which methotrexate-treated L1210 cells were incubated with 9,3',5'-[^{3}H]MeFH$_4$. In the absence of MTX, any folate derived from the thymidylate synthetase reaction would be quickly reduced to FH$_4$. However, since MTX inhibits DHFR, any FH$_2$ generated by whole cells would accumulate as such. In fact, of the total ^{3}H found in MTX-treated L1210 cells incubated for 1 hr with MeFH$_4$, 23 percent accumulated as FH$_2$. In contrast, when L1210R cells were used (these are known to be resistant to MTX by virtue of increased concentration of DHFR), no accumulation of FH$_2$ resulted. These data demonstrate the significance for MTX resistance of the increase of DHFR in the L1210R cells.

Folic Acid Transport

As mentioned above, folic acid either does not utilize the carrier present for the transport of reduced folates, or the affinity of folic acid for this carrier is very poor. Recent data from the laboratory of Huennekens (Rader *et al.*, 1974) indicate that these processes may be separable. For example, pCMB, an inhibitor of reduced folate transport in the L1210 cell, did not affect the uptake of folic acid by these cells. Clearly, mammalian cells transport the folic acid form extremely poorly and presumably depend upon intestinal and liver uptake and conversion to MeFH$_4$ for its transport into cells. As might be expected, growth of mammalian cells in culture requires large amounts of folic acid in the medium, but this may be replaced by small amounts of fFH$_4$ or MeFH$_4$. The latter compound also requires the presence of vitamin B$_{12}$ and a vitamin B$_{12}$ transport protein, transcobalamin II, for optimum utilization by cells (Chello and Bertino, 1973).

Structure Activity Relationships

Limited data are available regarding the nature of the carrier for reduced folates present in mammalian cells. Some structure activity studies carried out in L1210 cells in this laboratory (Nahas and Bertino, 1970) are summarized in Table 16-1. Fom these data the following conclusions can be made: (i) reduced folates are transported to a greater degree than are oxidized compounds; (ii) substitution of methyl or formyl groups at the N^5 position enhances transport of tetrahydrofolate; (iii) the addition of a 4-amino group, which replaces the 4-hydroxyl group in oxidized folate forms, also results in greater affinity for the carrier system present in these cells; (iv) the glutamate present in the terminal part of the folate molecule is also important for optimal transport; and (v) reduction of the pyrazine ring of the 2–4 diaminofolates such as aminopterin did not result in enhanced affinity for the transport system. Of interest is the finding that the N-4-dimethyl analogue of aminopterin is also a potent inhibitor of MTX and MeFH$_4$ transport. Unlike the enzyme DHFR, which binds this analogue less tightly, the transport carrier protein for folates can apparently tolerate bulk at the 4 position. These investigations raise the possibility of developing new inhibitors of folate transport that might be useful in chemotherapy.

TABLE 16-1   Inhibition of MeFH$_4$ and M T X by Folate
Analogues[a]

Compound	Inhibition, %	
	MeFH$_4$	MTX
Folate	None	None
Pteroate	None	None
10-methyl Folate	None	None
10-formyl Folate	None	None
Tetrahydrofolate	27	30
Tetrahydropteroate	8	None
10-methyl Tetrahydrofolate	32	26
10-formyl Tetrahydrofolate	30	28
5-methyl Tetrahydrofolate	75	56
5-methyl Tetrahydropteroate	88	77
5-formyl Tetrahydrofolate	68	48
Aminopterin	66	85
4-Aminopteroylaspartate	41	51
N^{10}-methyl Aminopterin (MTX)	59	94
N^{10}-ethyl Aminopterin	52	89
N^{10}-methyldichloro Aminopterin	63	74
N^2, N^2-dimethyl Aminopterin	56	53
N^4, N^4-dimethyl Aminopterin	39	29
Tetrahydroaminopterin	25	11
Tetrahydroamethopterin	73	74
Pyrimethamine	None	29
Quinazolinylmethylaminobenzoylaspartate	19	72

SOURCE: Nahas and Bertino (1970).
[a]MeFH$_4$ 3',5',9-tritium-labeled or 3',5',9-tritium-labeled MTX was
incubated with L-1210 cells in 10% horse serum in Eagles medium
at a concentration of 2×10^{-6} M in the absence or presence of the
compounds indicated at an equimolar concentration. Uptake of the
radioactive MeFH$_4$ or MTX was then measured for 60 min.

Active Metabolite Inhibitors and the Transport Process

While studying the transport of MTX into L1210 cells, Goldman *et al.*
(1968) made the surprising observation that metabolic inhibitors such
as sodium azide and iodoacetate augmented the accumulation of MTX.
Further work using L1210 cells and human erythrocytes resulted in the
conclusions that these compounds were inhibitors of MTX efflux,
therefore resulting in increased intracellular concentration of MTX.
More recently, Zager *et al.* (1973) have found that vincristine, an agent
used in the treatment of human malignant disease, increased the
intracellular concentration of MTX, also presumably by inhibiting

efflux. Similar results have been reported with human acute myelogenous leukemia cells (Bender *et al.*, 1975). However, it is not clear from these latter studies whether vincristine would augment MTX accumulation at concentrations of MTX that would completely saturate the uptake process. This augmentation of MTX could be of potential clinical usefulness.

Transport of Folates into the Central Nervous System

With the availability of doubly labeled reduced folates, we initiated several years ago studies of the transport and the metabolism of these compounds into cerebrospinal fluid (CSF) when given intravenously (Levitt *et al.*, 1971). The appearance and metabolism of MTX, folic acid, fFH_4, and $MeFH_4$ into the CSF of dogs after intravenous administration was studied. While it was well known that MTX was transported into the CSF very poorly, these studies demonstrated that folic acid was also transported poorly into the CSF. The small amount of radioactivity that did appear in the CSF after folic acid administration was in the form of $MeFH_4$. In contrast, both fFH_4 and $MeFH_4$ were rapidly transported across the brain into the CSF, achieving levels equivalent to those in the serum 2 hr following intravenous administration. When $MeFH_4$ was administered, the folate found in the CSF was identified as $MeFH_4$; however, after fFH_4 administration, the folate found in the CSF was also $MeFH_4$. Thus it seems clear that the transport process in the brain that results in high levels of folates in CSF, as compared to serum, is specific for reduced folates. Studies of transport of folates in the isolated choroid plexus indicate that MTX and folic acid have a high affinity for this tissue (Rubin *et al.*, 1968; Spector and Lorenzo, 1975). Therefore, it is not clear why these compounds are not accumulated in the CSF. One possibility may be that, although the affinity of these compounds for the choroid carrier is great, the ability of the carrier to transport these compounds across into the CSF may be limited, while CSF to choroid plexus transport may be active.

Transport of Folates and Monoglutamates into the Small Intestine

Several groups have studied the transport of folate monoglutamate and MTX in small intestine. While the exact mechanism of uptake remains controversial (reviewed elsewhere in this symposium), our studies (Strum *et al.*, 1971; Olinger *et al.*, 1973) agreed with those of Selhub *et al.* (1973) and indicate that folic acid given in small doses is converted largely to reduced folates by intestinal cells. The jejunum, because of its higher concentration of DHFR as compared to the ileum, appears to carry out this conversion more efficiently (Olinger *et al.*, 1973). In contrast to the carrier-mediated transport system described for the mouse lymphoma cells, folic acid, $MeFH_4$, fFH_4, and MTX all appear to be absorbed by the small intestine by a facilitated diffusion process. No competition for uptake of one folate form by another could be demonstrated in the presence of large amounts of a second folate form.

Studies of $MeFH_4$ Uptake and Conversion in B_{12}-Deficient and Replete Bone Marrow

$MeFH_4$ was found to be concentrated by normal bone marrow cells to a level severalfold higher than the external concentration (Corcino *et al.*, 1971). This is probably equal to the uptake of this compound in phytohemagglutinin-simulated lymphocytes (Das and Hoffbrand, 1970) and half that of murine lymphoma cells (Nahas *et al.*, 1969; unpublished studies from our laboratory). Utilizing doubly labeled $MeFH_4$, it was found that, of the $[^{14}C]CH_3$ group taken up by bone marrow cells in 15 min, only 22 percent was transferred to nonfolate compounds within that period. A similar value, 23 percent, was obtained in cells of marrow from a patient treated 7 days previously with 1,000 μg of cyanocobalamin for pernicious anemia. In the megaloblastic marrow obtained from the same untreated pernicious anemia patient, $[^{14}C]CH_3$ group transfer from $MeFH_4$ folate could not be detected, indicating that it was depressed to a value certainly less than 5 percent of the already exceptionally low amount of $MeFH_4$ folate that was taken up during incubation of the cobalamin-deficient marrow. The rate measured for normal marrow was quite significant, but it was much lower than that in L1210 murine lymphoma cells, in which 81 to 85 percent of the CH_3 group of $MeFH_4$ was transferred to nonfolate compounds within 5 min.

CONCLUSIONS

Data from our laboratory and others indicate that leukemia cells contain a carrier-mediated transport system for reduced folates that is also utilized by MTX. Transport of folates across other cell membranes may be different. Thus, different tissues utilize different transport mechanisms for these important compounds. The uptake and conversion of $MeFH_4$ by L5178Y cells appear to require the presence of vitamin B_{12} and a vitamin B_{12} transfer protein (TC II). This finding is consistent with the methyl trap hypothesis that requires that a functioning methionine synthetase enzyme be present in order to convert MeFH$_4$ to FH$_4$, thus allowing this important coenzyme to be utilized for purine and thymidylate synthetase within the cell. The demonstration that the uptake of MeFH$_4$ by human marrow cells and the transfer of the CH$_3$ group to methionine and macromolecular compounds are both markedly reduced by cobalamin deficiency is consistent also with the methyl trap hypothesis and is to date perhaps the most direct evidence for its existence.

ACKNOWLEDGMENTS

This work was supported by grants CA-08010 and CA-08341 from the National Cancer Institute. J. R. B. is a Research Professor of the American Cancer Society.

DISCUSSION

BLAKLEY: From the point of view of design of transport blockers of uptake, have you any molecular reconciliation of the fact that the oxidized 2,4-diamino compounds compete, whereas the oxidized 2-amino, 4-hydroxy compounds cannot compete?

BERTINO: No. It may be that conformation of the folate compound is important, and it would be worthwhile if we had some information on this point.

LITERATURE CITED

Baugh, C. M., and Krumdieck, C. L. 1971. Folate antagonists as chemotherapeutic agents. Ann. N.Y. Acad. Sci. *186*:7–28.
Bender, R. A., Bleyer, W. A., Fresby, S. A., and Oliverio, V. T. 1975. Alterations of methotrexate uptake in human leukemia cells by other agents. Cancer Res. *35*:1305–1308.
Bobzien, W. F., III, and Goldman, I. D. 1972. The mechanism of folate transport in rabbit reticulocytes. J. Clin. Invest. *51*:1688–1696.
Chello, P. L., and Bertino, J. R. 1973. Dependence of 5-methyltetrahydrofolate utilization by L5178Y mouse leukemia cells *in vitro* on the presence of hydroxycobalamin and transcobalamin II. Cancer Res. *33*:1898–1904.
Corcino, J. J., Waxman, S., and Herbert, V. 1971. Uptake of tritiated folates by human bone marrow cells *in vitro*. Br. J. Haematol. *20*:503.
Coward, J. K., Parameswaran, K. N., Cashmore, A. R., and Bertino, J. R. 1974. 7,8-Dihydropteroyl oligo-γ-L-glutamates: Synthesis and kinetic studies with purified dihydrofolate reductase from mammalian sources. Biochemistry *13*:3899–3903.
Coward, J. K., Chello, P. L., Cashmore, A. R., Paraweswaran, K. N., DeAngelis, L.

M., and Bertino, J. R. 1975. 5-methyl-5,6,7,8-Tetrahydropteroyl oligo-γ-L-glutamates: Synthesis and kinetic studies with methionine synthetase from bovine brain. Biochemistry *14*:1548–1552.

Das, K. C., and Hoffbrand, A. V. 1970. Studies of folate uptake by phyto-haemagglutinin-simulated lymphocytes. Br. J. Haematol. *19:*203–221.

Fischer, G. A. 1962. Defective transport of amethopterin (methotrexate) as a mechanism of resistance to the antimetabolite in L5178Y leukemia cells. Biochem. Pharmacol. *11*:1233–1234.

Goldman, I. D. 1971. The characteristics of the membrane transport of amethopterin and the naturally occurring folates. Ann. N.Y. Acad. Sci. *186*:400–422.

Goldman, I. D., Lichtenstein, W. S., and Oliverio, V. T. 1968. Carrier-mediated transport of the folic acid analog, methotrexate, in the L1210 leukemia cell. J. Biol. Chem. *243*:5007–5017.

Hakala, M. T. 1965a. On the role of drug penetration in amethopterin resistance of sarcoma-180 cells *in vitro*. Biochim. Biophys. Acta *102*:198–209.

Hakala, M. T. 1965b. On the nature of permeability of sarcoma-180 cells in amethopterin *in vitro*. Biochim. Biophys. Acta *102*:210–225.

Izak, G. M., Rachmilewitz, M., Grossowicz, W., Galewski, K., and Kraus, S. 1968. Folate activity in reticulocytes and the incorporation of tritiated pteroylglutamatic acid into red cells. Br. J. Haematol. *14*:447–452.

Kessel, D., and Hall, T. C. 1967. Amethopterin transport in Ehrlich ascites carcinoma and L1210 cells. Cancer Res. *27*:1539–1543.

Levitt, M., Nixon, P. F., Pincus, J. H., and Bertino, J. R. 1971. Transport characteristics of folates in cerebrospinal fluid: A study utilizing doubly labeled 5-methyltetrahydrofolate and 5-formyltetrahydrofolate. J. Clin. Invest. *50*:1301–1308.

Nahas, A., and Bertino, J. R. 1970. Common transport system for 4-aminofols and N⁵-substituted tetrahydrofolates in L1210 mouse leukemia cells. Pharmacologist *12*:303.

Nahas, A., Nixon, P. F., and Bertino, J. R. 1969. Transport of 5-methyltetrahydrofolate by L1210 mouse leukemia cells. Fed. Proc. *28*:389.

Nahas, A., Nixon, P. F., and Bertino, J. R. 1972. Uptake and metabolism of N⁵-formyltetrahydrofolate by L1210 leukemia cells. Cancer Res. *32*:1416–1421.

Nixon, P. F., and Bertino, J. R. 1970. Separation and identification of folate coenzymes on DEAE-sephadex, pp. 661–663. *In* Vitamins and coenzymes, D. B. McCormick and L. D. Wright, eds. Academic Press, New York.

Nixon, P. F., and Bertino, J. R. 1971. Enzymic preparations of radiolabeled (+), L-5-methyltetrahydrofolate and (+),L-5-formyltetrahydrofolate. Anal. Biochem. *43*:162–172.

Nixon, P. F., Slutsky, G., Nahas, A., and Bertino, J. R. 1973. The turnover of folate coenzymes in murine lymphoma cells. J. Biol. Chem. *248*:5932–5936.

Olinger, E. J., Bertino, J. R., and Binder, H. J. 1973. Intestinal folate absorption. II. Conversion and retention of pteroylmonoglutamate by jejunum. J. Clin. Invest. *52*:2138–2145.

Rader, J. I., Niethammer, D., and Huennekens, F. M. 1974. Effects of sulfhydryl inhibitors upon transport of folate compounds into L1210 cells. Biochem. Pharmacol. *23*:2057–2059.

Rubin, R., Owens, E., and Rall, D. 1968. Transport of methotrexate by the choroid plexus. Cancer Res. *28*:689–694.

Selhub, J., Brin, H., and Grossowiz, N. 1973. Uptake and reduction of radioactive folate by everted sacs of rat small intestine. Eur. J. Biochem. *33*:433–438.

Spector, R., and Lorenzo, A. V. 1975. Folate transport by the choroid plexus *in vitro*. Science *187*:540–542.

Strum, W., Nixon, P. F., Bertino, J. R., and Binder, H. J. 1971. Intestinal folate absorption. I. 5-Methyltetrahydrofolic acid. J. Clin. Invest. *50*:1910–1916.

Zager, R. F., Frisby, S. A., and Oliverio, V. T. 1973. The effects of antibiotics and cancer chemotherapeutic agents on the cellular transport and antitumor activity of methotrexate in L1210 murine leukemia. Cancer Res. *33*:1670–1676.

17

Physiology of Absorption of Monoglutamyl Folates from the Gastrointestinal Tract

BERNARD A. COOPER

This chapter summarizes the state of knowledge concerning absorption of monoglutamyl (unconjugated) folate from the intestinal tract. It is well established that most biological folate is polyglutamyl, but the presence of polyglutamyl folate conjugases active at various pH values in many raw foods (Baker *et al.*, 1965) and the fact that large meals may remain in the stomach at acid pH for considerable periods support the probability that much of the folate presented to the intestinal surface in the chyme has been completely or partially digested by conjugases.

Many studies of folate absorption have utilized folic acid—a form of folate not found in nature. It has been utilized because of its stability and availability, both with and without radioactive label. Use of this artificial folate may not reflect handling of biological folate unless other oxidized folates are handled in an identical fashion. Much of the formyltetrahydrofolate of food probably is oxidized to 10-formyldihydrofolate and to 10-formylfolic acid (Blakley, 1969) in the process of food preparation. Thus, a large proportion of the mono-glutamylfolate presented to the intestine may be oxidized (as 10-formylfolic acid), supporting the physiological relevance of studies of absorption of folic acid. A preliminary report has suggested that formylfolate may not enter the metabolic folate pool in man and the rat, although it is absorbed efficiently (Blair, 1975). This report requires corroboration and further study.

FATE OF FOLATE PRESENTED TO THE INTESTINE

Folate rapidly enters the human portal vein after feeding (Whitehead and Cooper, 1967; Whitehead *et al.*, 1972); the first identifiable folic acid appears in portal venous blood within 10 min of feeding 100 ml of folic acid solution (Figure 17-1). This study also demonstrates that

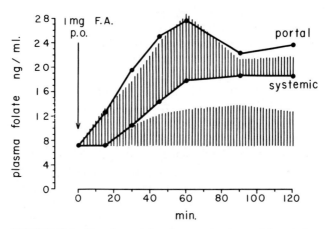

FIGURE 17-1 Hepatic portal and systemic plasma folate during folic acid absorption in man. Total portal and systemic plasma folate as measured by *L. casei* are depicted by the upper and lower lines, respectively. The lower shaded area represents systemic *S. faecalis*–active folate; the upper shaded area represents the difference between portal and systemic *S. faecalis*–active folate, shown to be composed of folic acid. The total *S. faecalis*–active folate in portal plasma is represented by the sum of the shaded areas. The unshaded wedge between the lower shaded area and the lower line was shown to represent 5-methyltetrahydrofolate displaced from the liver plus some formed from the folic acid absorbed (reprinted with permission from Br. J. Haematol. *13*:679, 1967).

there is an additional 10-min delay before folate levels in the peripheral venous blood increase and that some of the folate entering peripheral venous blood is not freshly absorbed folate but represents flushing from the liver of 5-methyltetrahydrofolate by the newly absorbed folic acid. Other studies have demonstrated that following this period there is a slow appearance of 5-methyltetrahydrofolate in plasma that has been formed from the absorbed folic acid.

When reduced folates are fed, the material absorbed does not traverse the intestine into the portal vein unchanged; most is converted to 5-methyltetrahydrofolate (Perry and Chanarin, 1970; Pratt and Cooper, 1971; Whitehead et al., 1972; Nixon and Bertino, 1972). This is true if the material administered is 5-formyltetrahydrofolate (folinic acid), dihydrofolate, or tetrahydrofolate. Conversion of 5-formyltetra-hydrofolate to methyltetrahydrofolate was not due to conversion of the 5-formyltetrahydrofolate to 5,10-methenyltetrahydrofolate by low pH in the stomach, since absorption was similar in two patients with pernicious anemia who were also studied (Pratt and Cooper, 1971). The conversion of 5-formyltetrahydrofolate to methyltetrahydrofolate in the intestine was elegantly studied by Nixon and Bertino (1972), who fed doubly labeled 5-formyltetrahydrofolate to subjects and compared its metabolism with that of the same material injected intravenously. By 90 min after intravenous injection, only 40 percent of the ^{14}C label from the formyl, and of the ^{3}H label from the PABA and C9 positions of folate, co-chromatographed with 5-formyltetrahydrofolate; whereas 60 percent of the ^{3}H, and a smaller proportion of the ^{14}C, co-chromato-graphed with 5-methyltetrahydrofolate. About 40 percent of the ^{14}C label was unassociated with folates. When the doubly labeled material was fed, no significant ^{14}C was found associated with 5-formylTHF, and about 20 percent co-chromatographed with 5-methyltetrahydrofolate. Seventy percent of the ^{14}C label was not associated with folates, and 8–9 percent of both labels eluted from the chromatograph in the position usually associated with 10-formyltetrahydrofolate; but, because micro-biological assays were not done, one cannot be sure that this was not an oxidation product of 5-methyltetrahydrofolate (Whiteley, 1971). It is apparent that the intestinal wall is an active site of conversion of reduced folates to 5-methyltetrahydrofolate—apparently more rapid in this conversion than nonintestinal tissues. Table 17-1 lists results of thin-layer chromatography–bioautography of human ileum obtained at operation. The analysis was performed by Tsukasa Abe, currently at Tokyo Medical and Dental University.

The striking observation is the absence of methylcobalamin. Methyl-cobalamin comprises a minority of the vitamin B_{12} present in tissues,

TABLE 17-1   Distribution of B_{12} Forms in Human Ileum[a]

Specimen No.	B_{12} Form	pg/Protein	pg/Alkaline Phosphatase
1	5'-Deoxyadenosylcobalamin	81.4	0.102
	Hydroxocobalamin	14.5	0.018
2	5'-Deoxyadenosylcobalamin	460	0.093
3	5'-Deoxyadenosylcobalamin	175	0.145

[a]Protein is expressed as milligrams; alkaline phosphatase is expressed as King Armstrong Units. No measurable spot of methylcobalamin or cyanocobalamin was detected in bioautograms of extracts of specimens of human ileum obtained at operation.

whereas it is the predominant cobalamin in plasma. It would be of interest to speculate that 5-methyltetrahydrofolate accumulates in intestine because the methylcobalamin-dependent homocysteine–methyltetrahydrofolate transferase enzyme is inactive, but data are not adequate to allow such speculation.

The different monoglutamates are absorbed with different effectiveness in man, measured by increase in peripheral venous folate level after feeding (Baker *et al.*, 1965a; Brown *et al.*, 1973). However, because the effect of liver trapping and flushing from liver of endogenous folates cannot be assessed, the slight advantage of some folates over others should not be overemphasized. The natural, biologically active isomer of 5-methyltetrahydrofolate appears to be better absorbed from human intestine than the unnatural isomer, indicating that the absorption process selectively transports the active isomer.

Recognizing that the human intestine can transfer folate, sometimes metabolizing it and sometimes not, what are the characteristics of the transport? The two major studies of quantitative aspects of folate absorption *in vivo* were reported by Burgen and Goldberg (1962) in rats and by Hepner *et al.* (1968) in man (Figure 17-2). In these studies, segments of intestine were perfused with folic acid solutions of known concentration, and their disappearance from the perfusate was measured relative to a nonabsorbable marker. Note that in these studies association of the folate with the wall of the intestine was considered to be absorption. Also note that the percentage of folate disappearing from the lumen per unit time was constant in both studies until the concentration was increased to about 10^{-6} M, above which it decreased rapidly. If there is no saturable intermediate step in the transport, the velocity of transport should be proportional to the concentration, and the same proportion should be absorbed irrespective of concentration. When the rate of transport is no longer proportional to concentration,

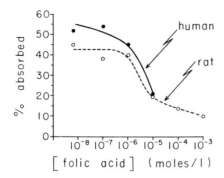

FIGURE 17-2 Absorption of folic acid from perfused intestine of man and rat. The percentage of folic acid absorbed from the perfused intestine during a fixed period of perfusion is plotted against the concentration of folic acid in the perfusing solution (redrawn from Burgen and Goldberg, 1962; and Hepner *et al.*, 1968).

because an intermediate step is partially saturated, the proportion of folate absorbed per unit time falls. If the limiting feature in the transport system is a folate binder required for transport, then the affinity of the binder for folate (its dissociation constant) can be expressed as the concentration of folate at which the percentage of absorption is reduced by 50 percent below the percentage absorbed at low concentrations. In the studies of Burgen and Goldberg (1962) and Hepner *et al.* (1968), these concentrations were 4×10^{-5} M and 1.8×10^{-4} M, respectively, for rat and man. If the saturating step in transport were the solubility of folic acid at the low pH of the unstirred water layer of the intestinal surface, then the pH of this layer must be about 3.5 in rats and slightly higher in man. (The limiting solubility of folic acid in water has been reported to be 10^{-6} M at pH 3.1 and 10^{-3} M at pH 4.8 [Hillcoat *et al.*, 1967].)

Burgen and Goldberg (1962) attempted to measure the direction of transport in the rat intestine and observed that the proportion of folic acid absorbed from the intestine was not affected by increasing the plasma folate concentration 1,000-fold with folic acid and that the rate of appearance of labeled folic acid in plasma from intestine was at least 14 times that appearing in intestine from plasma. The latter rate is probably a minimum, because their studies were not corrected for folate excretion in the bile (Baker *et al.*, 1965b; Pratt and Cooper, 1971). In a study of folic acid absorption in rats, Hepner (1969) observed that folic acid absorption was half saturated when about 10^{-6} mol was fed to the animals. If the material fed were diluted in 20 ml in the intestine and stomach, then the concentration at which absorption was half maximum would have been identical with that calculated by Burgen and Goldberg (1962).

A number of careful studies of the kinetics of folate transport have utilized everted sacs of intestine, and others have employed *in vitro* systems (Smith *et al.*, 1970; Olinger *et al.*, 1973; Selhub *et al.*, 1973; Bhan-thumnvavin *et al.*, 1974). In these, the folate concentration required for half-maximum transport appears to be considerably lower than in the *in vivo* studies (Table 17-2). In most *in vitro* studies, folate transport is mostly composed of radioactivity associated with the wall of the isolated intestinal preparation. In one *in vitro* study (Bhanthumnvavin *et al.*, 1974), a biphasic saturation curve of uptake of folic acid by the everted intestinal sacs was described, suggesting that there might be more than one saturable transport system.

The problem of uphill transport versus facilitated or other types of diffusion in folate transport has not been examined in any of these studies. In the *in vivo* studies, it is apparent that the body can accumulate folate from the gut. *In vitro* systems have not demonstrated uphill transport, suggesting that none occurs, or that they may not be valid systems for investigation of transport.

It has been suggested that folic acid and other folates may dissolve in the lipid surface layer of the cells and diffuse across in the unionized form. Even highly charged molecules can enter cells in this way if any significant proportion of the molecule is uncharged (Elsborg, 1974). The dissociation constants of folic acid are shown in Figure 17-3 (Blakley, 1969). Those for tetrahydrofolate are similar (Kallen and Jencks, 1966). Because some of the charged groups are acidic and some basic, it would be improbable that folic acid could exist in the un-charged state at any pH. In Figure 17-3, the proportion of molecules of folic acid in each charged state is plotted against pH. pH optimum for transport in everted sacs *in vitro* is about 6.0. In this system, some enhancement of folate transport by glucose is observed, but transport was not dependent on glucose. However, because the *in vitro* studies differ in important features from *in vivo* studies, data obtained about folate transport from *in vitro* studies should be considered preliminary until duplicated *in vivo*.

In vivo studies have demonstrated that folate transport in the jejunum is more rapid than in the ileum (Burgen and Goldberg, 1962; Hepner *et al.*, 1968; Hepner, 1969), that dilantin is a weak competitor of folate absorption (Hepner, 1969), that in malnourished alcoholics absorption of a small dose of folic acid is impaired (Halsted *et al.*, 1971), and that this is improved with refeeding but not following withdrawal of alcohol without restitution of nutrition.

The most powerful evidence that folate absorption involves a carrier mechanism is the selectivity of absorption of the natural isomer of 5-methyltetrahydrofolate from human intestine over the unnatural isomer and that several children unable to absorb any of the folates

TABLE 17-2   Apparent Association Constants for Transport of Folate from Intestine

Reference	K_t,[a] M	Preparation
Burgen and Goldberg (1962)	4 $\times$ 10^{-5}	Rat, intact
Hepner et al. (1968)	1.8 $\times$ 10^{-4}	Man, intact
Hepner (1969)	8.6 $\times$ 10^{-6}[b]	Rat, intact
Bhanthumnavin et al. (1974)	2.7 $\times$ 10^{-6}	Rat, everted sacs
Smith et al. (1970)	0.7 $\times$ 10^{-6}	Rat, everted sacs
Selhub et al. (1973)	1.55 $\times$ 10^{-6}[c]	Rat, everted sacs

[a]Concentration of folate for 50 percent maximum saturation of transport.
[b]Quantity of folic acid fed; not concentration.
[c]Half-maximum velocity of metabolic conversion, not transport.

have been described (Luhby et al., 1961; Lazkowsky et al., 1969; Santiago-Borrer et al., 1973). In some of these, folate transport into the spinal fluid was also impaired, but in others it was not. This suggests that the transport system across the intestine and in the choroid plexus are related and may be affected by genetic abnormality, but they are not identical since they may be affected independently. Leslie and Rowe (1972) have reported the isolation of a folate binder from intestinal brush border. The large number of folate binders described in cells and tissues preclude the assumption that the intestinal binder is the transport protein, but this awaits further investigation.

In summary, data obtained from studies of human subjects and animals indicate that the absorption of folic acid, and probably of other monoglutamates of folate, involves an intestinal transport system that is specific for the correct optical isomer, is related to but not identical with the system responsible for folate transport into spinal fluid, and does not require chemical or biological modification of the folate for transport to occur. Absorption in vivo may be carrier mediated, the carrier being half-saturated at between 10^{-5} and 10^{-4} M folic acid. Evidence of saturation could, however, reflect the limitation of solubility of folic acid in the unstirred water layer at the jejunal surface if the pH in this layer is about 4.1 in rats and 4.5 in man. Folic acid is rapidly transported into the portal vein, accumulated in the liver, and appears in the hepatic venous plasma after a slight delay. During this delay, endogenous 5-methyltetrahydrofolate is flushed from the liver into the hepatic venous plasma. Folate absorption is decreased in malnourished alcoholics and improves with refeeding, irrespective of continuation of alcoholic intake, is weakly inhibited by dilantin, and seems more active in the jejunum than in the ileum.

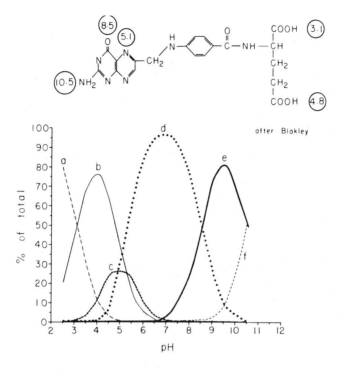

FIGURE 17-3 Ionized forms of folic acid: effect of pH. Based on the dissociation constants of the charged groups indicated in the formula, the proportion of folate molecules existing as each charged species of folic acid was calculated (vertical axis)/pH (horizontal axis).

| | Ionized groups: | | | | |
| | Alpha | Gamma | | | |
Species	COOH	COOH	OH-4	N5	NH2-2
a	No	No	No	Yes	Yes
b	Yes	No	No	Yes	Yes
c	Yes	Yes	No	Yes	Yes
d	Yes	Yes	No	No	Yes
e	Yes	Yes	Yes	No	Yes
f	Yes	Yes	Yes	No	No

LITERATURE CITED

Baker, H., Frank, O., Feingold, S., Ziffer, H., Gellene, R. A., Leevy, C., and Sobotka, H. 1965a. The fate of orally and parenterally administered folates. Am. J. Clin. Nutr. *17*:88–95.

Baker, S. J., Kumar, S., and Swaminathan, S. P. 1965b. Excretion of folic acid in bile. Lancet *i*:695.

Baugh, C. M., and Krumdieck, C. L. 1971. Naturally occurring folates. Ann. N.Y. Acad. Sci. *186*:7–28.

Bhanthumnvavin, K., Wright, J. R., and Halsted, C. H. 1974. Intestinal transport of tritiated folic acid (3H PGA) in the everted gut sac of different aged rats. Johns Hopkins Med. J. *135*:152–160.

Blair, J. A. 1975. The handling and metabolism of folates in the rat and man, with especial relationship to disease. Abstracts of the 5th Pteridine Symposium, Konstanz, pp. 45–46.

Blakley, R. L. 1969. The biochemistry of folic acid and related pteridines. Frontiers of biology series, North Holland Publishing Co., New York.

Brown, J. P., Scott, J. M., Foster, F. G., and Weir, D. G. 1973. Ingestion and absorption of naturally occurring pteroylmonoglutamates (folates) in man. Gastroenterology *64*:223–232.

Burgen, A. S. V., and Goldberg, N. J. 1962. Absorption of folic acid from the small intestine of the rat. Br. J. Pharmacol. Chemother. *19*:313–320.

Elsborg, L. 1974. Folic acid: A new approach to the mechanism of its intestinal absorption. Dan. Med. Bull. *21*:1–11.

Halsted, C. H., Robles, E. A., and Mezey, E. 1971. Decreased jujunal uptake of labeled folic acid (3H-PGA) in alcoholic patients: Roles of alcohol and nutrition. N. Engl. J. Med. *285*:701–706.

Hepner, G. W. 1969. The absorption of pteroylglutamic (folic) acid in rats. Br. J. Haematol. *16*:241–249.

Hepner, G. W., Booth, C. C., Cowan, J., Hoffbrand, A. V., and Mollin, D. L. 1968. Absorption of crystalline folic acid in man. Lancet *ii*:302–306.

Hillcoat, B. L., Nixon, P. F., and Blakley, R. L. 1967. Effect of substrate decomposition on the spectrophotometric assay of dihydrofolate reductase. Anal. Biochem. *21*:178–184.

Kallen, R. G., and Jencks, W. P. 1966. The dissociation constants of tetrahydrofolic acid. J. Biol. Chem. *241*:5845–5850.

Lazkowsky, P., Erlandson, M. E., and Bezan, A. I. 1969. Isolated defect of folic acid absorption with mental retardation and cerebral calcification. Blood *34*:452.

Leslie, G. I., and Rowe, P. B. 1972. Folate binding by the brush border membrane proteins of small intestinal epithelial cells. Biochemistry *11*:1696–1703.

Luhby, A. L., Eagle, F. J., Roth, E., and Cooperman, J. M. 1961. Relapsing megaloblastic anemia in an infant due to a specific defeat in gastrointestinal absorption of folic acid. Am. J. Dis. Child. *102*:482.

Nixon, P. F., and Bertino, J. R. 1972. Effective absorption and utilization of oral formyltetrahydrofolate in man. N. Engl. J. Med. *286*:175–179.

Olinger, E. J., Bertino, J. R., and Binder, H. J. 1973. Intestinal folate absorption. II. Conversion and retention of pteroylmonoglutamate by jejunum. J. Clin. Invest. *52*:2138–2145.

Perry, J., and Chanarin, I. 1970. Intestinal absorption of reduced folate compounds in man. Br. J. Haematol. *18*:329–339.

Pratt, R. F., and Cooper, B. A. 1971. Folates in plasma and bile of man after feeding folic acid-3H and 5-formyltetrahydrofolate (folinic acid). J. Clin. Invest. *50*:455–462.

Santiago-Borrer, P. J., Santini, R., Jr., Perez-Santiago, E., Maldonado, N., Millan, S., and Coll-Camalez, G. 1973. Congenital isolated defect of folic acid absorption. J. Pediatr. *82*:450–455.

Selhub, J., Brin, H., and Grossowicz, N. 1973. Uptake and reduction of radioactive folate by everted sacs of rat small intestine. Eur. J. Biochem. *33*:433–438.

Smith, M. E., Matty, A. J., and Blair, J. A. 1970. The transport of pteroylglutamic acid across the small intestine of the rat. Biochim. Biophys. Acta *219*:37–46.

Whitehead, V. M., and Cooper, B. A. 1967. Absorption of unaltered folic acid from the gastrointestinal tract in man. Br. J. Haematol. *13*:679–686.

Whitehead, V. M., Pratt, R., Viallet, A., and Cooper, B. A. 1972. Intestinal conversion of folinic acid to 5-methyltetrahydrofolate in man. Br. J. Haematol. *22*:63–72.

Whiteley, J. M. 1971. Some aspects of the chemistry of the folate molecule. Ann. N.Y. Acad. Sci. *186*:29–42.

18

Process of Digestion and Absorption of Pteroylpolyglutamate

CHARLES H. HALSTED, ANN REISENAUER, *and* GERALD S. GOTTERER

Natural folate occurs as pteroylmonoglutamate conjugated with as many as six additional glutamyl units in gamma peptide linkage (Butterworth *et al.*, 1963). Study of the process of absorption of conjugated folate has been facilitiated by the synthesis of spectrally pure pteroylpolyglutamates in the oxidized state (Krumdieck and Baugh, 1969). Chromatographic techniques have been developed that effectively separate the pteroylpolyglutamates, thus allowing for identification and quantitation of degradation products occurring during the process of deconjugation (Baugh and Krumdieck, 1971). Use of these compounds has allowed a partial definition of the process of intestinal absorption of pteroylpolyglutamate. Current evidence indicates that these compounds are hydrolyzed to pteroylmonoglutamate during the process of their intestinal absorption (Butterworth *et al.*, 1969; Baugh *et al.*, 1971; Halsted *et al.*, 1975a; Baugh *et al.*, 1975). The enzyme responsible for the hydrolysis of pteroylpolyglutamate is a γ-carboxypeptidase known as folate conjugase (Baugh and Krumdieck, 1971).

The possible sites of hydrolysis of pteroylpolyglutamate include the intraluminal contents, the brush border surface of the intestinal mucosa, or the interior of the mucosal cell. Very little activity of folate conjugase has been found in human intestinal juice (Klipstein, 1967; Hoffbrand and Peters, 1970; Graham and Godwin, 1975), including bile and pancreatic secretion collected after secretin–cholecystokinin stimulation (Graham and Godwin, 1975). By contrast, several studies have shown significant activity of folate conjugase in mammalian small-intestinal mucosa (Rosenberg et al., 1969; Hoffbrand and Peters, 1970; Graham and Godwin, 1975; Halsted et al., 1975c). Whereas a recent study of chick intestine suggests that there are at least two distinct peptidases responsible for the hydrolysis of pteroylpolygluta- mate (Rosenberg and Newmann, 1974), studies of mammalian liver (Baugh and Krumdieck, 1971) and small intestine (Halsted et al., 1975c) suggest a single γ-carboxypeptidase that cleaves the glutamyl units in a stepwise and progressive fashion. Two groups, using guinea pig (Hoffbrand and Peters, 1969) or rat (Rosenberg and Godwin, 1971) small-intestinal mucosa, have provided evidence that mucosal folate conjugase is an intracellular, probably lysosomal, enzyme with very little brush border activity. If these *in vitro* data are translated to the *in vivo* situation, the sequence of intestinal absorption of conjugated folate would appear to be mucosal uptake followed by hydrolysis to simple folate and subsequent exit of this compound from the mucosal cell.

In a recent series of experiments in human subjects, we used the method of jejunal perfusion to study the digestion and uptake of pteroylpolyglutamate (Halsted et al., 1975a). When a mixture of equimolar [^{3}H]pteroylmonoglutamate ([^{3}H]PG-1) and pteroyl- [^{14}C]glutamylhexaglutamate ([^{14}C]PG-7) was perfused in the normal human jejunum, the ^{3}H-labeled compound was taken up about one and one-half times as efficiently as the ^{14}C-labeled compound. Following column chromatography (Baugh and Krumdieck, 1971) of intestinal aspirates obtained during perfusion a complete spectrum of ^{14}C-labeled pteroylpolyglutamates was found, indicating that hydrolysis of [^{14}C]PG-7 occurred during the process of its absorption (Figure 18-1). *In vitro* experiments, in which intestinal aspirates obtained before folate perfusion or after saline perfusion were incubated with [^{14}C]PG-7, failed to reproduce the chromatographic spectrum of degradation products. This finding excluded the possibility that degradation of [^{14}C]PG-7 occurs as a result of reaction with an unbound intraluminal enzyme. The data showed that hydrolysis of [^{14}C]PG-7 occurs during perfusion and requires its contact with the intestinal mucosa.

In subsequent experiments, saline homogenates of surgically ob- tained human jejunal or ileal mucosal specimens were incubated with

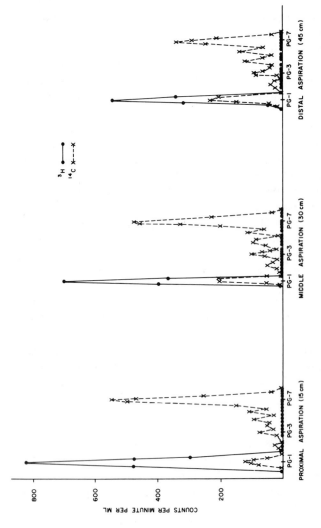

FIGURE 18-1 Chromatographic patterns of labeled folates in three intestinal aspirates obtained during jejunal perfusion of isotonic saline containing equimolar (2 µM) [³H]PG-1 and [¹⁴C]PG-7 in a normal subject (Halsted et al., 1975a). Aspirates were obtained 15, 30, and 45 cm downstream from the infusion port positioned at the ligament of Treitz and chromatographed on DEAE using a sodium chloride gradient. Nonradioactive markers identify peaks at the pteroylmono (PG-1), pteroyldi- (PG-2), and pteroyltri- (PG-3) positions. With passage of the solution, there was progressive decrease in concentration of [³H]PG-1 and [¹⁴C]PG-7 and the appearance of degradation products of [¹⁴C]PG-7, including increasing concentrations of [¹⁴C]PG-1 (reproduced with permission from Halsted et al., Gastroenterology 68:261–269, 1975a).

[^{14}C]PG-7 at 37° C for 15 min at pH 4.5 and pH 6.5, followed by column chromatography of the reactant mixture (Halsted *et al.*, 1975c). At each pH, the incubation resulted in a spectrum of [^{14}C]pteroylpoly-glutamates similar to that seen during jejunal perfusion, while a greater proportion of [^{14}C]pteroylmonoglutamate ([^{14}C]PG-1) was formed at the lower pH (Figure 18-2). These data confirm other evidence that the intestinal mucosa is the site of hydrolysis of pteroylpolyglutamate to pteroylmonoglutamate and that this hydrolytic reaction is an integral part of the absorptive process of pteroylpolyglutamate (Butterworth *et al.*, 1969; Rosenberg *et al.*, 1969; Baugh *et al.*, 1971, 1975; Halsted *et al.*, 1975a).

In evaluating our studies of human digestion and absorption of conjugated folate, it seemed most logical that hydrolysis of [^{14}C]PG-7 occurred on the brush border surface of the mucosa prior to absorption of the hydrolytic product. This sequence is analogous to that shown for disaccharide digestion and monosaccharide absorption (Gray and In-gelfinger, 1966) and would most easily explain the finding of in-traluminal degradation products of [^{14}C]PG-7 resulting from its contact with the jejunal mucosa during jejunal perfusion (Halsted *et al.*, 1975a). If this is the correct sequence, diseases affecting the brush border surface should result in decreased degradation of [^{14}C]PG-7. In order to evaluate this hypothesis, the digestion and absorption of [^{14}C]PG-7 was studied by the same technique of jejunal perfusion in a mucosal disease, tropical sprue, in collaboration with José Corcino at the University of Puerto Rico (Halsted *et al.*, 1975b). The luminal disap-pearance of [^{14}C]PG-7 was markedly decreased in six tropical sprue patients before treatment as compared to the findings after full clinical recovery. However, both before and after treatment, products of hydrolysis occurred in the luminal aspirates during perfusion with the same chromatographic patterns as shown earlier in the normal sub-jects. By direct measurement of enzymatic activity in small intestinal biopsies, mucosal folate conjugase was found to be greater in the pretreatment mucosa than in the postrecovery mucosa. These enzyme changes were the reverse of the activity of brush border disac-charidases, which were uniformly depressed in the untreated state. We also studied four patients with celiac sprue by the same techniques (unpublished data). The same chromatographic patterns appear in the luminal aspirates during perfusion of [^{14}C]PG-7. Like the mucosal enzymes in tropical sprue, the activity of folate conjugase did not parallel that of disaccharidase in pre- and postrecovery celiac sprue biopsies. These studies show that folate malabsorption in tropical or celiac sprue is not the result of deficient hydrolysis of pteroylpoly-

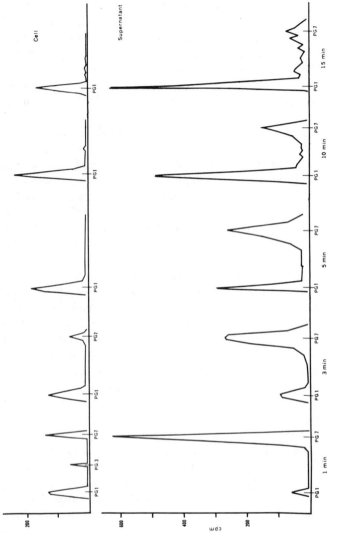

FIGURE 18-2 Chromatographs of cell and supernatant fractions after incubation of isolated cells with [^{14}C]PG-7 at timed intervals. Unlabeled markers identify certain peaks. Progressive conversion of [^{14}C]PG-7 to [^{14}C]PG-1 occurred over 15 min. [^{14}C]PG-7 in the cell fraction at 1 and 3 min represented contamination by supernatant fluid (reproduced with permission from Halsted *et al.*, J. Nutr. *106*:485–492, 1976).

glutamate. Since the activities of mucosal folate conjugase and brush border disaccharidase did not change in parallel before and after treatment, the digestion of conjugated folate is not analogous to that of disaccharide digestion. Mucosal folate conjugase is probably not similar to mucosal disaccharidase in its site of activity.

In order to define further the sequence of digestion and intestinal transport of pteroylpolyglutamate, we utilized two *in vitro* approaches with the small intestinal mucosa of the rat (Halsted *et al.*, 1976). In one set of experiments, the hydrolysis of pteroylpolyglutamate and the cellular and extracellular distribution of its degradation product, pteroylmonoglutamate, was studied in isolated small-intestinal epithelial cells prepared by a modification of a vibration technique (Harrison and Webster, 1969). In the other experimental set, the activity of folate conjugase was measured in whole and subcellular fractions of mucosal homogenates. In each set of experiments, synthetic and pure labeled folates were employed.

Epithelial cells were harvested from rat intestinal mucosa by an 8-min vibration of everted segments of small intestine in a 5-mM EDTA solution. On electron microscopy, the cells appeared as sheets of epithelium with clearly defined surface microvilli and intracellular organelles. The cells were incubated at varied time intervals in a Krebs–Ringer–phosphate buffer solution, pH 7.4, containing bovine serum albumin, 2 g/100 ml; glucose, 4 mM; [^{3}H]polyethylene glycol ([^{3}H]PEG) as an extracellular marker; [^{14}C]PG-7 (pteroyl-[^{14}C]glutamylhexaglutamate, synthesized and provided by Charles M. Baugh), 10 μM; and in certain experiments, [^{3}H]PG-1^2 (3,5,9-[^{3}H]pteroylmonoglutamate; Amersham/Searle, Arlington Heights, Ill.), 10 μM. Both folates were chromatographically pure. Cell viability was proven by a progressive decrease in glucose concentration in the incubation medium during incubation. Following incubation, the cell and supernatant fractions were separated and chromatographed on DEAE–cellulose chloride and a linear sodium chloride gradient to identify folates (Baugh and Krumdieck, 1971). Volumes were corrected and folates were quantitated by use of the extracellular [^{3}H]PEG marker, which was washed by buffer from each column prior to folate elution. These data were used to calculate the concentration of folates in the cellular and extracellular compartments.

Over a 15-min period, the cell preparation progressively converted [^{14}C]PG-7 in the incubation medium to [^{14}C]PG-1 (Figure 18-2). After correcting for volume and folate distribution, at each time interval between 1 and 15 min, cellular folate was almost entirely represented by [^{14}C]PG-1. When the concentration of [^{14}C]PG-1 was calculated in

the cellular and extracellular space, it was found that the concentration
of cellular [^{14}C]PG-1 increased progressively over 5 min, and then
equalized with extracellular [^{14}C]PG-1 by 15 min (Figure 18-3). The ratio
of cellular to extracellular concentration was 22:1 at 1 min, with a
progressive decline to unity by 15 min. When 3-min incubations were
performed with equimolar concentrations of [^{3}H]PG-1 and [^{14}C]PG-7 in
the incubation medium, the ratio of corrected cellular concentration of
[^{14}C]PG-1 to [^{3}H]PG-1 was 3.1 ± 0.23 (mean ± standard error of the
mean, n = 5). Thus, during incubation with [^{14}C]PG-7, the cells concentrated [^{14}C]PG-1 over extracellular [^{14}C]PG-1 and to a greater extent than

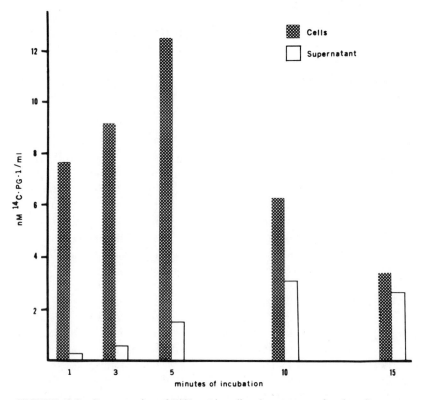

FIGURE 18-3   Concentration of [^{14}C]PG-1 in cell and supernatant fraction after correction using [^{3}H]PEG extracellular marker. Cellular concentration of [^{14}C]PG-1 increased
between 1 and 5 min and then equalized with extracellular concentration of
[^{14}C]PG-1 by 15 min. The ratio of concentrations in cell and extracellular space was
22:1 at 1 min and declined progressively to approach 1:1 by 15 min.

[^{3}H]PG-1. Two possible mechanisms could account for these findings. [^{14}C]PG-1 could have been formed within the cell after membrane transport of [^{14}C]PG-7 and then diffused to the extracellular space down a concentration gradient. Alternatively, [^{14}C]PG-1 could have been formed from [^{14}C]PG-7 at the cell surface at a site giving it kinetic advantage over free [^{3}H]PG-1 for active transport into the cell. These possibilities were examined by measurement of mucosal folate conjugase in whole homogenates and brush border fractions of the intestinal mucosa.

The charcoal precipitation method of Krumdieck and Baugh (1970) was used to measure folate conjugase with pure pteroyl-diglutamyl [^{14}C]glutamate (synthesized and provided by Carlos Krumdieck) as substrate. In preliminary experiments with saline homogenates of rat small intestinal mucosal scrapings, saturation kinetics were found, with a constant rate of hydrolysis at substrate concentrations between 10 and 30 nmol per 1.5-ml reaction tube. Using a substrate concentration of 20 nmol/1.5 ml, the reaction was linear with time to 15 min and at three enzyme concentrations. In whole homogenates of mucosal scrapings, the activity of mucosal folate conjugase as nanomoles hydrolyzed per milligram of protein (Lowry *et al.*, 1951) was significantly greater in the most proximal of five equal parts of the small intestine. Enzyme activity at pH 4.5 was consistently twice greater than that at pH 6.5 in each segment. The method of Forstner (1970) was used to prepare brush border fractions from whole homogenates of the small intestinal mucosa, using sucrase (Dahlqvist, 1964) as a marker enzyme. In five experiments at pH 4.5, the recovery of folate conjugase was only 5.5 ± 0.98 percent in the brush border fraction compared to 96.1 ± 4.83 percent in the combined supernatant and wash fractions, while the sucrase marker was recovered to 90.0 ± 6.9 percent in the brush border fraction. In each fraction, the ratios of activities of folate conjugase at pH 4.5 to pH 6.5 were similar, varying between 1.79 and 1.93, thus making unlikely the existence of two enzymes of different pH optima. Although our techniques did not distinguish between a truly soluble and lysosomal enzyme system, the findings are consistent with previous studies indicating that folate conjugase is an intracellular lysosomal enzyme (Hoffbrand and Peters, 1969; Rosenberg and Godwin, 1971).

Since only insignificant brush border activity of folate conjugase could be found, the possibility that [^{14}C]PG-7 is hydrolyzed on the surface of the cell prior to entry of [^{14}C]PG-1 seems unlikely. Correlation of the data from the isolated cell incubations and from the measurement of folate conjugase in brush border and supernatant fractions of the mucosa suggests that *in vitro* [^{14}C]PG-7 is transported into the cell prior to its enzymatic hydrolysis to [^{14}C]PG-1 by an intracellular folate conjugase.

Thus, our *in vivo* data have shown that hydrolytic products of [^{14}C]PG-7 occur in the intestinal lumen as a result of contact of [^{14}C]PG-7 with the intestinal mucosa. In either tropical or celiac sprue, the hydrolysis of [^{14}C]PG-7 appears to proceed normally, implying that folate conjugase is not a brush border enzyme. *In vitro*, the data suggest that [^{14}C]PG-7 enters the mucosal cell intact prior to intracellular hydrolysis. If the conclusion from the *in vitro* data is applied to the *in vivo* observations, one must suppose that degradation products seen in the lumen during perfusion of [^{14}C]PG-7 are the result of a cumbersome process of transport of [^{14}C]PG-7 into the epithelial cell followed by efflux of degradation products to the lumen. On the other hand, the data do not exclude the possibility that *in vivo*, in health or mucosal disease, a lysosomal folate conjugase arrives on the mucosal surface by a process of secretion or cell degradation. The activity of other lysosomal enzymes has been shown to be increased in celiac sprue (Peters *et al.*, 1975). A loosely adherent enzyme system permitting contact digestion (Ugolev, 1972) might be undetected by the rigorous methodology of brush border separation but at the same time could account for *in vivo* jejunal perfusion findings. Additional studies using a variety of experimental models are required to establish definitively the mechanism by which conjugated folate is digested and absorbed by the small intestine.

SUMMARY

The digestion and absorption of ^{14}C-labeled pteroylheptaglutamate ([^{14}C]PG-7) was studied *in vivo* in man by jejunal perfusion and *in vitro* in the rat using mucosa from the small intestine. The *in vivo* data show that during the process of its absorption [^{14}C]PG-7 is hydrolyzed in a progressive fashion to [^{14}C]pteroylmonoglutamate ([^{14}C]PG-1) by mucosal folate conjugase present in health and in mucosal disease. The *in vitro* data suggest that [^{14}C]PG-7 enters the mucosal epithelial cell prior to its hydrolysis to [^{14}C]PG-1. Further studies are required to define the sequence of *in vivo* digestion and absorption of [^{14}C]PG-7.

ACKNOWLEDGMENTS

This work was supported by clinical Investigator Award 1 KO8 AM 70293, Grants 1 RO1 AM 18330 and 5RO1 AM 08644 from the National Institutes of

Health, Award No. 465 from The Nutrition Foundation, New York, N.Y., Grant 1C-3M from The American Cancer Society, and Grant BM 574-17348 from The National Science Foundation.
The technical assistance of Carolyn Back is appreciated.

LITERATURE CITED

Baugh, C. M., and Krumdieck, C. L. 1971. Naturally occurring folates. Ann. N.Y. Acad. Sci. *186*:7–28.
Baugh, C. M., Krumdieck, C. L., Baker, H. J., and Butterworth, C. E., Jr. 1971. Studies on the absorption and metabolism of folic acid. Folate absorption in the dog after exposure of isolated intestinal segments to synthetic pteroylpolyglutamates of various chain lengths. J. Clin. Invest. *50*:2009–2021.
Baugh, C. M., Krumdieck, C. L., Baker, H. J., and Butterworth, C. E., Jr. 1975. Absorption of folic acid poly-γ-glutamates in dogs. J. Nutr. *105*:80–89.
Butterworth, C. E., Santini, R., and Frommeyer, W. S. 1963. The pteroylglutamate components of American diets as determined by chromatographic fractionation. J. Clin. Invest. *42*:1929–1939.
Butterworth, C. E., Jr., Baugh, C. M., and Krumdieck, C. 1969. A study of folate absorption and metabolism in man utilizing carbon 14-labeled polyglutamates synthesized by the solid phase method. J. Clin. Invest. *48*:1131–1142.
Dahlqvist, A. 1964. Method for assay of intestinal disaccharidases. Anal. Biochem. *7*:18–24.
Forstner, G. G. 1970. [1-¹⁴C]glucosamine incorporation by subcellular fractions of small intestinal mucosa. J. Biol. Chem. *245*:3584–3592.
Graham, D. Y., and Godwin, H. A. 1975. Investigation of folate polyglutamate hydrolysis in man: Comparison of proximal small intestinal contents with mucosal homogenates. Clin. Res. *23*:249A. (Abstract)
Gray, G. M., and Ingelfinger, F. J. 1966. Intestinal absorption of sucrose in man; interrelations of hydrolysis and monosaccharide product absorption. J. Clin. Invest. *45*:388–398.
Halsted, C. H., Baugh, C. M., and Butterworth, C. E., Jr. 1975a. Jejunal perfusion of simple and conjugated folates in man. Gastroenterology *68*:261–269.
Halsted, C. H., Reisenauer, A. M., and Corcino, J. J. 1975b. Effect of tropical sprue on hydrolysis and absorption of conjugated folate. Gastroenterology *68*:908a. (Abstract)
Halsted, C. H., Reisenauer, A. M., and Corcino, J. J. 1975c. Studies of human folate conjugase. Clin. Res. *23*:250A. (Abstract)
Halsted, C. H., Reisenauer, A., Back, C., and Gotterer, G. S. 1976. *In vitro* uptake in metabolism of pteroylpolyglutamate by rat small intestine. J. Nutr. *106*:485–492.
Harrison, D. D., and Webster, H. L. 1969. The preparation of isolated crypt cells. Exp. Cell Res. *55*:257–260.
Hoffbrand, A. V., and Peters, T. J. 1969. The subcellular localization of pteroylpolyglutamate hydrolase and folate in guinea pig intestinal mucosa. Biochim. Biophys. Acta *192*:479–485.
Hoffbrand, A. V., and Peters, T. J. 1970. Recent advances in knowledge of clinical and biochemical aspects of folate. Schweiz. Med. Wochenschr. *100*:1954–1960.
Lowry, O. H., Rosenbrough, N. J., Farr, A. L., and Randall, R. J. 1951. Protein measurement with the Folin phenol reagent. J. Biol. Chem. *193*:265–275.

Klipstein, F. A. 1967. Intestinal folate conjugase activity in tropical sprue. Am. J. Clin. Nutr. *20*:1004–1009.

Krumdieck, C. L., and Baugh, C. M. 1969. The solid phase synthesis of polyglutamates of folic acid. Biochemistry *8*:1568–1572.

Krumdieck, C., and Baugh, C. M. 1970. Radioactive assay of folic acid polyglutamate conjugase(s). Anal. Biochem. *35*:123–129.

Peters, T. J., Heath, J. R., Wansbrough-Jones, M. H., and Doe, W. F. 1975. Enzyme activities and properties of lysosomes and brush borders in jejunal biopsies from control subjects and patients with celiac disease. Clin. Sci. Mol. Med. *48*:259–267.

Rosenberg, I. H., and Godwin, H. A. 1971. The digestion and absorption of dietary folate. Gastroenterology *60*:445–463.

Rosenberg, I. H., and Newmann, H. 1974. Multi-step mechanism in the hydrolysis of pteroylpolyglutamates by chicken intestine. J. Biol. Chem. *249*:5126–5130.

Rosenberg, I. H., Streiff, R. R., Godwin, H. A., and Castle, W. B. 1969. Absorption of polyglutamic folate: Participation of deconjugating enzymes of the intestinal mucosa. N. Engl. J. Med. *280*:985–988.

Ugolev, A. M. 1972. Membrane digestion. Gut *13*:735–747.

19

Introduction to Discussion of Human Requirements for Folic Acid

WILLIAM J. DARBY

The Chairman of the opening session of this Workshop challenged us with a series of direct questions, which restated are:

- What should the Recommended Dietary Allowance for folic acid be?
- How do we assess nutriture relating to the folates?
- What are the consequences of folate deficiency in man?
- What are the effects of folate excess in man?
- How can we best standardize assay techniques for this group of dietary essentials?
- Should standardizations of data on food composition be based on total folate content?
- Can we identify a system of biological or nutritional equivalents for describing folate activity?
- How should new tables of folate content of foods be developed?

The charge to us through this series of questions is to provide a summary of the current scientific knowledge that can serve as a

209

reasoned basis for considering revision of the present Recommended Dietary Allowances for this nutrient and to identify needs for, and set directions of, future developments, including research.

Man's knowledge concerning any subject is always fragmentary. But application cannot await the ultimate perfection. Indeed it was Francis Bacon who stated that the goal of Science is not to make imperfect man perfect, but rather to make imperfect man healthy, happy, and comfortable.

It behooves us today to focus our discussions increasingly sharply upon the nutritional implications of our current understanding of the folates. In order to begin to put this into focus, perhaps I may say that, to prepare it for low-power examination, it may be useful to recall some of the earliest efforts to set needed guidelines and approximations of requirements. Indeed much of what I shall review of these beginnings was published in *Vitamins and Hormones,* volume V (Darby, 1947), and based upon the state of knowledge up to the autumn of 1946—almost 30 years ago.

The period from the early 1930's to the late 1940's was noteworthy for the remarkable rate and variety of advances in knowledge concerning dietary essentials required for hematopoiesis in man. Early clinical and experimental observations suggested that at least two distinct vitamins were involved, substances that are familiar today as vitamin B_{12} and folic acid. It is with the latter that we are here concerned.

The clinical identification and synthesis in 1945 of pteroylglutamate permitted the rapid clarification of an accumulated diversity of observed growth, hematologic, or other histological effects—effects earlier attributed to "vitamin N," "factor U," "vitamin B_c," "Norit eluate factor," "*L. casei* factors," "folic acid," "extrinsic factor," etc.

The initial clinical studies utilizing the chemically identifiable materials were not models of experimental design for determination of nutritional requirements. They were efforts to ascertain whether various clinical syndromes would respond to these newly discovered vitamins. Relatively little attention was given to quantitative considerations and even less to dietary control during the periods of treatment. Indeed, seeming indifference to this latter aspect of experimental design of nutritional studies aimed at quantitating requirements has persisted for an unjustifiable length of time in the history of studies of the folates.

Despite these limitations, careful examination of certain of the earliest observations led a few workers to begin to estimate "orders of magnitude" of requirements. Thus, by the autumn of 1946 a review of evidence justified the conclusions that:

The 'potential folic acid(s)'—mono-, tri-, and heptaglutamates—were all active in Paul L. Day's 'Vitamin N-deficient monkeys' and predictably so in man. [A prediction subsequently validated.] The problems of bioassay were complex. Estimates of requirements of the folates could not be obtained from studies of patients with pernicious anemia, but observations on a variety of other macrocytic anemias could provide valid information.

Indeed it was suggested (Darby *et al.*, 1946) that therapeutic doses of pteroylglutamic acid in sprue and related syndromes might be of the order of 1.0 mg daily, and that 0.1–0.2 mg daily might suffice for maintenance requirements in man. Some early crude approximations were attempted based upon clinical assessment of length of time of relapse following response to known total doses of pteroylglutamate. Such reasoning by Goldsmith (1946) and by the Vanderbilt group again led to estimated limits for the adult patient of "the order of from 0.1–1.0 mg; probably about midway would be a reasonable estimate. . . ." it was stated. Day and Totter (1946) estimated the requirement of the young monkey as between 50 and 100 μg/day when consuming 325 kcal. If one reasoned by analogy upon a proportionate basis of average intake, man might be estimated to need 300–600 μg.

Again the tenuous nature of these early estimates was obvious to the investigators who suggested them, as was the complexity of the problem of estimating the distribution in foods and the availability and utilization of the then recognized several conjugates. But such estimates did provide some guide to the range of levels that should be explored in investigations designed to quantitate requirements.

The earliest such studies of which I am aware that were designed to ascertain minimal dose responses, and thereby approximate requirements, were those of Woodruff *et al.* (1951). They observed responses of cases of megaloblastic anemia in infancy to 200 μg of folate (i.e., PGA) per day and reported the effectiveness of low parenteral and oral doses of "citrovorum factor" equivalent in activity to 75 to 200 μg of folic acid.

These early clinical efforts, recognizably limited in their sophistication of approach, did provide quantitative limits as guides for later more crucially designed investigations.

Another, and perhaps more general, observation is pertinent here. Each time a new nutrient is recognized as essential for man and identified, the scientific and medical community goes through much this same pattern of approaching requirements from an initial safe and usually excessive therapeutic level. Accordingly, initial estimated standards of needed intake for essential nutrients have almost invariably been lowered as a result of subsequent, more critically designed studies. This has occurred repeatedly for nutrient after nutrient listed in the table of Recommended Dietary Allowances since the first edition in 1941. Now, as to folates, it is evident that the discrepancy between the current allowances for folates and present evidence pertaining to usual dietary intake of seemingly healthy persons required reconciliation. Does the evidence indicate that our current allowances are too high?

Other considerations arising from the earlier studies pertain to functions other than hemapoiesis and must be considered in setting allowances. Some of these have been touched upon so far in this Workshop, but they must be put into sharper focus as we strive to improve our present estimates of allowances. These considerations include, *inter alia*, the long-recognized physiology of gastrointestinal absorption, the metabolism of estrogens, the resistance to certain infections, the dependence of folate requirement or function upon ascorbate nutriture, the effect of folate upon hydroxyphenyl metabolism, the level of maternal nutriture at which fetal development is impaired—indeed the extension of much of the discussion at this meeting to the physiology of the whole organism throughout the life cycle.

Perhaps, then, the most that we as a workshop group can do today is to provide the best knowledge base for a later group to utilize in revising allowances with judgmental consideration of these other influences.

LITERATURE CITED

Darby, W. J. 1947. The physiological effects of the pteroylglutamates in man—with particular reference to pteroylglutamic acid, pp. 119–161. *In* Vitamins and hormones, Vol. V. Academic Press, Inc., New York.

Darby, W. J., Jones, E., and Johnson, H. C. 1946. Effect of synthetic *Lactobacillus casei* factor in treatment of sprue. J. Am. Med. Assoc. *130*:780–786.

Goldsmith, G. A. 1946. Report at the AAAS Conference on Vitamins at Gibson Island, Md., July 23–27.

Day, P. L., and Totter, J. R. 1946. Reported at the AAAS Conference on Vitamins at Gibson Island, Md., July 23–27.

Woodruff, C. W., Peterson, J. C., and Darby, W. J. 1951. Citrovorum factor and folic acid in treatment of megaloblastic anemia of infancy. Proc. Soc. Exp. Biol. Med. 77:16–19.

20

Detection of Folic Acid Deficiency in Populations

HOWERDE E. SAUBERLICH

In recent years, folic acid (folacin, folate) nutriture has received increased interest and attention. Although the prevalence of folic acid deficiency throughout the world remains uncertain, recent reports would indicate that the incidence and importance of megaloblastic anemia and folic acid deficiency have been underestimated (WHO Report, 1968; Blakley, 1969; FAO/WHO Report, 1970; Streiff, 1970; Cook *et al.*, 1971; WHO Report, 1972; Sauberlich *et al.*, 1974). Nutritional megaloblastic anemia is the result of folic acid deficiency far more commonly than of vitamin B_{12} deficiency. Megaloblastic anemia resulting from folic acid deficiency may be noted in 2.5 to 5.0 percent of pregnant women in developed countries; a considerably higher incidence is observed in pregnant women of developing countries (WHO Report, 1968; Blakley, 1969; Rothman, 1970; FAO/WHO Report, 1970; Streiff, 1970; Sauberlich *et al.*, 1974). In many of the developing countries, and to a lesser extent in the developed countries, folic acid deficiency may also occur in children, men, and nonpregnant women (WHO Report, 1968; Blakley, 1969; FAO/WHO Report, 1970; Rothman, 1970). Although folic acid deficiency occurs most commonly from

213

inadequate intakes of the vitamin, a deficiency may result from impaired absorption, metabolic derangements, and excessive demands by the tissues of the body (Herbert, 1968; Blakley, 1969; Chanarin, 1969; Kahn, 1970; Rothman, 1970; Streiff, 1970; Doscherholmen, 1971; Rowe, 1971; WHO Report, 1972; Herbert, 1973; Sauberlich *et al.*, 1974).

Nutritional status for a given nutrient usually may be assessed by the following general approaches: (i) observations for clinical signs and symptoms; (ii) obtaining dietary intake information concerning the nutrient by either direct methods or dietary recall procedures; and (iii) utilization of biochemical and histological techniques. It is exceedingly difficult to diagnose clinically a folic acid deficiency. Hence, dietary intake information and biochemical procedures are employed to evaluate the nutritional status with regard to this vitamin.

Although folic acid occurs in most foodstuffs, reliable tables listing values for either "free" folates or "total" folates are limited. Although not well-established, "free" folate is considered to be readily absorbed from the intestinal tract, perhaps to the same extent as pteroylglutamic acid. However, for the majority of foods, most of the vitamin is present as polyglutamates, which require the action of conjugase to free the vitamin for absorption and metabolic activity. The amount of the "total" folic acid made available and absorbed is uncertain. As a result, few attempts have been made to obtain dietary intake information for folic acid.

In Table 20-1 are listed folate intakes for a few countries as summarized by FAO/WHO (1970). The values represent mainly "free" folic acid as determined by *Lactobacillus casei* on samples without pretreatment with conjugase. Even for these few figures, folic acid intake per day per person varied over a wide range and represents inadequate intakes as judged by recommended daily intakes or allowances of the nutrient (FAO/WHO Report, 1970; WHO Report, 1972; NRC–NAS Report, 1974).

Table 20-2 depicts the 1970 World Health Organization recommended daily intakes for "free" folate (FAO/WHO Report, 1970). In 1972, the World Health Organization (WHO Report, 1972) stated that "Such adults receive not only pteroylmonoglutamic acid: their diet also supplies them with an undetermined amount of polyglutamate forms of folate, which should be taken into account in evaluating the requirements of total folate and not only those of 'free' folate as was done by the FAO/WHO Expert Group" (FAO/WHO Report, 1970).

Table 20-3 presents the WHO recommended daily intakes of "total" folate. Total folate includes both "free" and polyglutamate forms. These values are similar to the 1974 NRC–NAS Food and Nutrition

TABLE 20-1   Folic Acid Intake in Certain Countries

Country	Folic Acid Intake, μg/person/day
Libya (1957)	40–64
Jordan (1962)	50–79
Bolivia (1964)	41–92
Nigeria (1967)	46–138
United States (1968)	37–297
United Kingdom (1968)	53–296

SOURCE: WHO Technical Report Series No. 452 (1970).

TABLE 20-2   WHO Recommended Daily Intakes of "Free" Folate

Age or Status	Recommended Daily Intake, μg/day
0–6 months	40
7–12 months	60
1–12 years	100
13 years and over	200
Pregnancy	400
Lactation	300

SOURCE: FAO Nutrition Meetings Report Series No. 47 (1970).

TABLE 20-3   WHO Recommended Daily Intakes of Folate

Age or Status	Total Folate,[a] μg/day
0–6 months	40–50
7–12 months	120
1–12 years	200
13 years and over	400
Pregnancy	800
Lactation	600

SOURCE: WHO Technical Report Series No. 503 (1972).
[a]Total folate includes free and bound or polyglutamate forms.

Board Recommended Daily Dietary Allowances (NRC–NAS Report, 1974) for folacin (Table 20-4).

Thus, folic acid dietary intake information may be evaluated in terms of either "free" folate requirements or "total" folate requirements. However, until the extent of absorption of food folacin is known with certainty and reliable folic acid food values are available, folate dietary intake information will be difficult to interpret and of limited use.

Folic acid nutritional status can be evaluated with reasonable reliability by biochemical techniques. Although a number of procedures have been proposed (Sauberlich et al., 1974), measurements of serum and red blood cell folate levels are the most commonly performed and most practical for application to population studies. It is generally considered that low serum folate levels may not necessarily be associated with megaloblastic anemia nor with any abnormal biochemical changes (Hall et al., 1975). Low serum levels may be a reflection of only recent low dietary intakes of folic acid and provide little information concerning tissue reserves. Nevertheless, continued low serum folic acid levels would eventually be accompanied by signs of megaloblastic anemia and megaloblastic bone marrow changes.

Red blood cell folic acid levels have been regarded as a more accurate and less variable quantitative index of the severity of folacin deficiency than serum folate (Sauberlich et al., 1974). The red blood cell folic acid levels reflect the body folacin status at the time the red cells were formed. The assessment requires that both serum and whole blood folic acid levels be measured and the folate level in the red blood

TABLE 20-4   NRC-NAS Food and Nutrition
Board Recommended Daily Dietary Allowances
for Folacin

Group	Age, years	Folacin, μg/day[a]
Infants	0–1	50
Children	1–3	100
	4–6	200
	7–10	300
Males	≥11	400
Females	≥11	400
Pregnancy	–	800
Lactation	–	600

SOURCE: NRC–NAS Report (1974).
[a]The folacin allowances are based in dietary sources of folacin as determined by Lactobacillus casei assay.

TABLE 20-5 WHO Guidelines for Evaluating
Nutritional Data

Nutrient	Normal Range	Probable Deficiency
Serum B_{12}, pg/ml	150–1,000	<100
Serum folate, ng/ml	6–20	<3
Red cell folate, ng/ml	150–700	<100

SOURCE: WHO Technical Report Series No. 503 (1972).

cells be calculated on the basis of the hematocrit value. A simplified, but less precise, procedure involves the measurement of whole blood folic acid levels only. The results are expressed in terms of folic acid per milliliter of red blood cells calculated on the basis of the hematocrit value for the blood sample and ignoring the folic acid contributed by the serum.

In controlled human folic acid deficiency studies (Herbert, 1967; Sauberlich *et al.*, 1974), serum folic acid levels fell rapidly to below normal levels well before the appearance of hematological changes. Low red blood cell folate levels were encountered only shortly before the appearance of a megaloblastic bone marrow (Herbert, 1967). Based largely on the results of such controlled studies and on the treatment of folacin-deficient patients, guidelines have been developed and used in evaluating serum and red blood cell folic acid data. Tables 20-5, 20-6, and 20-7 depict several guidelines that have been used for the interpretation of serum and red blood cell folic acid levels.

Fasting serum folic acid levels of less than 3.0 ng/ml have been

TABLE 20-6 INCAP Suggested Guide to
Interpretation of Serum Folic Acid Levels
(All Ages)

Category	Serum Folate Level, ng/ml
Deficient	<3.0
Low	3.0–4.9
Acceptable or high	>5.0

SOURCE: G. Arroyave, *Metabolic Adaptation and Nutrition*, p. 98. Pan American Health Organization Scientific Publication No. 222, 1971.

218   HOWERDE E. SAUBERLICH

TABLE 20-7   Guidelines for the Interpretation of Serum and Red Blood
Cell Folacin Levels

| Measurement | Less than Acceptable (at Risk), ng/ml | | Acceptable (Low Risk), ng/ml |
	Deficient (High Risk)	Low (Medium Risk)	
Serum folacin (all ages)	<3.0	3.0–5.9	≥6.0
Red blood cell folacin (all ages)	<140	140–159	≥160

SOURCE: Sauberlich *et al.* (1974).

considered "deficient," levels from 3.0 to 5.9 ng/ml have been considered "low," and values of 6.0 ng/ml and above have been considered "acceptable." Red blood cell folic acid levels less than 140
ng/ml of cells have been considered "deficient," levels from 140 to 159
ng/ml have been considered "low," and values of 160 ng/ml and above
have been considered "acceptable" (Sauberlich *et al.*, 1974). Microbiological assay procedures have been used almost entirely to measure folic acid levels in serum and red blood cells. *Lactobacillus casei*
has been the organism of choice since it responds to the major folic acid
analogues present in serum. In serum, the main folates are N^5-
methylfolates, which support the growth of *L. casei*. A majority of the
folic acid activity in red blood cells is derived from a conjugated form
that must be deconjugated prior to assay. Recently, isotopic assay
procedures have been developed for measuring folic acid in serum
(Rothenberg *et al.*, 1972; Waxman and Schreiber, 1973; Dunn and
Foster, 1973; Tajuddin and Gardyna, 1973; Rothenberg and da Costa,
1973; Shaw, 1973; Skelly *et al.*, 1973; Kamen and Caston, 1974;
Sauberlich *et al.*, 1974). Sex of the subjects appears to have little
influence on folic acid levels in serum and red blood cells. The effect of
age on these levels has been observed as variable. In Table 20-8 are
presented folacin levels in serum and red blood cells of subjects of
various ages obtained in survey samples obtained from several states.
Mean folacin levels were observed to be in excess of 6.0 ng/ml of serum
and 300 ng/ml of red blood cells for all age groups (Table 20-8). In the
Ten-State Nutrition Survey, the mean serum folic acid levels were
generally higher in the groups under 12 years of age than in the older
ages (Table 20-9). As shown in Figure 20-1, little difference was
observed between the mean serum folate levels of males and females.
These unpublished findings from the Ten-State Nutrition Survey did
indicate ethnic differences in both serum and red blood cell folate
levels (Figure 20-1; Tables 20-9 and 20-10. Folate nutritional status ap-

TABLE 20-8 Serum and Red Blood Cell Folacin Levels by Age Groups for Populations Studied in Five States[a]

Age Group	Sample	Folacin Level, ng/ml, in:					
		Arizona	Colorado	Kentucky	New York	West Virginia	All States
0–5 months	Serum	—	7.6 (13)	—	4.4 (1)	5.5 (5)	6.9
	RBC	—	329.5 (13)	—	488.0 (1)	270.1 (5)	322.2
6–11 months	Serum	—	8.6 (21)	—	—	8.9 (7)	8.8
	RBC	—	392.5 (19)	—	—	383.3 (7)	387.9
1–5 years	Serum	8.0 (19)	10.9 (246)	10.6 (52)	8.2 (15)	8.3 (5)	9.0
	RBC	377.4 (17)	406.6 (245)	325.8 (51)	296.4 (15)	306.3 (5)	334.2
6–17 years	Serum	7.9 (232)	12.2 (24)	8.9 (188)	6.9 (218)	7.9 (274)	8.4
	RBC	396.7 (209)	398.0 (24)	304.7 (181)	282.0 (207)	280.9 (261)	319.0
≥18 years	Serum	5.7 (168)	—	7.0 (285)	7.0 (550)	6.9 (342)	6.8
	RBC	347.8 (156)	—	287.0 (280)	324.0 (536)	313.1 (326)	316.0

[a]Values in parentheses represent the number of samples assayed.

TABLE 20-9   Mean Serum Folate Values by Age, Sex, Ethnic Group, and
Low- and High-Income Ratio States[a]

| Ethnic Group and Age, years | Mean Serum Folate Levels, ng/ml, in: | | | |
| | Low-Income States | | High-Income States | |
	Male	Female	Male	Female
White				
<13	7.5 (288)	7.5 (223)	8.8 (943)	8.8 (751)
⩾13	5.8 (484)	6.3 (704)	7.7 (2,254)	7.5 (3,181)
Black				
<13	5.3 (365)	5.3 (384)	5.3 (231)	5.9 (238)
⩾13	4.6 (867)	5.0 (867)	5.5 (375)	5.8 (655)
Spanish–American				
<13	5.9 (190)	5.3 (166)	6.6 (212)	6.3 (191)
⩾13	4.8 (222)	5.0 (398)	5.6 (282)	5.3 (469)

[a]Values in parentheses indicate number of subjects studied in the Ten-State Nutrition
Survey. Low-income states: Texas, Louisiana, Kentucky, West Virginia, and South
Carolina; high-income states: Massachusetts, New York, Michigan, California, and
Washington.

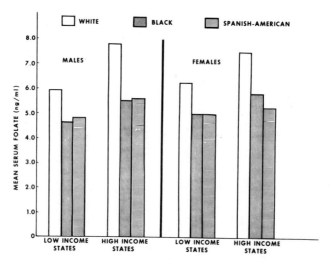

FIGURE 20-1   Mean serum folate values (nanogram/milliliter) for
subjects 13 years of age and over by sex, income, and ethnic
grouping as observed in the Ten-State Nutrition Survey (1968–1970).
Low-income states: Texas, Louisiana, Kentucky, West Virginia,
and South Carolina; high-income states: Massachusetts, New York,
Michigan, California, and Washington.

TABLE 20-10   Red Blood Cell Folate Levels by Sex
and Ethnic Group (All Age Groups)[a]

Group	Mean RBC Folate, ng/ml		
	Male	Female	All
Black	194	216	207
	(549)	(806)	(1,355)
Spanish–American	233	223	227
	(453)	(595)	(1,048)
White	244	241	242
	(2,009)	(2,404)	(4,413)

[a]Values in parentheses indicate number of subjects studied.
Data are from low-income states studied in the Ten-State
Nutrition Survey (Texas, Louisiana, Kentucky, West
Virginia, and South Carolina).

peared to be related to income level. Whether these differences were a reflection of differences in dietary intake of folic acid is uncertain. The mean serum folate levels of subjects from the low-income states (Texas, Louisiana, Kentucky, West Virginia, and South Carolina) fell below those of subjects from the high-income states (Massachusetts, New York, Michigan, California, and Washington) (Table 20-9).

The ethnic differences in red blood cell folates are demonstrated in Figure 20-2 for subjects from the high-income states studied in the Ten-State Nutrition Survey. The percent of subjects with red blood cell folate levels of less than 160 ng/ml was approximately 15 percent for the White population compared to over 30 percent for the Black and Spanish-American groups.

Similar observations were noted in the Ten-State Nutrition Survey regarding serum folate levels for the same ethnic groups (Table 20-9). Cumulative percentage distribution of serum folate values for persons either under or over 13 years of age by ethnic group is illustrated in Figures 20-3 and 20-4.

Distribution plots for serum and red blood cell folic acid levels obtained from a study on adult female subjects are shown in Figures 20-5 and 20-6. Subjects with low serum and red blood cell folic acid levels were encountered. One subject had a serum folic acid level of less than 3.0 ng/ml, while 66 individuals (19 percent) had values of less than 6.0 ng/ml. Four subjects had red blood cell folic acid levels of less than 160 ng/ml. Subjects with unusually high folic acid levels in both serum and red blood cells were observed in this study and in other

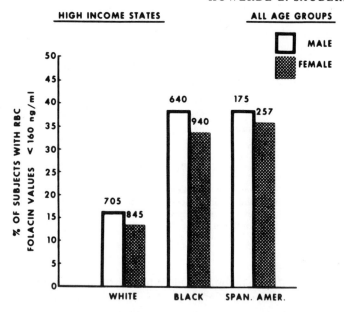

FIGURE 20-2 Percent of subjects with red blood cell folacin
values of less than 160 ng/ml as relates to sex and ethnic grouping.
All age groups included. Numbers on graph indicate number of
subjects observed in the Ten-State Nutrition Survey (1968–1970).
High-income states: Massachusetts, New York, Michigan, California, and Washington.

population surveys. The significance of these high values remains
unclear.

Red blood cell folic acid measurements do not distinguish between
megaloblastic anemia due to vitamin B_{12} deficiency and that due to a
folacin deficiency (Hoffbrand et al., 1966). Thus, in individuals with a
primary vitamin B_{12} deficiency, folic acid levels in the serum may be
elevated, while low levels may be encountered in the red cells. However, a low folic acid value for both red blood cells and serum is strong
evidence that a folic acid deficiency exists. Nevertheless, during
nutrition surveys an occasional subject is encountered with a low
serum vitamin B_{12} level. This is exemplified in Figure 20-7, where two
subjects with serum vitamin B_{12} levels of less than 150 pg/ml are noted.
Serum vitamin B_{12} levels of less than 150 pg/ml have been considered to
indicate inadequate vitamin B_{12} nutrition (Sauberlich et al., 1974).
Whenever feasible, serum vitamin B_{12} measurements should be performed in conjunction with folic acid nutritional assessments.

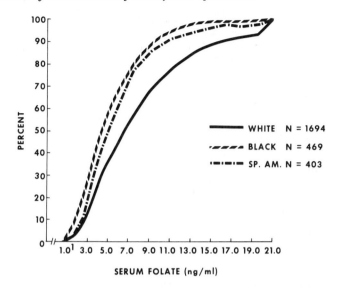

FIGURE 20-3   Cumulative percentage distribution of serum folate values for persons under 13 years of age by ethnic group. Values on figure indicate the number of subjects observed in the Ten-State Nutrition Survey (1968–1970). Values for subjects studied in the high-income states of Massachusetts, New York, Michigan, California, and Washington.

Several recent reports provide additional evidence of the existence of poor folic acid nutrition in population groups. A rural Negro population in South Africa subsisting on a predominantly maize-meal diet had an incidence of folic acid deficiency of 43.8 percent in nonanemic women in late pregnancy, 33.1 percent in nonpregnant women, and 18.6 percent in adult men (Colman *et al.*, 1975). More than one-third of all subjects older than 60 years were deficient in folic acid. Normal red blood cell folate levels were stated to range from 160 to 640 ng/ml of cells. It should be noted that the Negro population studied consumes a traditional alcoholic maize brew. The effect of the consumption of this beverage on red blood cell folate levels is unknown. Of interest, however, was the observation that fortification of the maize diet to provide an additional daily intake of 300 μg of folic acid prevented the progressive folate depletion in late pregnancy (Colman *et al.*, 1975).

Daniel *et al.* (1975) studied the dietary intakes of folic acid and the concentration of folate in plasma of healthy adolescents. Of those

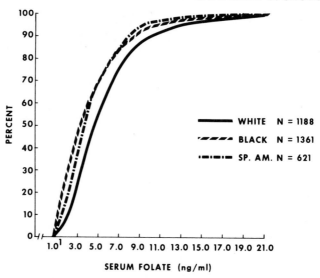

FIGURE 20-4   Cumulative percentage distribution of serum folate
values for persons 13 years of age and over by ethnic group. Values
on figure indicate the number of subjects observed in the Ten-State
Nutrition Survey (1968–1970). Values for subjects studied in the
low-income states of Texas, Louisiana, Kentucky, West Virginia,
and South Carolina.

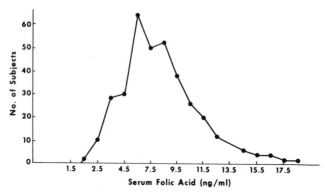

FIGURE 20-5   Distribution plot of serum folic acid values for 348
females age 18–28 years. Mean serum folic acid value was 8.2 ± 2.8
ng/ml. Range, 2.5–18.0 ng/ml. One subject had a value of less than
3.0 ng/ml, while 66 had values less than 6.0 ng/ml.

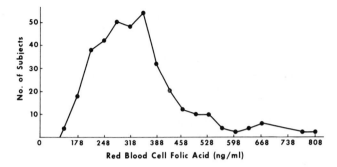

FIGURE 20-6   Distribution plot of red blood cell folic acid values for 347 females age 18–28 years. Mean red blood cell folic acid value was 330 ± 108 ng/ml. Range, 125–825 ng/ml. Four subjects had values of less than 160 ng/ml.

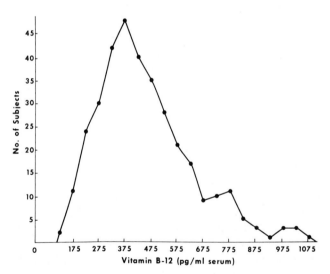

FIGURE 20-7   Distribution plot of serum vitamin B_{12} levels for 348 females age 18–28 years. Mean serum vitamin B_{12} values was 458 ± 200 pg/ml. Range, 100–1,350 pg/ml. Two subjects had values of less than 150 pg/ml.

studied (total of 459), 9.4 percent of the adolescent males and 4.7 percent of the adolescent females had plasma folate concentrations below 2.0 ng/ml. Plasma folic acid concentrations were greater in girls than in boys, and there was a decrease in values in both sexes as they matured. The investigators suggested that the decrease in plasma folate concentrations with increasing maturity may represent greater tissue and cellular demands for folic acid, more in boys than girls. In a study on 97 9-year-old girls, Riester and Waslien (1975) observed a mean serum folic acid level of 8.0 ng/ml (range, 2.4–16.9 ng/ml). They did not observe any significant correlations between various nutrient intakes, serum folate levels, or hemoglobin and hematocrit.

In addition to a dietary deficiency of folic acid, a number of other factors may influence folate metabolism. The effect of vitamin B_{12} deficiency was noted above. Numerous drugs will interfere in the absorption and/or utilization of folic acid (Waxman et al., 1970; Herbert, 1973). Examples are the folate antagonists (diphenylhydantoin, dilantin, and primidone), oral contraceptive agents, and alcohol. However, probably few of the low serum or red blood cell folate values encountered in nutrition surveys are the sole result of the use of these drugs and agents.

Alcohol is recognized as a folic acid antagonist blocking the effect of this vitamin at several stages, including the production of malabsorption of folates and decreasing serum and liver folate levels (Eichner and Hillman, 1973; Hillman, 1975; Herbert and Tisman, 1975; Hines, 1975). Thus, folic acid-deficiency anemia may commonly be secondary to alcoholism. Alcoholic subjects usually have serum folic acid levels below normal that respond to increased folic acid intakes and cessation of alcohol.

Iron deficiency may lead to decreased serum folate levels in the rat (Toskes et al., 1974). Perhaps some of the low serum folate levels observed in the human subject are associated with iron deficiency (Saraya et al., 1973). In several population studies, however, we could not find any correlations between folic acid nutriture and iron status.

Numerous reports have appeared on the effects of oral contraceptive agents on serum and red blood cell folic acid levels (Lindenbaum et al., 1975; Shojania and Hornady, 1973; Streiff, 1970; Paine et al., 1975). The findings have been variable. Recently Smith et al. (1975) observed that serum folic acid levels were reduced in subjects taking oral contraceptive agents. Of the 80 women on oral contraceptive agents, 71 percent had serum folate levels of less than 5 ng/ml, and 17 percent were below 3 ng/ml. In the 71 non-oral contraceptive agent users, 48 percent had serum folate less than 5 ng/ml, and 14 percent had levels of less than 3 ng/ml. The mean serum folate level for the oral contraceptive agent users was 4.5 ng/ml; it was 5.4 ng/ml for the nonusers. Thirty percent of the oral contraceptive agent users had a red blood cell folate level of less than 140 ng/ml, while only 9 percent of the nonusers had values below this level (mean, 173 versus 199 ng/ml).

Prasad *et al.* (1975) also reported recently that the use of oral contraceptive agents lowered plasma and red blood cell folate levels in some of their subjects. In the higher socioeconomic group studied, the mean erythrocyte folic acid level was 303 ng/ml in the non-oral contraceptive agent users in comparison to 175 ng/ml in the oral contraceptive agent users. The subjects were reported to ingest only 86–93 μg of folic acid per day.

As noted above, in population studies a significant number of individuals are observed with low serum and erythrocyte folate levels. Do these low values indicate inadequate intakes of folic acid in the diet or are they the result of other unknown factors? What is the clinical significance of these low values? Are the guidelines used in assessing folic acid nutritional status too high or inadequate? Can the guides be applied equally to all ages and to both sexes? Do folic acid supplements reverse or change the serum and red blood cell folate levels in those subjects with low folate values? Would food fortification with folic acid prove beneficial? Are the Recommended Dietary Allowances for folic acid too high? Tables of folic acid contents of foods and dietary information on folate intakes are inadequate. In summary, the most practical procedure to evaluate folic acid nutritional status in population groups or in clinical patients is the measurement of folate levels in the serum and red blood cells. Whenever possible, serum vitamin B_{12} analyses should be performed in conjunction with the folate measurements in order to identify cases that may be complicated with pernicious anemia or a dietary vitamin B_{12} deficiency.

DISCUSSION

COOPER: A major study of the nutritional adequacy of the Canadian population that was initiated some years ago has been partially published in the report "Nutrition Canada." Included in this study are dietary histories, blood samples, medical evaluation, and a large number of other data. The initial report concerning folate sufficiency in Canada revealed that median serum folate in Canadian males ranged between 4.0 and 4.2 ng/ml in approximately 4,000 subjects, and between 3.8 and 4.4 in women in a study utilizing a similar number of subjects. There has been considerable concern about the apparent folate deficiency in the normal population, although the other major findings of the study were that obesity was common and that aging women developed obesity on diets of approximately 1,400 calories per day. Apparent folate deficiency was no worse in census tracts selected for having a mean income below the poverty line (1,500 dollars for a single person and 3,000 dollars for a couple), nor was there a significant difference between the location of the census tract (metropolitan, urban, or rural) or whether the survey was done in winter or summer. Median serum folates in native peoples in Canada (Inuit and Indians) were considerably lower than in the Caucasian population.

We have undertaken to determine if the serum folate values reported represent a serious incidence of folate deficiency, or whether the normal values in government assay were aberrant. Our data on a group of volunteer blood donors donating blood in Montreal reveal the serum folate distributions listed in Table 20-11. In our experience, megaloblastic anemia due to folate deficiency is restricted to patients with serum folate less than 4.0. It is apparent that among Montreal residents voluntarily donating blood, the incidence of folate deficiency is extremely low. We shall be matching the blood donors with subjects in the "Nutrition Canada" study based on income, location of residence, employment, education, etc., and expect to provide evidence that the apparent folate deficiency in Canada was due to a different range of normal values for the folate assay.

We have been doing hematocrits and red blood cell folates on these subjects simultaneously. We find that the erythrocyte folate is surprisingly low when taken from the blood transfusion bag and have not yet solved this technical problem. Erythrocyte folates were not done as part of the "Nutrition Canada" survey. We compared serum folates on blood donors with the serum folates of patients assayed in our laboratory and referred primarily from in-patient populations of several Montreal hospitals. Comparison between these two groups is listed in Table 20-11. It is apparent that the populations are similar, but that a larger proportion of low serum folates is observed in the hospital patients. Because serum folate decreases during a short period of decreased folate intake, this relationship would be expected.

TABLE 20-11   Plasma and Serum Folates in
Volunteer Blood Donors and in Patients
Referred for Folate Level Studies

	Plasma or Serum Folate, μg/l	
Percentile	Blood Donors	Patients
5	2.7	1.2
25	5.2	2.6
50	6.9	4.4
75	9.7	6.3
95	14.3	11.4

The data that we have obtained with blood donors and hospital patients in Montreal are virtually superimposable on those reported here today by Dr. Sauberlich for white Americans. The Black and Latin American populations in Canada are extremely small and have not been specifically identified in the "Nutrition Canada" survey or in our studies. Dr. Sauberlich's data and ours suggest that folate deficiency is a trivial problem in the Caucasian populations of Canada and the United States, whereas his data and the "Nutrition Canada" studies suggest that it may be a serious problem in the Black and Spanish American populations in the United States and in the Inuit and Indian populations in Canada.

LITERATURE CITED

Blakley, R. L. 1969. *The biochemistry of folic acid and related pteridines.* Frontiers of biology, Vol. 13, A. Neuberger and E. L. Tatum, eds., North-Holland Publishing Co., Amsterdam (J. Wiley & Sons, Inc., New York, distributors).

Chanarin, I. 1969. The megaloblastic anaemias. Blackwell Scientific Publ., Oxford, England.

Colman, N., Barker, E. A., Barker, M., Green, R., and Metz, J. 1975. Prevention of folate deficiency by food fortification. IV. Identification of target groups in addition to pregnant women in an adult rural population. Am. J. Clin. Nutr. 28:471–476.

Cook, J. D., Alvarado, J., Gutnisky, A., Jamra, M., Labardini, J., Layrisse, M., Linares, J., Loria, A., Maspes, V., Restrepo, A., Reynafarje, C., Sanchez-Medal, L., Valez, H., and Viteri, F. 1971. Nutritional deficiency and anemia in Latin America: A collaborative study. Blood 38:591–603.

Daniel, W. A., Jr., Gaines, E. G., and Bennett, D. L. 1975. Dietary intakes and plasma concentrations of folate in healthy adolescents. Am. J. Clin. Nutr. 28:363–370.

Doscherholmen, A. 1971. Folate deficiency, absolute and relative. Minn. Med. 54:909–911.

Dunn, R. T., and Foster, L. B. 1973. Radioassay of serum folate. Clin. Chem. 19:101–110.

Eichner, E. R., and Hillman, R. S. 1973. Effect of alcohol on serum folate level. J. Clin. Invest. 52:584–591.

FAO/WHO Report. 1970. Requirements of ascorbic acid, vitamin B$_{12}$, folate, and iron. Report of a Joint FAO/WHO Expert Group, FAO nutrition meetings report series No. 47. Food and Agriculture Organization of the United Nations, Rome.

Hall, C. A., Bardwell, S. A., Allen, E. S., and Rappazzo, M. E. 1975. Variation in plasma folate levels among groups of healthy persons. Am. J. Clin. Nutr. 28:854–857.

Herbert, V. 1967. Biochemical and hematologic lesions in folic acid deficiency. Am. J. Clin. Nutr. 20:562–569.

Herbert, V. 1968. Nutritional requirements for vitamins B$_{12}$ and folic acid. Am. J. Clin. Nutr. 21:743–752.

Herbert, V. 1973. The five possible causes of all nutrient deficiency: Illustrated by deficients of vitamin B$_{12}$ and folic acid. Am. J. Clin. Nutr. 26:77–86.

Herbert, V., and Tisman, G. 1975. Hematologic effects of alcohol. Ann. N.Y. Acad. Sci. 252:307–315.

Hillman, R. S. 1975. Alcohol and hematopoiesis. Ann. N.Y. Acad. Sci. 252:297–306.

Hines, J. D. 1975. Hematologic abnormalities involving vitamin B$_6$ and folate metabolism in alcoholic subjects. Ann. N.Y. Acad. Sci. 252:316–327.

Hoffbrand, A. V., Newcombe, B. F. A., and Mollin, D. L., 1966. Method of assay of red cell folate activity and the value of the assay as a test for folate deficiency. J. Clin. Pathol. 19:17–28.

Kahn, S. B. 1970. Recent advances in the nutritional anemias. Med. Clin. North Am. 54:631–645.

Kamen, B. A., and Caston, J. D. 1974. Direct radiochemical assay for serum folate: Competition between ³H-folic acid and 5-methyltetrahydrofolic acid for a folate binder. J. Lab. Clin. Med. 83:167–174.

Lindenbaum, J., Whitehead, N., and Reyner, F. 1975. Oral contraceptive hormones, folate metabolism, and the cervical epithelium. Am. J. Clin. Nutr. 28:346–353.

NRC–NAS Report. 1974. Recommended Dietary Allowances, 8th Ed. Food and Nutrition Board, National Research Council–National Academy of Sciences, Washington, D.C.

Paine, C. J., Grafton, W. D., Dickson, V. L., and Eichner, E. R. 1975. Oral contraceptives, serum folate, and hematologic status. J. Am. Med. Assoc. 231:731–733.

Prasad, A. S., Lei, K. Y., Oberleas, D., Moghissi, K. S., and Stryker, J. C. 1975. Effect of oral contraceptive agents on nutrients. II. Vitamins. Am. J. Clin. Nutr. 28:385–391.

Riester, P. T., and Waslien, C. I. 1975. Folacin status of nine year old girls in Alabama. Fed. Proc. 34:904. (Abstract)

Rothenberg, S. P., and da Costa, M. 1973. Radioassay of folate. Clin. Chem. 19:785–786.

Rothenberg, S. P., da Costa, M., and Rosenberg, Z. 1972. A radioassay for serum folate: Use of a two-phase sequential-incubation, ligand-binding system. N. Engl. J. Med. 286:1335–1339.

Rothman, D. 1970. Folic acid in pregnancy. Am. J. Obstet. Gynecol. 108:149–175.

Rowe, P. B. 1971. Inborn errors of folic acid metabolism—the regulation of the interconversion of active derivatives of folic acid. Minn. Med. 54:391–396.

Saraya, A. K., Singla, P. N., Ramchandran, K., and Ghai, O. P. 1970. Nutritional macrocytic anemia of infancy and childhood. Am. J. Clin. Nutr. 23:1378–1384.

Saraya, A. K., Choudhry, V. P., and Ghai, P. P. 1973. Interrelationships of vitamin B_{12}, folic acid, and iron in anemia of infancy and childhood: Effect of vitamin B_{12} and iron therapy on folate metabolism. Am. J. Clin. Nutr. 26:640–646.

Sauberlich, H. E., Dowdy, R. P., and Skala, J. H. 1974. Laboratory tests for the assessment of nutritional status, p. 49. CRC Press, Inc., Cleveland, Ohio.

Shaw, W. 1973. Radioassay of serum folate: Some criticisms. Clin. Chem. 19:281–282.

Shojania, A. M., and Hornady, G. J. 1973. Oral contraceptives and folate absorption. J. Lab. Clin. Med. 82:869–875.

Skelly, D. S., Brown, L. P., and Besch, P. K. 1973. Radioimmunoassay. Clin. Chem. 19:146–186.

Smith, J. L., Goldsmith, G. A., and Lawrence, J. D. 1975. Effects of oral contraceptive steroids on vitamin and lipid levels in serum. Am. J. Clin. Nutr. 28:371–376.

Streiff, R. R. 1970. Folate deficiency and oral contraceptives. J. Am. Med. Assoc. 214:105–108.

Streiff, R. R. 1970. Folic acid deficiency anemia. Semin. Hematol. 7:23–39.

Tajuddin, M., and Gardyna, H. A. 1973. Radioassay of serum folate, with use of a serum blank and nondialyzed milk as folate binder. Clin. Chem. 19:125–126.

Toskes, P. P., Smith, G. W., Bensinger, T. A., Giannella, R. A., and Conrad, M. E. 1974. Folic acid abnormalities in iron deficiency: The mechanism of decreased serum folate levels in rats. Am. J. Clin. Nutr. 27:355–361.

Waxman, S., and Schreiber, C. 1973. Measurement of serum folate levels and serum folic acid-binding protein by ³H-PGA radioassay. Blood 42:281–290.

Waxman, S., Corcino, J. J., and Herbert, V. 1970. Drugs, toxins and dietary amino acids affecting vitamin B_{12} or folic acid absorption or utilization. Am. J. Med. *48*:599.

WHO Report. 1968. Nutritional anaemias, report of a WHO Scientific Group, WHO technical report series no. 405. World Health Organization, Geneva, Switzerland.

WHO Report. 1970. Requirements of ascorbic acid, vitamin D, vitamin B_{12}, lalate, and iron. WHO technical report series no. 452.

WHO Report, 1972. Nutritional anaemias, report of a WHO Group of Experts, Geneva, Switzerland, October 11–15, 1971, WHO technical report series no. 503. Geneva, Switzerland.

21

Folacin Requirement of Infants

CAROL I. WASLIEN

The folacin requirements of infants and children established by the Joint FAO/WHO Expert Group (FAO/WHO, 1970) and the Food and Nutrition Board of the National Academy of Sciences (FNB, 1974) are based on studies of three children with goat's milk megaloblastic anemia (Sullivan *et al.*, 1966) and of seven children with the megaloblastic anemia of severe protein–calorie malnutrition (Velez *et al.*, 1963). In the first study, one 12-month-old infant failed to show a reticulocyte response to daily oral administration of 10 or 20 μg of pteroylglutamic acid (PGA) but did respond to 50 μg. Two other infants, 6 and 9 months of age, also responded to 50 μg of oral PGA by an increase in reticulocytes, red and white blood cells, and platelets. From the total intake of PGA and the folacin content of milk plus a rough approximation of milk consumption, 52 to 60 μg of total folacin or 7.6 to 9.4 μg/kg was shown to be needed to elicit hematological recovery. Initial serum folacin levels were low in the three children (1.0–1.5 ng/ml), but no mention was made of other indices that are better indicators of folacin status, and no information was given regarding folacin status subsequent to the PGA administration. Thus, it is not possible to judge the severity of the initial folacin deficiency or its correction by PGA. Although serum vitamin B_{12} levels were normal, no mention was made of iron or ascorbic acid status, deficiencies of which may influence folacin metabolism.

In the second investigation (Velez *et al.*, 1963), seven malnourished children were fed a diet low in folacin. An additional 5 to 20 μg of oral PGA were sufficient to correct megaloblastic bone marrows, elicit a reticulocyte response, and increase hemoglobin levels. The diets were said to contain less than 10 μg of folacin, but no analyses of the diets were performed, nor was folacin status of these children assessed before or after PGA administration. It is likely that they were deficient in other nutrients since iron, ascorbic acid, and vitamin B complex were added to the diets of some children. Thus it is difficult to say how much folacin was actually needed other than that required to elicit hematological recovery in this study.

A subsequent investigation by the same laboratory (Ghitis and Tripathy, 1970) was made on two malnourished infants with megaloblastic anemia. The children received either a whole milk diet or milk treated with activated charcoal to remove free folacin. Doses of 15 to 35 μg or 3.7 and 5.9 μg/kg body weight free folacin from whole milk or supplemental oral PGA was needed to elicit a reticulocyte response, increase hemoglobin and platelet levels, and correct megaloblastic bone marrows. Folacin status subsequent to whole milk or PGA was not measured so it is difficult to judge if these relatively low intakes were indeed adequate to meet all metabolic needs for folacin. The weight of one child stabilized for 4.5 months, suggesting either that the diet was inadequate in nutrients other than folacin, possibly as a result of their removal by the charcoal treatment, or that the level of folacin was inadequate for complete recovery from folacin deficiency.

In another study (Robinson, 1965), a 6-month-old infant with megaloblastic anemia and rapid folacin clearance was fed a diet entirely free of dietary folacin but supplemented with 50 μg of PGA, or approximately 8 μg/kg body weight. The child responded with a restoration of a normoblastic bone marrow, a decrease in hypersegmentation of polymorphonuclear neutrophils, and an increase in reticulocytes and hemoglobin. No additional reticulocyte response to 100 μg of PGA was observed, further indicating that 50 μg was adequate. Unfortunately, no lower doses of PGA were evaluated, nor was folacin status re-evaluated after PGA administration, so it is not possible to determine if 50 μg of PGA really represented the actual folacin requirement.

A series of studies has been conducted to determine the folacin requirement of Egyptian children recovering from protein–calorie malnutrition. In the first study (Halsted *et al.*, 1969), a diet consisting of whole milk and cookies was administered to malnourished anemic children for 2 weeks along with sufficient intramuscular iron to restore hemoglobin levels. Fifteen children who were still anemic were then given 75 μg of PGA subcutaneously. Five of these children showed a reticulocyte response with restoration of a normoblastic bone marrow, while six additional children had restoration of their bone marrow without a reticulocytosis, and four showed no response to PGA. Vitamin B_{12} levels were normal or high throughout the study, and protein, albumin, iron, and iron-binding-capacity levels were probably corrected by the time of folacin administration; but vitamin E levels remained low, and no mention was made of ascorbic acid status. Although it is difficult to calculate the absolute folacin intake required to initiate the hematologic response in these children since the total folacin intake was not recorded, approximately 119 μg of folacin or 15 μg/kg body weight came from milk and PGA each day. It is possible that larger doses of PGA would have resulted in a reticulocyte response in more children, or that lesser doses would have been equally effective in some children. However, it is unlikely that the whole milk and biscuits, supplying at least 44 μg of folacin, or 5 μg/kg, contained adequate amounts of folacin since bone marrows of five children continued to be megaloblastic until PGA was administered, and their serum folate levels remained as low as on admission.

As a continuation of this study (Waslien *et al.*, 1972), a special formula with controlled folacin content (CF), designed by Ross Laboratories to be high in protein and minerals and moderate in folacin (Table 21-1), was used to quantitate carefully the folacin requirement in another group of malnourished Egyptian children (Kamel *et al.*, 1972). Although this diet contained adequate levels of all vitamins and minerals, it was supplemented with additional oral vitamins and trace elements since these malnourished children probably had deficiencies of numerous nutrients that could influence their response to folacin. In addition, 50 mg of iron as iron dextran was administered each day for the first 6 days of the study.

Immediately following administration of parenteral iron and the CF diet, which contained 26 μg/l and contributed 6.3 μg/kg total folacin daily, patients responded clinically by improvement in appetite and loss of edema and by increases in total protein, albumin, iron, and E serum levels. A reticulocyte response occurred on an average of 10.2 days in 21 of the 23 children and resulted in a slight increase in hemoglobin. However, there was also a slight intensification of the megaloblastic character of the bone marrow and an increase in the

TABLE 21-1 Composition of CF Formula

Proximate Analysis	Amount
Protein, g/l	24
Fat, g/l	34
Carbohydrate, g/l	68
Ash, g/l	8
kcal/l	676
Calcium, g/l	1.08
Phosphorus, g/l	0.66
Potassium, g/l	1.64
Sodium, g/l	0.48
Magnesium, g/l	0.07
Chloride, g/l	0.79
Iron, g/l	0.014
Vitamins	
A, IU/l	3,100
D, IU/l	420
E, IU/l	1.37
B_1, mg/l	1.35
B_2, mg/l	1.29
B_6, μg/l	205
C, mg/l	71
Niacin, mg/l	2.93
Folacin	
Total, μg/l	27
Free, μg/l	25

incidence of hypersegmented polymorphonuclear neutrophils as well as decreases in serum and red blood cell folacin levels, indicating that the CF diet did not contain adequate folacin. When the reticulocyte response to iron and the CF diet had ended after the first 2 to 3 weeks, or when it was apparent that there would be no response, each of the 23 children was given 20, 30, 40, or 50 μg of PGA intramuscularly per day until the reticulocyte response to these doses of PGA had ended, or again when it was clear that a response would not occur. The parenteral dose was then increased by an additional 50 μg of PGA/day for all children and the existence of a second reticulocyte response to folacin was detected.

Mean serum folacin levels increased, but not in relation to the level of PGA administered, and RBC folacin levels did not change at all (Table 21-2). A reticulocyte response occurred in all but one or two children in

TABLE 21-2 Serum and Red Blood Cell Folate Levels with Various Doses of Folic Acid

Group	Dose of Folic Acid, μg/day	No.	Serum and Red Blood Cell Folate Levels, ng/ml							
			Admission		After Low-Folate Diet		After Initial Folic Acid Dose		After Additional Folic Acid Dose, 50 μg/day	
			Serum	RBC	Serum	RBC	Serum	RBC	Serum	RBC
I	20	5	3.3 ± 2.7	189 ± 140	1.8 ± 1.4	119 ± 34	3.5 ± 1.7	123 ± 22	4.7 ± 2.6	118 ± 38
II	30	6	2.5 ± 1.9	122 ± 54	2.6 ± 2.0	100 ± 35	4.5 ± 2.7	154 ± 86	9.4 ± 4.0	237 ± 95
III	40	5	2.3 ± 1.3	224 ± 54	1.5 ± 0.6	171 ± 96	2.8 ± 0.9	138 ± 58	5.3 ± 1.3	132 ± 51
IV	50	7	3.1 ± 0.9	230 ± 153	1.5 ± 1.4	180 ± 130	3.7 ± 2.3	128 ± 40	5.4 ± 2.2	107 ± 36
AVERAGE		23	3.0 ± 2.2	209 ± 141	1.8 ± 1.2	144 ± 95	3.7 ± 2.2	136 ± 58	5.8 ± 3.4	140 ± 74

each group, but the incidence of responses was not related to the level of PGA administration (Table 21-3). Reticulocyte levels in the 50 μg group were triple those of the other groups, but there was no difference in the number of days taken to reach a maximum or in the number of children showing a second reticulocyte response to an additional 50 μg of PGA.

A high proportion of the children receiving CF plus 50 μg of PGA (12.8 μg/kg body weight) showed a distinct reticulocyte peak, an increase in hemoglobin concentration to above 11 g/100 ml of blood, a decrease in hypersegmentation bone marrow conversions, and a meaningful increase in serum folacin levels (Table 21-4). Similarly, there was little difference in the number responding at the lowest level (CF plus 20 μg added PGA, i.e., a total folacin intake of 9.0 μg/kg body weight). This negligible difference in response makes it difficult to state that an intake above 9.0 μg/kg is, in fact, more beneficial than 9.0 μg. However, since all indices of folacin status deteriorated on the CF diet, it can be concluded that 6.3 μg folacin/kg is not sufficient. These intakes are not unlike those found by previous investigators (Robinson, 1965; Sullivan *et al.*, 1966).

It is possible that malnourished children cannot absorb oral folic acid. Lesions of the intestinal mucosa are not uncommon in PCM and may interfere with folic acid absorption. In order to translate the recommended intake of 9.0 μg/kg from diet and parenterally administered PGA into a dietary folacin recommendation, the nature of folic acid absorption in 15 malnourished children was determined using tritiated PGA (Mahran *et al.*, 1975). Three-day stool collections were assayed for unabsorbed folate. Absorption was within normal limits in all children, averaging 77 percent. Those with diarrhea had significantly poorer absorption, 69 percent as compared with 83 percent, but

TABLE 21-3 Adequacy of Primary Doses of Folic Acid as Indicated by Double Reticulocyte Response

Group	No. with Reticulocytosis to Initial Dose/ Total No. Receiving Dose	Maximum Primary Response, Reticulocyte %	Days to Attain Peak	No. Showing Second Reticulocyte Response
I, 20 μg of folic/day	3/5	12.1	5	1
II, 30 μg of folic/day	4/6	15.5	8	1
III, 40 μg of folic/day	4/5	15.5	5	2
IV, 50 μg of folic/day	5/7	40.0	11	1

TABLE 21-4   Patients Showing Positive Response on Graded Dosage of PGA

Response	No. Showing Positive Response/Total			
	20^a	30	40	50
Distinct reticulocyte peak	3/5	4/6	4/5	5/7
Increase in hemoglobin concentration to >11 g/100 ml	1/5	4/6	2/5	4/7
Decrease in PMN hypersegmentation	3/4	1/1	3/4	2/2
Conversion to normoblastic bone marrow	2/4	3/4	2/5	3/6
Conversion of low-serum folate to levels above 3 ng/100 ml	3/4	3/5	3/5	4/5

[a]Folic acid administered, micrograms/day.

PGA absorption was not related to serum or RBC folacin or bone marrow morphology. If one corrects the previous minimum intake of folacin for the average malabsorption, the folacin requirements would increase from 9 to 9.6 μg folacin/kg body weight. If, in addition, one assumes that none of the polyglutamate is absorbed and that only half of the free folacin present in milk can be absorbed as has been suggested by the NRC (FNB, 1974), the folacin dietary requirement would increase to 13.9 μg/kg.

Recently, the same CF diet as was previously used to measure the folacin requirements of malnourished children has been fed to a group of Lebanese infants without overt malnutrition in an effort to determine the requirements of this vitamin in healthy children (Asfour et al., 1975). Although the children chosen for the study exhibited the best growth and development of all the orphanage children, five were below the third percentile of the growth standards based on North American children.

The infants received intramuscular injections of iron dextran and oral alpha-tocopherol prior to the study since earlier studies on this group of children revealed that inadequacy of these two nutrients was common. They were then subdivided into three groups comparable in age and sex. During the next 8 months all three groups received the CF diet with added vitamins and trace elements and either 0, 5, or 10 μg of oral PGA each day, making daily intakes of 3.6, 4.3, and 5.0 μg of folacin/kg body weight. Three of the originally selected infants were adopted within the first 2 months of the observation period and another was adopted at a later date. Four children were added to replace the adopted children. In total, seven children were observed for an 8-month period and five were observed for 5–6 months.

Although initial biochemical assessment of the children indicated that total serum protein and albumin were within normal limits, there was a significant increase in albumin during the first 3 months and a further increase during the next 5 months (Table 21-5). Serum vitamin B_{12} and ascorbic acid values were normal for all children in the study, but the majority of children had initial serum tocopherol values of less than 0.5 mg/100 ml. The initial 200-mg tocopherol supplement and daily intakes of 5 mg resulted in serum levels of 0.3–0.4 mg/100 ml, indicating either that normal serum levels are less than 0.5 mg/100 ml or that the recommended intake of 5 mg may need to be reconsidered.

Serum iron levels were low in five of six children measured prior to iron administration, and unsaturated iron binding capacity (UIBC) values were low in two. After the fourth month of the CF diet plus trace element supplements supplying a total of approximately 14 mg of iron per day (which alone more than fulfilled recommended iron intakes) plus the additional intramuscular iron, serum iron levels were still low in 6 of 10 subjects, but in no case were UIBC values elevated. The normal UIBC, the increases in hemoglobin levels, and other evidence make it unlikely that these low serum levels represent an iron deficiency state.

Initial serum and RBC folacin for all children studied averaged 4.9 and 299 ng/ml, respectively (Tables 21-6 and 21-7). Four children had initial serum levels of less than 3.0, but only two had an RBC value of less than 150 ng/ml. Any slight differences in average serum folates between the groups receiving added PGA and those on CF alone appeared very slowly. There was no significant difference in serum folacin values until the fifth or sixth month of supplementation. At that time children receiving the 5- and 10-μg PGA supplements had significantly ($P > 0.05$) higher levels (4.5 and 4.8 ng/ml, respectively) than did the unsupplemented group (3.5 ng/ml of serum). The limited data available for the 7- to 8-month period are insufficient to allow conclusions as to their significance, although they appear to be in the direction that suggests a continuation of this separation of the levels between unsupplemented versus supplemented children.

Statistically significant higher RBC folacin values occurred at the second month in the supplemented group, but at other months there were no significant differences between groups. Part of the explanation for this apparent similarity in RBC values may be the differences between mean initial values for the groups and the initial wide ranges of values reflected in the large standard deviations. The variations are related to the initial iron nutriture of the children. High values of RBC folate occur in iron deficiency, a condition that was present initially in many of the children. This and the subsequent rates of response to

TABLE 21-5 Biochemical Assessment of Nutritional Status of Infants Receiving Experimental Diets

Month of Study	Protein		Vitamins			Iron		
	Total, g/100 ml	Albumin, g/100 ml	B_{12}, pg/ml	E, mg/100 ml	C, mg/100 ml	Iron, mg/100 ml	UIBC, μg/100 ml	Saturation Index
0	(20) 6.9 ± 0.9	(20) 3.6 ± 0.6	(17) 375 ± 95	(10) 0.24 ± 0.14	(10) 0.45 ± 0.22	(6) 37 ± 4	(6) 226 ± 64	(6) 15.0 ± 3.9
3	(10) 6.6 ± 0.6	(10) 4.1 ± 0.4	(9) 473 ± 116	(12) 0.72 ± 0.18	—	(14) 53 ± 32	(8) 160 ± 33	(8) 22.6 ± 7.9
8	(3) 6.8 ± 0.4	(3) 4.7 ± 0.1	—	(4) 0.34 ± 0.15	—	(4) 40 ± 9	—	—

Folacin Requirement of Infants   241

TABLE 21-6   Serum Folacin Levels with Varying PGA Intakes

| Month | Serum Folacin Level, ng/ml | | |
	CF	CF + 5 μg of PGA	CF + 10 μg of PGA
0	5.0 ± 3.4	4.5 ± 1.1	5.2 ± 3.1
1	3.9 ± 1.7	3.4 ± 2.2	4.3 ± 2.1
2	4.6 ± 0.9	6.7 ± 1.9	5.4 ± 1.8
3	3.1 ± 1.0	3.4 ± 0.8	5.0 ± 2.1
4	3.9 ± 1.6	5.1 ± 1.7	4.9 ± 2.2
5–6	3.5 ± 0.4	4.5 ± 0.4	4.8 ± 0.4
7–8	3.2 ± 1.1	5.7 ± 6.0	4.5 ± 6.6

administered iron give a logical explanation for the behavior of the RBC folates. The variations in RBC folate content decreased during the study.

There was a tendency for both mean serum and RBC folacin values to decrease in only the CF group, but no change was apparent in these values for the PGA-supplemented groups. It is of especial significance that at no time during the study did any child exhibit a megaloblastic marrow.

Graphic presentation of serum and RBC folacin values illustrate the individual variation observed among these infants receiving the CF diet. Child 16 had initially high serum folacin (10.0 ng/ml) and RBC folacin (470 ng/ml) and exhibited a pronounced decrease in both levels with ultimate stabilization after 3 months at 4.2 ng/ml and 200 ng/ml, respectively. Simultaneous with the continuous increase in hemoglobin, there was gain in body weight. Child 6 initially had intermediate RBC and serum folacin values, with the latter remaining relatively stable at approximately 4 ng/ml throughout. He exhibited a decrease in RBC

TABLE 21-7   RBC Folacin Levels with Varying PGA Intakes

| Month | RBC Folacin Level, ng/ml | | |
	CF	CF + 5 μg of PGA	CF + 10 μg of PGA
0	325 ± 148	259 ± 62	314 ± 207
1	196 ± 77	247 ± 94	286 ± 136
2	204 ± 11	267 ± 24	361 ± 93
3	147 ± 46	202 ± 51	259 ± 104
4	162 ± 68	247 ± 78	261 ± 112
5–6	224 ± 80	197 ± 48	230 ± 122
7–8	175 ± 74	142 ± 227	275 ± 280

levels to 170 ng/ml at 3 to 4 months and a subsequent increase to 320 at 6 months.

A significant increase in hemoglobin levels and weight gain occurred in all children on the unsupplemented CF diets, representing a folacin intake of 3.5 μg/kg body weight or 70 percent of the FAO/WHO recommended amount. Children 1, 8, and 16 had increases in hemoglobin to over 12 g/100 ml of blood, and child 6 showed an increase to 11.2 g after the first month, where the level remained for the remainder of the study (Figure 21-1). Continuous increments of body weight occurred in children 6, 8, and 16; child 1, the oldest, experienced a plateau in body weight at 17 months of age but subsequently resumed an increase in body weight. Two of the four children maintained both serum and RBC folacin levels within acceptable normal limits, and two had serum and RBC folacin levels below the lower limit for normal. Closer examination of these last two children shows that they had low folacin levels prior to the study. Thus, even these two children could maintain their folacin levels and still gain weight and increase their hemoglobin levels with no display of clinical or hematological evidence of folacin inadequacy.

All three children who received CF plus 5 μg of PGA, representing 4.3 μg/kg body weight or 85 percent of the FAO/WHO recommended intake, experienced definite increments in hemoglobin concentration and good weight gains (Figure 21-2). All had hemoglobin concentrations above 12 g/100 ml by 3 to 6 months. All three had normal serum folacin, and two had normal RBC folacin levels after 5 to 8 months of this diet.

All children on the CF plus 10 μg of PGA diet had good weight gains and progressive increases in hemoglobin concentrations (Figure 21-3).

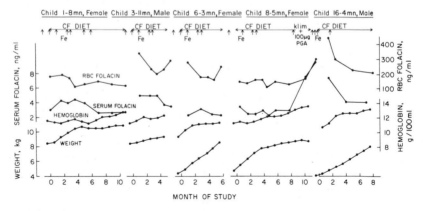

FIGURE 21-1   Changes in weight, hemoglobin, and folacin in children fed the CF diet.

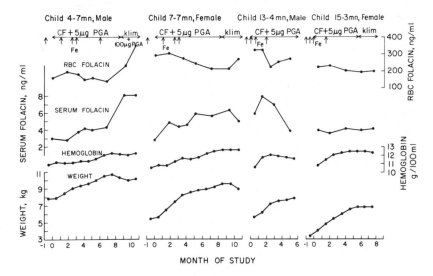

FIGURE 21-2   Changes in weight, hemoglobin, and folacin in children fed the CF + 5 μg of PGA diet.

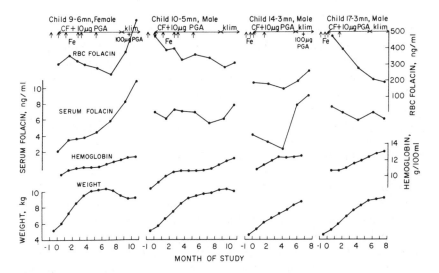

FIGURE 21-3   Changes in weight, hemoglobin, and folacin in children fed the CF + 10 μg of PGA diet.

Two had hemoglobin levels above 12 g/100 ml, and two had levels that rose from 8.8 and 10.4 to 11 and 11.7 g, respectively.

In order to judge the nutritional adequacy of the CF diet and to determine if minimal changes detected in the peripheral blood levels of some infants were due to folacin intake, a whole milk formula (Klim) was given to eight of the infants from the preceding study and three additional infants who had not received CF diet, while two infants continued to receive the CF diet. Four of the original 8 infants transferred to whole milk received, in addition, 100 μg of PGA daily (Klim plus 100 μg of PGA).

Children 1 and 16, continued on the CF diet, showed no further change in serum or RBC folacin and body weight and hemoglobin continued to increase. (Figure 21-1). Children 5 and 15, who were changed from CF plus 5 μg of PGA to whole milk (Figure 21-2), showed no meaningful increase in serum and RBC folacin or hemoglobin, nor did children 10 and 17, who were transferred from CF plus 10 μg of PGA (Figure 21-3) to the whole-milk formula. Child 8 from the CF diet (Figure 21-1), child 4 from the CF plus 5 μg of PGA diet (Figure 21-2), and children 9 and 14 from the CF plus 10 μg of PGA diet (Figure 21-3) had definite increases in serum and RBC folacin but no apparent change in rate of growth or hemoglobin increment when changed to Klim plus 100 μg of PGA.

Throughout the study, no megaloblastosis of the bone marrow was noted. Three children had elevated polymorphonuclear (PMN) lobe counts in the peripheral blood on admission. These same children had normal serum and RBC folacin levels. There was a random occurrence of increased lobe counts in the children throughout the study, with three of five children on the CF diet, two of four on the CF plus 5 μg of PGA diet, and one of five on the CF plus 10 μg of PGA diet having two or more instances of elevated counts. Administration of Klim or Klim plus 100 μg of PGA did not alter the character of the PMN values.

In conclusion, it appears that, for a child less than 2 years of age, diets providing 3.5 μg of folacin/kg body weight are sufficient to maintain growth, hemopoiesis, and clinical well-being for at least 6 to 9 months despite the presence of serum and RBC folacin levels widely regarded as indicating borderline deficiency. Slightly higher intakes, 4.3 and 5.0 μg/kg, similarly supported growth, hemopoiesis, and clinical well-being and resulted in higher serum and RBC folacin concentrations. Thus 3.5–5.0 μg of folacin/kg body weight, and the FAO/WHO recommendation of 5.0 μg, are adequate for the normal child. It is also apparent that the requirement of the healthy child is one-third to one-half the amount needed for maximal repletion of the child recovering from protein–calorie malnutrition.

Some questions that remain to be answered in assessing folacin requirements in infants include:

1. How much of the folacin in different foods is actually absorbed and utilized?
2. What is the requirement for folacin for maintaining functions other than hemopoiesis?
3. What kind of variation in requirements occurs during stress other than protein–calorie malnutrition?

DISCUSSION

HALSTED: At the time you gave graded amounts of folic acid, were all your patients protein repleted?

WASLIEN: Yes, they were repleted with respect to protein. Serum levels of vitamins B_{12} and E were also normal, and we gave adequate ascorbic acid, so they were probably not deficient in this nutrient as well.

HERBERT: I think the conclusions with controlled folate milk preparations have to be restricted to their own facts. By that I mean the requirement is applicable only to a milk diet that probably has high folate binder concentration and that may render substantial amounts of folate unabsorbable. The folate requirement, that is the amount absorbed, is almost certainly lower than the amount shown as fed.

WASLIEN: However, with infants, milk is usually the major food item. On the other hand, the amount of binder could vary with the kind of milk fed.

WAXMAN: Was your CF diet like Similac?

WASLIEN: Yes.

WAXMAN: I ask this because we have looked at Similac for unsaturated folate binding protein and have not found it. Most of the prepared baby foods do not have detectable exogenous folate binding capacity.

WASLIEN: Well, that might explain why normal children required so much less folate.

CHANARIN: I think that when one does a study to determine the amount of folate that gives a hematological response, that is all that has been determined. Levels that give a hematological response are not necessarily the dose of the nutrient required each day. I think there is a danger of thinking they are one and the same thing.

BUTTERWORTH: Is there any evidence that the milk binder does in fact, in a dose relationship, reduce the availability of folate? Is it not digested, inactivated, or destroyed? Can you say categorically that the existence of a binder in the diet renders folate unavailable?

246

HERBERT: I think we may be able to say it with data in the very near future. ROTHENBERG: Indirect data are available. The lowest absorbability is seen with goat's milk, which has a higher concentration of binder than other milk.

LITERATURE CITED

Asfour, R., Wahbeh, N., Waslien, C. I., Guindi, S., and Darby, W. J. Folacin requirements of children. III. Normal infants. Submitted to Am. J. Clin. Nutr.

FAO/WHO (Food and Agriculture Organization/World Health Organization). 1970. Requirements of ascorbic acid, vitamin D, vitamin B_{12}, folate and iron. Report of a FAO/WHO Expert Committee. WHO technical report series no. 452. World Health Organization, Geneva, Switzerland. 77 pp.

FNB (Food and Nutrition Board, National Research Council). 1974. Recommended dietary allowances, 8th ed. National Academy of Sciences, Washington, D.C. 129 pp.

Ghitis, J., and Tripathy, K. 1970. Availability of milk folate. Studies with cow's milk in experimental folic acid deficiency. Am. J. Clin. Nutr. 23:141-146.

Halsted, C. H., Sourial, N., Guindi, S., Maurad, K. A. H., Khattab, A.-K., Carter, J. P., and Patwardhan, V. N. 1969. Anemia of kwashiorkor in Cairo: Deficiencies of protein, iron and folic acid. Am. J. Clin. Nutr. 22:1371-1382.

Kamel, K., Waslien, C. I., El-Ramly, Z., Guindy, S., Mourad, K. A., Khattab, A.-K., Hashem, N., Patwardhan, V. N., and Darby, W. J. 1972. Folate requirements of children. II. Response of children recovering from protein–calorie malnutrition to graded doses of parenterally administered folic acid. Am. J. Clin. Nutr. 25:152-165.

Mahran, A. B., Gabr, M. K., Guindi, S., Waslien, C. I., and Monsour, M. M. Folacin requirements of children. IV. Folic acid absorption in children with protein–calorie malnutrition. Submitted to Am. J. Clin. Nutr.

Robinson, M. G. 1965. Megalobastic anemia of infancy. Minnesota Med. 48:1623-1628.

Sullivan, L. W., Luhby, A. L., and Streiff, R. R. 1966. Studies of the requirement for folic acid in infants and the etiology of folate deficiency in goat's milk megaloblastic anemia. Am. J. Clin. Nutr. 18:311.

Velez, H., Ghitis, J., Pradilla, A., and Vitale, J. J. 1963. Cali-Harvard Nutrition Project. I. Megaloblastic anemia in kwashiorkor. Am. J. Clin. Nutr. 12:54-61.

Waslien, C. I., Kamel, K., El-Ramly, Z., Carter, J. P., Mourad, K. A., Khattab, A.-K., and Darby, W. J. 1972. Folate requirements of children. I. A formula diet low in folic acid for study of folate deficiency in protein–calorie malnutrition. Am. J. Clin. Nutr. 25:147-151.

22

Folic Acid Requirement in Adults (Including Pregnant and Lactating Females)

VICTOR HERBERT

DEFINITION OF REQUIREMENT

Requirement, as used in this presentation, means "minimal daily requirement" (MDR) from exogenous sources required to sustain normality. Normality is defined as that state of well-being, in the absence of medication, in which there exists no biochemical hypofunction produced by an inadequate dietary supply of the vitamin and correctable by increasing the supply (Herbert, 1973).

The MDR can be reduced to a formula (Herbert, 1971) applicable generally to essential (i.e., required from exogenous sources) nutrient deficiency, as follows:

$$\text{MDR (units/day)} = \frac{\text{UBS (units)}}{\text{D (days)}}$$

where:

MDR = Minimal daily requirement of nutrient from exogenous sources;

247

UBS = utilizable body stores of nutrient; and

   D = number of days required to develop tissue deficiency after cessation of absorption from exogenous sources of nutrient (with appropriate correction for *incomplete* cessation of absorption).

The above formula may also be written as:

$$D = \frac{UBS}{MDR}$$

or

$$UBS = D \times MDR$$

Note that the MDR is stated in units per day absorbed from exogenous sources. Thus, MDR is most easily ascertained by shutting off all food sources of the nutrient and supplying it parenterally in a free form guaranteeing "total" absorption. When the nutrient is supplied orally, the form or forms in which it is supplied and the nature of the foods in which it is supplied or with which it is mixed may substantially affect absorbability. As applied to folic acid, the relatively high absorbability of pharmaceutical folic acid (pteroylglutamic acid) (Herbert, 1970), which is rapidly absorbed (primarily from the proximal small intestine, although it is capable of being absorbed from the entire length of the small intestine), has made PGA the preferred form of folate fed (Bernstein *et al.*, 1970; Gerson *et al.*, 1971) in studies to determine MDR for folate. Other presentations at this workshop deal with the factors making more difficult determination of MDR using various food folates, which are primarily in polyglutamate forms (see Chapters 3, 5, 9–11, 14, 16–18).

FOLIC ACID REQUIREMENTS IN ADULTS

This section will deal with the MDR considered as that quantity of nutrient that will sustain normality in healthy adult male and nonpregnant female subjects without excess deposits of the nutrient (i.e., subjects with "low" body stores). Normality is considered as absence of any clinical symptoms or signs and absence of any laboratory evidence of deficiency of the nutrient. The folic acid requirement in pregnancy is discussed in a separate section below, and the requirement in situations of increased need will be separately discussed by Dr. Lindenbaum (Chapter 23).

The adult MDR for folic acid is about 50 μg (Herbert, 1968). This is the quantity of PGA that, when administered orally or parenterally daily to patients with folate deficiency uncomplicated by other systemic disease and not ingesting more than 5 μg of other dietary folate, will produce a relatively rapid return toward hematologic normality, accompanied by reticulocytosis and rise of hematocrit toward normal. Serum folate levels do not rise appreciably on this dose of folic acid given for periods of up to 1 month, despite conversion of bone marrow morphology from megaloblastic to normoblastic and marked hematologic improvement (Zalusky and Herbert, 1961). A larger daily dose of PGA (0.1–0.2 mg) will cause the serum folate level in such subjects to rise to normal within a month (Herbert, 1963). Even smaller daily doses of PGA (25 μg) have been reported to produce responses where the folate deficiency was not strictly dietary in origin, i.e., in sprue (Sheehy et al., 1961) and anticonvulsant-associated megaloblastic anemia (Druskin et al., 1962).

It should be noted that patients with sprue (Sheehy et al., 1961) and anticonvulsant-associated megaloblastic anemia (Druskin et al., 1962) who had hematologic response to 25 μg of PGA daily had this PGA superimposed on normal diets rather than diets deficient in folate. It is a reasonable assumption, therefore, that those subjects absorbed approximately another 25 μg of folate from their normal diets, adding up to a total of about 50 μg.

When a healthy normal adult male with a normal folate intake was switched to a daily folate intake of approximately 5 μg/day, folate deficiency megaloblastic anemia developed in approximately 4.5 months (Herbert, 1962a). Dividing the 4.5 months required to develop megaloblastic anemia on the diet containing approximately 5 μg of folate per day into the middle-class New England adult male "average" tissue folate store of 7.5 ± 2.5 mg (Herbert, 1971), one arrives at a rough estimate of approximately 50 μg of folic acid per day as the MDR. Similar calculation of a 50-μg MDR for folic acid can be found in the study of O'Brien (1968), who found it took 5 months after the onset of acquired acute miliary tropical sprue in healthy people resident in the tropics (seen at Singapore) for folate deficiency anemia to develop. In sprue, food folate absorption is reduced rather than abolished, but there is also reduction of reabsorption of the approximately 0.1 mg of folate excreted daily in the bile (Herbert, 1970).

Chronic alcoholic subjects, taken off alcohol but not allowed to build their body folate stores to normal, may develop folate deficiency megaloblastosis within only 5 to 10 weeks of reinduction of inadequate folate intake (Eichner *et al.*, 1971; Herbert, 1971). However, alcohol has direct toxic effects on hematopoiesis, that which reduces the value of alcoholic subjects as models for helping to delineate MDR for normal individuals (Eichner and Hillman, 1973; Wu *et al.*, 1975).

Chanarin (1971) has pointed out that, in the absence of direct measurement of tissue folate store, as exemplified by hepatic folate, an MDR derived by placing a normal individual with presumably normal stores on a folate-deficient diet would only be an approximation of requirement. One can agree with this caveat but nevertheless point out that liver folate is closely reflected by red cell folate (Herbert, 1968a; Wu *et al.*, 1975). Normal red cell folate thus should generally mean normal body folate stores, and total body stores of folate in healthy well-fed adult males generally appear to fall between 5 and 12 mg (Herbert, 1962b; Waters, 1963; FAO/WHO Expert Group, 1970; Chanarin, 1971).

It should be noted that the studies cited above indicated that 50 μg of PGA daily would restore adults with subnormal folate status toward normal, thus indicating that such doses may actually slightly exceed the MDR, which is the amount required to *sustain* normality rather than the possibly greater amount necessary to return an individual from subnormal toward normal.

That 50 μg of PGA daily will *sustain* normality is supported by a study of three healthy adult female medical research technicians who were given a diet containing approximately 5 μg of total folate daily, supplemented with a single daily oral tablet of PGA. In the space of slightly more than a month, a clear fall of the serum folate from 10.3 ng/ml to 4.2 ng/ml occurred in the technician whose daily tablet contained 25 μg of PGA. However, the normal serum folate level of 6.5 ng/ml of the subject receiving a daily tablet containing 50 μg of PGA was essentially unchanged (6.2 ng/ml) at the end of the study, and the normal serum folate of 11 ng/ml in a subject receiving a daily tablet containing 100 μg of PGA was also essentially the same (9.4 ng/ml at the end of the study) (Herbert, 1962b).

Furthermore, Fleming *et al.* (1963) noted that a supplement of approximately 50 μg of food folate per day prevented the appearance of elevated formiminoglutamate in the urine of a patient on a folate-deficient diet that had led to abnormally high formiminoglutamate excretion in the urine of three patients who did not receive this supplement. It should be noted that the absorbability of the food folate was probably less than the absorbability of PGA, and thus the study of Fleming *et al.* (1963) indicated that less than 50 μg of PGA equivalent would prevent the appearance of elevated urine formiminoglutamate. This is in accord with the unpublished observations of Chanarin (1971), who found that 10 to 20 µg of PGA daily by injection would restore formiminoglutamate excretion to normal in patients with megaloblastic anemia due to folate deficiency associated with gluten-sensitive enteropathy or partial gastrectomy (Chanarin, 1971).

In one case (Sullivan and Herbert, 1964), a woman with folate-deficiency megaloblastic anemia was sustained on a diet almost devoid of folate for 2 years, supplemented by 75 µg of PGA daily. On this diet, macrocytosis disappeared after 214 days, and neutrophil nucleus hypersegmentation disappeared after 282 days. Since her tissue folate stores were gradually replenished on this dose, 75 µg of PGA daily can be considered as probably greater than required to sustain normality (since sustaining normality does not require increasing the level of tissue stores).

The recommended dose of PGA for therapeutic trials in subjects with suspected folate deficiency who do not have an increased folate requirement is 100 µg daily, orally or intramuscularly (Herbert, 1963). This dose produces a gradual rise toward normal in the serum folate level over a period of 2 to 4 weeks, accompanied by a sharp return toward hematologic normality. Since a gradual increase in tissue folate stores accompanies this therapy, it must be considered as in excess of the MDR to sustain normality.

FOLATE REQUIREMENTS IN PREGNANCY

The MDR for folic acid is increased by any increase in the daily metabolic rate or cell turnover rate (Herbert, 1968; see Chapter 23) and therefore is increased in pregnancy. In fact, folate deficiency of varying degrees of severity may encompass up to one-third of all the pregnant women in the world (WHO Scientific Group, 1968; FAO/WHO Expert Group, 1970; Pritchard, 1970; Herbert, 1972; WHO Group of Experts, 1972; Colman *et al.*, 1974; Committee on Dietary Allowances, 1974; Herbert *et al.*, 1975).

Assuming adequate folate stores at the start of pregnancy, the MDR to sustain normality in pregnancy appears to be in the range of 100 µg of PGA, ingested from the start of pregnancy. Assuming lesser stores at the start of pregnancy, and supplementation beginning later than the start of pregnancy, this figure may rise to 200–300 µg. Chanarin *et al.* (1968) found a daily supplement of 25 µg PGA insufficient to prevent megaloblastosis, although 100 µg was adequate to keep the red cell folate normal at the end of pregnancy and in the early days of the puerperium. Hansen and Rybo (1967) obtained similar results. However, the quantity of supplementation necessary to sustain normal folate metabolism in pregnancy varies with differences in quantity and absorbability of folate from the diets of different population groups and quantity of folate stores at the start of pregnancy. Thus, Willoughby and Jewell (1966) found that their population group required a larger daily supplementation (300 μg of PGA) to assure adequate folate stores. Chanarin (1969) and Cooper (1973) have reviewed the folate intake required to prevent all manifestations of deficiency. The data they review, plus those of other studies (Pritchard, 1970; Herbert, 1972; WHO Group of Experts, 1972; Colman et al., 1974; Committee on Dietary Allowances, 1974; Herbert et al., 1975) suggest that all manifestations of folate deficiency could be prevented, in women who start pregnancy with moderate folate stores, by diets containing the equivalent of 200 μg of PGA per day, i.e., 200 μg of variably absorbed folate per day, of which about 1/4 to 1/2 was "free" folate.

Colman et al. (1974) have demonstrated that folate deficiency in pregnancy may be prevented by food fortification. They have also demonstrated that maize meal containing a daily supplement of 500 μg of PGA produced an effect similar to that of 300 μg of PGA daily in tablet form, namely progressive rise in red cell and serum folate levels despite continuation of pregnancy (Colman et al., 1975). They point out that, "It is questionable whether it would ever be necessary to fortify any food with the intention of providing a folic acid supplement greater than the equivalent of 300 μg PGA in tablet form" (i.e., 500 μg of PGA as food fortification, with decreased folate absorption from the maize [N. Colman, personal communication] bringing the level down to the equivalent of 300 μg of PGA daily in tablet form).

The therapeutic dose to treat folate deficiency megaloblastosis in pregnancy may at times be greater than 0.4 mg of PGA daily, since some pregnant women with folate deficiency megaloblastosis may not respond to therapeutic trial with 0.1–0.2 mg of PGA daily (Alperin et al., 1966; Herbert, 1968b), and some may respond poorly to 0.4 mg (Pritchard, 1970). The average Asian pregnant woman, being smaller than the average American pregnant woman, may respond more frequently to therapeutic trial with 0.1 mg of PGA daily (Izak et al., 1963).

FOLATE REQUIREMENTS IN LACTATION

About 50 μg of folate per day is lost in the breast milk during lactation (FAO/WHO Expert Group, 1970), and there appears to be selective ability of breast milk to take up folate from the plasma of the mother (Metz *et al.*, 1968). Thus, the MDR for the lactating woman appears to be in the range of 100 µg of PGA equivalent daily.

NOTE

The Recommended Dietary Allowances (RDA) (National Academy of Sciences–National Research Council, 1974), designed for the maintenance of good nutrition of practically all healthy people in the United States, is 400 µg of folate daily for all males and females aged 11 or older, with 800 µg for pregnant and 600 µg for lactating women. These allowances are set at a level sufficiently above the top level of the range of individual human variability so as to allow a margin of safety to encompass such factors as variable absorption of folates from different foodstuffs, variable inhibition of absorption by conjugase inhibitors in foodstuffs, and other factors touched on in the discussion of "folacin" that occupies pages 71–74 of the RDA Eighth Edition (NAS–NRC, 1974). For these reasons the RDA is always greater than the MDR. It is this latter index with which this work is concerned.

ACKNOWLEDGMENT

This work was supported by a Veterans Administration Medical Investigatorship (3570-01 and -02), Public Health Service grant AM15163 from the National Institute of General Medical Sciences, and Health Research Council of the City of New York Career Science Award I-683.

LITERATURE CITED

Alperin, J. B., Hutchinson, H. T., and Levin, W. C. 1966. Studies of folic acid requirements in megaloblastic anemia of pregnancy. Arch. Intern. Med. *117*:681–688.
Bernstein, L. H., Gutstein, S., Weiner, S., and Efron, G. 1970. The absorption and malabsorption of folic acid and its polyglutamates. Am. J. Med. *48*:570–579.
Chanarin, I. 1969. The megaloblastic anaemias. Blackwell Scientific Publications, Oxford.
Chanarin, I. 1971. Folic acid and derivatives, pp. 71-152. *In* International encyclopedia of pharmacology and therapeutics, Section 36, Hematopoietic agents, Vol. I, Hematinic agents, J. C. Dreyfus, ed. Pergamon Press, Oxford and New York.
Chanarin, I., Rothman, D., Perry, J., and Stratfull, D. 1968. Normal dietary folate, iron, and protein intake, with particular reference to pregnancy. Br. Med. J. *2*:394–397.
Colman, N., Barker, M., Green, R., and Metz, J. 1974. Prevention of folate deficiency in pregnancy by food fortification. Am. J. Clin. Nutr. *27*:339–344.
Colman, N., Larsen, J. V., Barker, M., Barker, E. A., Green, R., and Metz, J. 1975.

Prevention of folate deficiency by food fortification. III. Effect in pregnant subjects of varying amounts of added folic acid. Am. J. Clin. Nutr. 28:465–470.

Committee on Dietary Allowances. 1974. Recommended dietary allowances. Food and Nutrition Board, National Research Council, National Academy of Sciences, Washington, D.C.

Cooper, B. A. 1973. Folate and vitamin B₁₂ in pregnancy. Clin. Haematol. 2:461–476.

Druskin, M. S., Wallen, M. H., and Bonagura, L. 1962. Anticonvulsant-associated megaloblastic anemia. Response to 25 microgm. of folic acid administered by mouth daily. N. Engl. J. Med. 267:483–485.

Eichner, E. R., and Hillman, R. S. 1973. Effect of alcohol on serum folate level. J. Clin. Invest. 52:584–591.

Eichner, E. R., Pierce, H. I., and Hillman, R. S. 1971. Folate balance in dietary-induced megaloblastic anemia. N. Engl. J. Med. 284:933–938.

FAO/WHO Expert Group. 1970. Requirements of ascorbic acid, vitamin D, vitamin B₁₂, folate, and iron. WHO technical report series no. 452.

Fleming, A., Knowles, J. P., and Prankerd, T. A. 1963. Pregnancy anemia. Lancet i:606.

Gerson, C. D., Cohen, N., Hepner, G. W., Brown, N., Herbert, V., and Janowitz, H. D. 1971. Folic acid absorption in man: Enhancing effect of glucose. Gastroenterology 61:224–227.

Hansen, H., and Rybo, G. 1967. Folic acid dosage in prophylactic treatment during pregnancy. Acta Obstet. Gynecol. Scand. 46(Suppl. 7):107–112.

Herbert, V. 1962a. Experimental nutritional folate deficiency in man. Tr. Assoc. Am. Physicians 75:307–320.

Herbert, V. 1962b. Minimal daily adult folate requirement. Arch. Int. Med. 110:649–652.

Herbert, V. 1963. Current concepts in therapy. Megaloblastic anemia. N. Engl. J. Med. 268:201–203, 368–371.

Herbert, V. 1968a. Folic acid deficiency in man, p. 525. In Vitamins and hormones, Vol. 26. Academic Press, New York.

Herbert, V. 1968b. Nutritional requirements for vitamin B₁₂ and folic acid. Am. J. Clin. Nutr. 21:743–752.

Herbert, V. 1970. Drugs effective in megaloblastic anemias, pp. 1414–1444. In The pharmacologic basis of therapeutics, 4th ed., L. S. Goodman and A. Gilman, eds. The Macmillan Co., New York.

Herbert, V. 1971. Predicting nutrient deficiency by formula. N. Engl. J. Med. 284:976–977.

Herbert, V. 1972. Folate metabolism; folate deficiency in developing populations. In Lectures, XIV International Congress of Hematology, Sao Paulo, Brazil, July 16–21, 1972. Published by the Secretariat of Culture, Sports and Tourism, Government of the State of Sao Paulo.

Herbert, V. 1973. Folic acid and vitamin B₁₂, pp. 221–244. In modern nutrition in health and disease, R. S. Goodhart and M. E. Shils, eds. Lea & Febiger, Philadelphia.

Herbert, V., Colman, N., Spivack, M., Ocasio, E., Ghanta, V., Kimmel, K., Brenner, L., Freundlich, J., and Scott, J. (In press). Folic acid deficiency in the United States: Folate assays in a prenatal clinic. Am. J. Obstet. Gynecol.

Izak, G., Rachmilewitz, M., Zan, S., and Grossowicz, N. 1963. The effect of small doses of folic acid in nutritional megaloblastic anemia. Am. J. Clin. Nutr. 13:369–377.

Metz, J., Zalusky, R., and Herbert, V. 1968. Folic acid binding by serum and milk. Am. J. Clin. Nutr. 21:289–297.

National Academy of Sciences–National Research Council. 1974. Recommended Dietary Allowances, 8th ed. Publ. no. 2216.

O'Brien, W. 1968. Acute military tropical sprue in Southeast Asia. Am. J. Clin. Nutr. *21*:1007–1012.

Pritchard, J. A. 1970. Anemias complicating pregnancy and the puerperium. *In* Maternal nutrition and the course of pregnancy. Committee on Maternal Nutrition, Food and Nutrition Board, National Research Council, National Academy of Sciences, Washington, D.C.

Sheehy, T. W., Rubini, M. E., Perez-Santiago, E., Santini, R., Jr., and Haddock, J. 1961. The effect of "minute" and "titrated" amounts of folic acid on the megaloblastic anemia of tropical sprue. Blood *18*:623–636.

Sullivan, L. W., and Herbert, V. 1964. Suppression of hematopoiesis by ethanol. J. Clin. Invest. *43*:2048–2062.

Waters, A. H. 1963. Folic acid metabolism in the megaloblastic anaemias. Thesis, London.

WHO Group of Experts on Nutritional Anaemias. 1972. Nutritional anaemias. WHO technical report series no. 503.

WHO Scientific Group on Nutritional Anemias. 1968. WHO technical report series no. 405.

Willoughby, M. L. N., and Jewell, F. J. 1966. Investigation of folic acid requirements in pregnancy. Br. Med. J. *2*:1568–1571.

Wu, A., Chanarin, I., Slavin, G., and Levi, A. J. 1975. Folate deficiency in the alcoholic—its relationship to clinical and haematological abnormalities, liver disease and folate stores. Br. J. Haematol. *29*:469–478.

Zalusky, R., and Herbert, V. 1961. Megaloblastic anemia in scurvy with response to fifty micrograms of folic acid daily. N. Engl. J. Med. *265*:1033–1038.

23

Folic Acid Requirement
in Situations of
Increased Need

JOHN LINDENBAUM

Folate stores in man are so rapidly depleted (in a period of a few months) (Herbert, 1962a; Eichner and Hillman, 1971) that conditions in which there is an increased need for the vitamin may precipitate megaloblastic anemia, particularly when dietary intake is borderline. In reviews of this subject it has been customary to produce a long list of conditions felt to be associated with increased folate requirements (sometimes resembling the table of contents of a textbook of medicine). Increased folate requirement can be defined as that demonstrated by failure of folate deficiency megaloblastic anemia to respond to small doses of pteroylmonoglutamic acid (PGA) in the range of 50 to 100 μg daily in an adult, with subsequent response to pharmacologic amounts of PGA. If such a conservative definition is employed, it will be found that there are very few conditions in which an actual increase in requirement for the vitamin has been proved. The conditions for which increased folate requirement has been demonstrated are:

- Pregnancy and lactation
- Infancy

- Hemolytic anemias
- Alcohol ingestion
- Dihydrofolate reductase inhibitors

If more liberal definitions are used, such as an association with decreased serum folate levels, a longer list of conditions can be assembled. Increased folate requirement is suspected but has not been demonstrated for the following:

- Homocystinurias
- Infections and other inflammatory disorders
- Anticonvulsant drug therapy
- Myelofibrosis
- Sideroblastic anemias (nonalcoholic)
- Malignancies
- Iron deficiency anemia
- Ascorbic acid deficiency

Disturbance of folate balance has been demonstrated for the following, but it is of uncertain clinical significance.

- States of Increased Excretion
  Skin
  Urine
  Dialysis
  Bile
  Intestine
- Hyperthyroidism

And there is a question of localized increased folate utilization caused by oral contraceptive agents.

However, the interpretation of serum folate concentrations as a true indicator of folate deficiency is uncertain, especially in view of their early sensitivity to fluctuations in dietary vitamin intake (Herbert, 1962a, 1962b). Decreased red cell folate concentrations may be taken as a more reliable reflection of depleted vitamin stores, but they do not indicate increased coenzyme requirements in a given condition unless it can be shown (as has rarely been possible) that dietary folate supply has been adequate. Thus a discussion of many situations in which increased folate requirement has been suspected is inevitably a mixture of hard and soft data and more or less elegant speculation as to underlying mechanisms. We will attempt to review the current state of understanding of increased folate needs, with an emphasis, wherever possible, on separating what little has been established in this area from what is speculative and on the few controlled or experimental approaches to the problem.

PREGNANCY AND LACTATION

The increased requirements for folate during pregnancy and the puerperium are discussed in Chapter 22. Several cases with megaloblastic anemia that have required more than 100–200 μg for adequate response have been documented by Alperin et al. (1966) and Lowenstein and co-workers (1966). The amount of supplemental folate required to prevent megaloblastosis and maintain normal serum and red cell folate values is in the range of 100 to 200 μg daily (Hansen and Rybo, 1967; Chanarin et al., 1968; Chanarin, 1969). Factors postulated to be responsible for increased demands for folate include the requirements of the developing fetus and placenta, the increasing red cell mass, and, during the postpartum period, further folate losses via lactation (Chanarin, 1969).

INFANCY

In Chapter 21, Dr. Waslien reviews the evidence, that on a microgram per kilogram basis, folate requirements in infancy are increased, which is based on studies of patients with megaloblastic anemia in infancy occurring in association with poor dietary intake.

HEMOLYTIC ANEMIAS

An increased incidence of folate-deficiency megaloblastic anemia appears to be well established in patients with chronic hemolytic anemias (Lindenbaum and Klipstein, 1963; Chanarin, 1969). Most commonly this has been manifest clinically by an increase in severity of anemia beyond that characteristic for a given patient due to the hemolytic state alone (Lindenbaum and Klipstein, 1963). Reticulocytosis may persist in varying degree in many patients despite the development of the superimposed megaloblastic state (Lindenbaum and Klipstein, 1963). One or more of a variety of other factors adversely affecting folate balance has been present in at least 80 percent of the reported patients with hemolytic anemias associated with a megaloblastic bone marrow. These factors include poor diet, pregnancy, infancy, the administration of folate antagonists, infection, malabsorption, and alcohol ingestion (Lindenbaum and Klipstein, 1963). In a small number of well-studied patients, no cause of folate deficiency other than the hemolytic state has been identified (Lindenbaum and Klipstein, 1963; Alperin, 1967; Lopez *et al.*, 1973). In addition, some of the reported cases have been associated with a transient acute hemolytic anemia (Baikie and Pirrie, 1956; Pritchard *et al.*, 1965) or with a very mild chronic hemolytic state (Lindenbaum and Klipstein, 1963). The best evidence that folate requirement is indeed increased in certain patients with chronic hemolysis has been the failure of the megaloblastic changes to respond to doses of 50–200 μg of PGA given along with a folate-rich normal hospital diet (Lindenbaum and Klipstein, 1963; Alperin, 1967) with subsequent responses to doses of 300–1,000 μg daily (Lindenbaum and Klipstein, 1963; Alperin, 1967; Boineau and Coltman, 1967).

Those who develop superimposed megaloblastosis appear to represent a small fraction of patients with hemolytic anemias, perhaps of the order of 1 percent, at least in Western countries. An incidence of 5.8 percent was reported in sickle disease in Nigeria (Watson-Williams, 1965). More subtle disturbances of folate balance have been detected in a larger percentage of patients. In most surveys, substantial numbers of patients have had low serum folate concentrations (Lindenbaum and Klipstein, 1963; Pearson and Cobb, 1964; Jimenez *et al.*, 1966; Vinke *et al.*, 1969; Purugganan *et al.*, 1971; Lui, 1974, 1975; Hoffbrand, 1974) and rapid clearances of intravenously administered PGA (Chanarin *et al.*, 1959; Hogan *et al.*, 1964; Watson-Williams, 1965), findings of uncertain significance. The increased urinary formiminoglutamic acid excretion in many patients with hemolysis, even though reported to be responsive to treatment with large doses of folic acid, may not necessarily indicate significant folate deficiency (Pearson and Cobb, 1964). Red cell folate concentrations, a better indication of folate stores, but one that would tend to be elevated in patients with reticulocytosis, have been reported to be low in 0 to 18 percent of patients with hemolytic anemias (Purugganan *et al.*, 1971; Hoffbrand, 1974; Lui, 1974). It is apparent that the patient who develops megaloblastosis in the absence of other precipitating factors has an unusually high requirement for folate compared to the average patient with chronic hemolysis for reasons that have not been determined. This is supported by the tendency for folate deficiency to recur in such patients after withdrawal of therapy with pharmacologic doses of PGA (Luhby and Cooperman,

1961; Alperin, 1967; Lopez et al., 1974). In one patient, folic acid clearance remained abnormally rapid after 37 days of treatment with pharmacological doses of the vitamin (Lindenbaum and Klipstein, 1963).

It has been postulated that the tendency to develop folate deficiency in such patients is due to the increased need for folate for DNA synthesis by the hyperactive bone marrow (Chanarin et al., 1959; Lindenbaum and Klipstein, 1963). Eichner and Hillman (1971) attempted to develop an experimental model in man to test this hypothesis. Two volunteers were subjected to frequent phlebotomies and given iron supplementation to induce marrow red cell production levels of three to four times normal. They were then placed on a low-folate diet for 4 weeks with continuous daily phlebotomy. Serum folate levels fell at a rate similar to that in other subjects on the same diet who were not phlebotomized and did not reach the range of serious deficiency (below 3 ng/ml). Marrow morphology remained normoblastic (Eichner and Hillman, 1971). It is also of interest that polycythemia vera is not associated with an increased incidence of folate deficiency (Kremenchuzky and Hoffbrand, 1965).

ALCOHOL INGESTION

Megaloblastic anemia due to folate deficiency is common in chronic alcoholics who are ingesting a folate-poor diet (Herbert et al., 1963; Deller et al., 1965; Kimber et al., 1965; Klipstein and Lindenbaum, 1965; Hines, 1969; Eichner and Hillman, 1971; Lindenbaum, 1974). While almost all of the reported patients with megaloblastic anemia have had some form of alcoholic liver disease, the correlation of megaloblastic changes with severity of hepatic dysfunction has been poor (Deller et al., 1965; Klipstein and Lindenbaum, 1965), and megaloblastic anemia has only very rarely been encountered in cirrhotic patients who are teetotalers (Klipstein and Lindenbaum, 1965; Kimber et al., 1965). There is a very strong association between decreased dietary folate intake and the presence of megaloblastosis (Herbert et al., 1963; Deller et al., 1965; Klipstein and Lindenbaum, 1965; Hines, 1969; Eichner and Hillman, 1971; Lindenbaum, 1974). Certain patients, for unknown reasons, appear to be especially prone to recurrent episodes of severe folate deficiency (Lindenbaum, 1974). Many alcoholics who do not have megaloblastic changes have low serum folate concentrations (Herbert et al., 1963; Klipstein and Lindenbaum, 1965; Hines, 1969; Eichner and Hillman, 1971).

The experimental studies of Sullivan and Herbert (1964) clearly established that alcohol ingestion increases folate need. When alcohol was administered to three patients with megaloblastic anemia due to folate deficiency, the response to orally or parentally administered doses of 75 μg of folic acid was prevented or interrupted by the coadministration of alcoholic beverages or ethanol. The hematosuppressive effect of ethanol could be overcome with folate doses in the range of 150 to 500 μg. (Sullivan and Herbert, 1964). Subsequent investigators have confirmed the development of megaloblastic marrow abnormalities when alcohol and a folate-poor diet were given to human volunteers (Hines, 1969; Hines and Cowan, 1970; Eichner and Hillman, 1971; Cowan, 1973; Eichner and Hillman, 1973). In addition, Eichner and Hillman (1971, 1973) found that, when alcohol was given along with a low-folate diet, megaloblastic marrow conversion occurred much more rapidly than when on the diet alone. Megaloblastic changes did not occur when alcohol was given with folate supplements to well-nourished volunteers (Lindenbaum and Lieber, 1969; Cowan, 1973).

The manner in which alcohol increases folate requirements has not been established. Folate malabsorption may be contributory but is not the primary mechanism. Impaired jejunal uptake of folate has been demonstrated clinically in malnourished, folate-deficient alcoholics (Halsted *et al.*, 1971, 1973) and experimentally when alcohol was administered along with a folate-deficient diet (Halsted *et al.*, 1973) but not when alcohol was given with a nutritious diet (Lindenbaum and Lieber, 1971; Halsted *et al.*, 1973). In this situation, folate malabsorption may be the result rather than the cause of folate deficiency (Halsted *et al.*, 1971; Lindenbaum and Pezzimenti, 1973). Furthermore, ethanol blocked the effects of parenteral as well as oral folic acid in the studies of Sullivan and Herbert (Sullivan and Herbert, 1964).

Eichner and Hillman reported that alcohol administration to normal volunteers along with a folate-deficient diet caused a striking fall in serum folate levels within 6–8 h (Eichner and Hillman, 1973; Paine *et al.*, 1973). Since urinary folate levels remained constant, the rapid drop was interpreted as most likely due to a block in the delivery of storage methyl folate from the liver into the circulation (Eichner and Hillman, 1973).

Few other studies have been done to determine the effects of alcohol on folate metabolism. *In vitro* inhibitory effects of ethanol were found on the formate-activating liver enzyme tetrahydrofolate formylase and on formate incorporation into bone marrow cells, but the concentrations of alcohol utilized were well above those encountered clinically (Bertino *et al.*, 1965), and the importance of the enzyme in mammalian systems is uncertain. Ethanol and folate have been found to have opposite effects on the activity of several jejunal glycolytic enzymes in man (Greene *et al.*, 1974), but the significance of these observations is unknown. Hines has recently reported a reversal of the ratio of bound to free serum folate as measured by radiochemical assay in a subject receiving ethanol (Hines, 1975). In rats, Brown and colleagues (1973) recently found decreased incorporation of tritiated folic acid into hepatic polyglutamate derivatives after ethanol administration for 2 weeks.

The high incidence of serious folate deficiency in alcoholics as well as the demonstrated normal absorption of folate given with ethanol when folate deficiency is prevented (Lindenbaum and Lieber, 1971; Halsted *et al.*, 1973) would appear to be a strong argument in favor of legislation for the addition of folate to alcoholic beverages that are likely to be consumed by the population at risk.

DIHYDROFOLATE REDUCTASE INHIBITORS

The effects of these agents, which produce a cellular deficiency of reduced forms of folate, have been recently reviewed (Stebbins *et al.*, 1973).

HOMOCYSTINURIAS

In the commonly reported form of homocystinurias due to cystathionine synthase deficiency, low serum and red cell folate concentrations and rapid clearances of intravenously injected PGA are common findings (Carey *et al.*, 1968; Hoffbrand, 1974). In two patients, folic acid therapy caused a reduction in urinary homocystine excretion and an increase in methionine excretion, consistent with enhanced conversion of homocysteine to methionine (Carey *et al.*, 1968). While the evidence for an increased folate requirement seems fairly persuasive, megaloblastic anemia requiring increased amounts of therapeutic PGA has not been documented. One case of recurrent megaloblastic anemia responsive to "small doses" of folic acid has been described in this disorder, although this patient may also have had celiac disease (Butterworth *et al.*, 1971).

A very interesting patient with a less common form of homocystinuria due to deficient 5,10-methylenetetrahydrofolate reductase activity, with low serum folate concentrations in the absence of a megaloblastic anemia, has recently been reported by Freeman and co-workers (1975). Recurrent episodes were noted of a schizophrenia-like illness apparently responding to pharmacologic doses of PGA and perhaps requiring maintenance with large doses (Freeman *et al.*, 1975).

INFLAMMATORY DISEASES

Many clinicians have observed that infections often seem to precipitate megaloblastic anemia, and abnormal biochemical tests for folate deficiency have been reported in patients with tuberculosis (Roberts *et al.*, 1966; Klipstein *et al.*, 1967; Line *et al.*, 1971), regional enteritis (Hoffbrand *et al.*, 1968b), and rheumatoid arthritis (Gough *et al.*, 1964). Decreased dietary intake appears to play an important role in many cases (Klipstein *et al.*, 1967). Malabsorption during intestinal (Lindenbaum, 1965) or even systemic infections (Cook *et al.*, 1974), as well as in a minority of cases of regional enteritis (Hoffbrand *et al.*, 1968b), may be contributory. None of the reported cases with megaloblastic anemia in these disorders has been shown to require more than minute doses of folic acid, although most have been treated initially with large doses. May and colleagues (1952) reported many years ago that the experimental production of turpentine abscesses in growing monkeys receiving a diet containing borderline quantities of folate accelerated the development of megaloblastic change. Since the abscesses were associated with anorexia and decreased food intake, these studies did not unequivocally show an increased folate need. No changes in serum folate concentrations during the course of experimental sandfly fever in seven human volunteers were noted by Beisel and co-workers (1972). However, these studies involved a mild, self-limited illness in young healthy adult males who were maintained on a constant daily supplement of 500 μg of PGA (Beisel *et al.*, 1972).

ANTICONVULSANT DRUG THERAPY

Much evidence suggests an association between folate deficiency megaloblastic anemia and therapy with hydantoins and barbiturates for epilepsy (Klipstein, 1964; Chanarin, 1969; Norris and Pratt, 1974). While megaloblastic anemia is relatively rare in such patients, a high proportion has decreased serum folate concentrations and there is an increased incidence of lowered red cell folates (Klipstein, 1964;

Chanarin, 1969; Teasdale and Pearce, 1972; Hoffbrand, 1974; Norris and Pratt, 1974). Nonetheless, an increased folate requirement has not been demonstrated. Only one patient has been reported who was treated with minute doses of PGA (Druskin et al., 1962). This patient responded to 25 μg daily after not responding to diet alone during the first week in the hospital. However, she experienced a febrile illness during the first week that may have interfered with the response. Furthermore, the patient was an alcoholic on a marginal diet (Druskin et al., 1962), and the role of the anticonvulsants in causing her megaloblastic anemia is arguable.

The mechanism of anticonvulsant-associated folate deficiency has not been established. Earlier reports of inhibition of polyglutamyl folate absorption have not been confirmed, but it is possible that diphenylhydantoin may impair monoglutamyl uptake by the small bowel (Gerson et al., 1972; Stebbins et al., 1973). The hypothesis that anticonvulsants may induce an enzyme that accelerates folate metabolism (Maxwell et al., 1972) has not yet been adequately tested. While folic acid therapy may lower anticonvulsant serum levels, no effect on fit frequency or behavior has been demonstrated in controlled trials (Norris and Pratt, 1974).

MYELOFIBROSIS

A strikingly increased incidence of megaloblastic change, low serum and red cell folate levels, and increased urinary formiminoglutamic excretion was reported by Hoffbrand and colleagues (1968a) in English patients with myelofibrosis. Folate deficiency has also been reported in this disorder in the United States, but the incidence appears to be less frequent (Hogan et al., 1964; Hoffbrand, 1974). Several of the patients studied by Hoffbrand et al. (1968a) showed hematologic responses to large doses of folic acid, while one responded to 200 μg daily. In another patient who did not show any improvement in hemoglobin concentration, the bone marrow remained megaloblastic on 100 μg but became normoblastic on 500 μg (Hoffbrand et al., 1968a), suggesting an increased requirement for folate. Infection and poor diet appeared to be precipitating factors in these cases, and a mechanism whereby the presence of myelofibrosis might contribute to folate deficiency was not established, although by analogy with hemolytic anemias it is possible that there are increased folate requirements due to ineffective erythropoiesis (Hoffbrand et al., 1968a).

SIDEROBLASTIC ANEMIA

An increased incidence of folate deficiency, with megaloblastic marrow abnormalities and partial responses to folic acid therapy, has been reported in a high percentage of patients seen in England with primary sideroblastic anemias (MacGibbon and Mollin, 1965). It has been postulated that there is an increased requirement for folate by the hyperactive marrow as a result of ineffective erythropoiesis. MacGibbon and Mollin (1965) have described two patients with sideroblastic anemia, low serum folate concentrations, and megaloblastic bone marrows that did not respond to therapy with 100 μg of folic acid but who became normoblastic on pharmacologic doses. The incidence of low serum folate levels and partial responsiveness to folic acid has been much less in patients studied in the United States (Kushner *et al.*, 1971; J. Lindenbaum, unpublished observations).

MALIGNANCIES

Cases of megaloblastic anemia in association with solid tumors and hematopoietic malignancies have been reported, although the incidence of this complication appears to be less than in patients with hemolytic anemias or pregnancy (Rose, 1966; Hoffbrand *et al.*, 1967; Chanarin, 1970). The degree of megaloblastic change has often not been severe (Hoffbrand *et al.*, 1967). In a few cases, responses to PGA have been reported (Rose, 1966; Hoffbrand *et al.*, 1967; Chanarin, 1970; Alperin *et al.*, 1971). However, there has not been a clear-cut demonstration of an increased requirement for the vitamin by therapy with titrated doses of increasing amounts of folate, and several patients have responded to doses in the order of 50–200 μg daily* (Hoffbrand *et al.*, 1967; Chanarin, 1970; Alperin *et al.*, 1971). Decreased dietary folate intake and, in occasional cases, malabsorption (Rose, 1966) may have been of paramount importance in the development of megaloblastic anemia in these patients, and the etiologic role of increased folate utilization by the tumor, while an attractive concept, has not yet been demonstrated in man (Alperin *et al.*, 1971).

---

*One patient, mentioned by Hoffbrand and colleagues (1967), with multiple myeloma and intermediate megaloblastic changes, was said to show successive "small reticulocyte responses" without other hematologic improvement during therapy with 0.2 and 15 mg doses of PGA.

266 JOHN LINDENBAUM

A high incidence of low serum folate levels, rapid clearances of intravenously administered PGA, and increased excretion of urinary formiminoglutamic acid have been reported by many observers in patients with malignant disease (Chanarin, 1969). Even after repeated pharmacologic doses of folic acid, the clearance of the vitamin has remained rapid (Chanarin and Bennett, 1962). On the other hand, a much lower incidence of decreased red cell folate values (8–16 percent) has been reported in patients with cancer (Magnus, 1967; Hoffbrand, 1974).

An attempt by Gailani and colleagues (1970) to treat seven patients with advanced cancer with a folate-deficient diet for periods of 25 to 140 days was of interest, though not a therapeutic success. The rate of development of folate deficiency in these patients appeared to be similar to that reported in normal subjects (Herbert, 1962a, 1962b). Tumor folate levels fell at a similar rate to hepatic and erythrocyte concentrations (Gailani et al., 1970).

Reports in the literature of the acceleration of leukemia by the administration of folic acid have been anecdotal and incompletely documented (Farber et al., 1948; Heinle and Welch, 1948). The observation that folic acid administration and withdrawal is associated with exacerbation and remission in chronic myelogenous leukemia (Heinle and Welch, 1948) was made before the phenomenon of spontaneous cyclic leukocytosis in this disease was recognized (Morley et al., 1967).

IRON DEFICIENCY

In view of the frequent association of folate and iron deficiency in clinical practice, a number of authors have speculated that iron deficiency may increase folate requirements. The evidence for this at present is equivocal and unconvincing (Chanarin and Rothman, 1971; Lui, 1975).

ASCORBIC ACID DEFICIENCY

Whether the association of scurvy and megaloblastic anemia is due to increased folate requirements secondary to ascorbate lack or is merely a result of a double nutritional deficiency state is a subject of unresolved controversy (Chanarin, 1969).

INCREASED FOLATE EXCRETION

Increased folate losses via desquamated skin in patients with extensive dermatologic disorders such as exfoliative dermatitis and psoriasis have been documented (Hild, 1969; Touraine *et al.*, 1973), and serum and red cell folates are decreased in a number of these patients (Shuster *et al.*, 1967; Hild, 1969; Touraine *et al.*, 1973), but it is doubtful whether the amounts of folate lost via this route could cause megaloblastic anemia in the absence of other disturbances of vitamin balance. The same can be said of the well-documented small folate losses occurring during hemodialysis or peritoneal dialysis in patients with renal disease (Whitehead *et al.*, 1968; Sevitt and Hoffbrand, 1969), and of the increased urinary folate excretion in liver disease (Retief and Huskisson, 1969), congestive heart failure (Retief and Huskisson, 1969), and pregnancy (Fleming, 1972). Folate coenzymes appear to undergo an extensive enterohepatic recirculation, and folate concentrations in bile are severalfold higher than those in serum (Baker *et al.*, 1965). It is therefore conceivable that extensive folate losses might occur with prolonged vomiting, nasogastric suction, or in malabsorption syndromes in which the enterohepatic circulation is interrupted. In the latter situation, folate loss in desquamated intestinal cells might also contribute to a folate-losing enteropathy (Baker, 1968). A patient was reported recently with severe prolonged vomiting due to pancreatitis in whom folate deficiency megaloblastic anemia developed over a period of several weeks of continuous removal of gastroduodenal fluids by suction while receiving parenteral hyperalimentation with folate-free solutions (Ballard and Lindenbaum, 1974).

THYROTOXICOSIS

Animals made hyperthyroid by the administration of thyroid hormone have decreased hepatic stores of folate (Noronha and Sreenivasan, 1959). Low serum folate concentrations, rapid folic acid clearances, and increased urinary formiminoglutamic acid excretion have been reported in patients with untreated thyrotoxicosis (Lindenbaum and Klipstein, 1964; Mohamed and Roberts, 1965; Rigas *et al.*, 1968). In two recent series, however, decreased serum folate levels were not encountered (Elman *et al.*, 1970; Caplan *et al.*, 1975). If a disturbance in folate balance related to increased metabolic requirements occurs in the hyperthyroid state, it appears to be a mild one, since megaloblastic anemia due to folate deficiency has not been reported. The tendency to hyperphagia in this disorder (Thomas et al., 1973) may result in compensatory increases in folate intake in many patients.

ORAL CONTRACEPTIVE AGENTS

The possible relationship of therapy with oral contraceptive agents (OCA) with disturbances in folate metabolism has been the subject of a recent review (Lindenbaum et al., 1975). Thirty-one case reports of folate deficiency megaloblastic anemia in women taking OCA have been reported in the literature since 1969 (Lewis, 1974; Green, 1975; Lindenbaum et al., 1975). In several of the reported cases, other factors causing folate lack, such as poor dietary intake or occult celiac disease, have been present, or the folate deficiency has persisted or recurred after cessation of therapy with OCA (Green, 1975; Lindenbaum et al., 1975). In view of the extensive use of OCA and the rarity of this complication, the role of OCA in the etiology of megaloblastic anemia is not yet established. Several reports of decreased serum and/or red cell folate concentrations in women taking OCA have conflicted with those of other groups (Davis and Smith, 1974; Lindenbaum et al., 1975; Paine et al., 1975; Prasad et al., 1975; Smith et al., 1975). Earlier claims of impairment of pteroylpolyglutamate absorption by OCA have also not been confirmed by subsequent workers (Lindenbaum et al., 1975). Shojania (1975) has recently reported rapid clearances of intravenously administered folic acid in a small group of women on OCA. He also found that women taking OCA excreted more folate in the urine for a given level of serum or red cell folate than controls (Shojania, 1975). This is of interest in view of Fleming's finding (1972) of increased urinary folate excretion in pregnancy.

N. Whitehead and colleagues (1973) have recently demonstrated abnormal cytologic findings on Papanicolaou-stained cervicovaginal smears in 19 percent of a group of 115 women taking OCA. The cytologic changes resembled those described (Van Niekerk, 1966) in folate deficiency megaloblastic anemia but were generally less florid (Whitehead et al., 1973). The changes were seen in women on a variety of estrogen–progestin combinations as well as on progestins only. They were not associated with anemia, increased neutrophil lobe counts, macrocytosis, or decreased serum folate levels. However, after therapy with pharmacological doses of PGA, the cervical abnormalities reverted to normal (Whitehead et al., 1973). These changes tended to recur on OCA after withdrawal of folate therapy (Lindenbaum et al., 1975). We have postulated that these "megaloblastic" cervicovaginal abnormalities are the result of a localized increased need for folate coenzymes at the target organ level in women taking sex steroids (Whitehead *et al.*, 1973; Lindenbaum *et al.*, 1975). A localized disorder of folate transport into cervical cells is another possibility. Much further work needs to be done to test these hypotheses.

The concept of a folate deficiency state localized to a particular cell line is not a new one. Hoffbrand and Newcombe (1967), for example, reported an interesting group of patients with gastrointestinal disorders whose bone marrows showed normoblastic erythropoiesis but megaloblastic granulocytopoiesis. Several of these patients had normal urinary formiminoglutamic acid excretion and red cell folate concentrations while leukocyte folate levels were decreased, suggesting a deficiency state localized to white cells (Hoffbrand and Newcombe, 1967).

CONCLUSIONS

1. Clearcut evidence of increased folate requirement is present in conditions where megaloblastic anemia is not responsive to doses of PGA similar to the minimal daily requirement and subsequently is corrected by pharmacologic doses.

2. This stringent criterion for increased folate need has been met in patients with megaloblastic anemia associated with pregnancy, infancy, hemolytic anemias, and alcohol intoxication. While it has been speculated that folate deficiency occurs in hemolytic anemias because of increased coenzyme utilization by the hyperactive marrow, no evidence to support this hypothesis has been produced to date.

3. In the homocystinurias, megaloblastic anemia requiring pharmacologic doses of PGA has not been reported, but the high incidence of folate deficiency and the fall in urinary homocystine excretion following folic acid therapy are suggestive of a state of increased folate utilization.

4. Despite suggestive clinical observations, an increased folate need has not been clearly demonstrated in inflammatory disorders or in patients taking anticonvulsant drugs.

5. In rare patients with myelofibrosis and sideroblastic anemias, morphologic responses to titrated doses of PGA (without improvement in hemoglobin levels) have been reported.

6. There is no evidence in man that malignancies increase folate requirement.

7. It has not yet been proven that folic acid need is increased in either iron deficiency anemia or scurvy.

8. Increased folate excretion may occur via the skin, urine, hemodialysis or peritoneal dialysis, bile, or gastrointestinal tract, but it is doubtful whether the magnitude of vitamin losses by any of these routes would be great enough to result in severe folate deficiency in the absence of other causes.

9. While it is possible that mild folate deficiency occurs in some patients with hyperthyroidism, no cases have been reported in which megaloblastic anemia due to folic acid deficiency has developed.

10. The concept that folate deficiency may be localized to certain tissues requires further testing. Megaloblastic cervical abnormalities in women taking oral contraceptive agents that disappear after treatment with PGA and folate-deficient megaloblastic leukopoiesis associated with normal erythrocyte morphology and folate concentrations may be examples of such disorders.

11. A critical review of the current status of knowledge of disorders of folate utilization thus demonstrates how little has been established. Many widely accepted assertions in this area remain speculative. Progress in our understanding of these disorders will no doubt be accelerated when reliable methods for studying folate catabolism and reutilization are developed.

DISCUSSION

HERBERT: There is at least one direct test for measuring localized folate deficiency, the so-called deoxyuridine (dU) suppression test (i.e., the ability of nonradioactive dU to suppress the incorporation of subsequently added radioactive thymidine into human cells *in vitro*). We applied this test to several women on oral contraceptives. In one woman, who, before she began taking oral contraceptives had normal vaginal epithelium, we found, after she had been taking oral contraceptives for 3 months, a vaginal epithelium as described by Dr. Lindenbaum. This woman, at that time, had a dU suppression, normal serum and red cell folate, megaloblastic vaginal epithelium, normal bone marrow dU suppression test, but subnormal lymphocyte dU suppression test, which was corrected to normal by adding folate.

We have extended this observation to iron deficiency because of the reports in the literature of some patients with iron deficiency who have hypersegmentation. It has been noted that in four patients with iron deficiency, who had neutrophil hypersegmentation but normal serum and red cell folate levels, all four had subnormal dU suppression tests in their lymphocytes, which were corrected to normal by adding folate *in vitro*, but normal bone marrow du suppression tests. So this is further evidence that there is localized folate deficiency in some cell lines and not in others. In the oral contraceptive patient, the affected cell lines may include the vaginal epithelium and the white cell lines, but not the red cell lines. Again with iron deficiency, the white cell line may have folate deficiency and the red cell line not have folate deficiency.

cooper: The problem of the use of the du suppression test for folate deficiency in lymphocytes is a difficult one. Barbara Bain has found that the folate requirements for lymphocytes in culture may be greatly in excess of those generally considered adequate for the intact human. In her study the quantity of DNA synthesized by lymphocytes in mixed lymphocyte culture, and the number of cells generated, was directly proportional to the folic acid present in the medium between 10 and 120 ng/ml. She and we were able to demonstrate that folate in the medium was not depleted during incubation, and that the requirement for methyltetrahydrofolate was similar to that for folic acid. From our studies with du penetration into lymphocytes, as a measure of DNA synthesis, and with Dr. Bain's studies with folate requirement in lymphocytes, it has become apparent that du does not penetrate lymphocytes nearly as readily as does thymidine or that iododeoxyuridine incorporation into DNA is decreased. We have not yet determined if this is due to competition for transport or to dilution of the thymidylate pool in the cells.

Because the PHA response does not require cellular proliferation, Dr. Hoffbrand and others have demonstrated that it is not significantly altered by methotrexate. Thymidine incorporation into lymphocytes stimulated by PHA is variably affected by folic, but in most it is decreased. Because the lymphocyte is relatively impermeable to du, and because of its peculiar folate requirements in culture, it is our conviction that the du suppression test, which has been so successful and so well documented for study of bone marrow, requires considerable investigation and evaluation before it can be applied to lymphocytes in culture.

LITERATURE CITED

Alperin, J. B. 1967. Folic acid deficiency complicating sickle cell anemia. Arch. Intern. Med. *120*:298–306.

Alperin, J. B., Hutchinson, H. T., and Levin, W. C. 1966. Studies of folic acid requirements in megaloblastic anemia of pregnancy. Arch. Intern. Med. *117*:681.

Alperin, J. B., Haggard, M. E., and Levin, W. C. 1971. The effects of disseminated malignancies on folic acid (FA) requirements in man. Clin. Res. *19*:36.

Baikie, A. G., and Pirrie, R. 1956. Megaloblastic erythropoiesis in idiopathic acquired haemolytic anaemia. Scott. Med. J. *1*:330–334.

Baker, S. J. 1968. Discussion of Dr. Herbert's paper. Vitam. Horm. *26*:537–538.

Baker, S. J., Kumar, S., and Swaminathan, S. P. 1965. Excretion of folic acid in bile. Lancet *i*:685.

Ballard, H. S., and Lindenbaum, J. 1974. Megaloblastic anemia complicating hyperalimentation therapy. Am. J. Med. *56*:740–742.

Beisel, W. R., Herman, Y. F., Sauberlich, H. E., Herman, R. H., Bartelloni, P. J., and Canham, J. E. 1972. Experimentally induced sandfly fever and vitamin metabolism in man. Am. J. Clin. Nutr. 25:1165–1173.

Bertino, J. R., Ward, J., Sartorelli, A. C., and Silber, R. 1965. An effect of ethanol on folate metabolism. J. Clin. Invest. 44:1028.

Boineau, M. C., and Coltman, C. A., Jr. 1967. Titrated folic acid requirement in the hemolytic anemia associated with an intracardiac prosthetic device. Clin. Res. 15:272.

Brown, J. P., Davidson, G. E., Scott, J. M., and Weir, D. G. 1973. Effect of diphenylhydantoin and ethanol feeding on the synthesis of rat liver folates from exogenous pteroylglutamate [3H]. Biochem. Pharmacol. 22:3287–3289.

Butterworth, C. E., Jr., Krumdieck, C. L., and Baugh, C. M. 1971. Studies on the absorption and metabolism of folic acid II. Homocystinuria. Ala. J. Med. Sci. 8:30–43.

Caplan, R. H., Davis, K., Bengston, B., and Smith, M. J. 1975. Serum folate and vitamin B_{12} levels in hypothyroid and hyperthyroid patients. Arch. Intern. Med. 135:701–704.

Carey, M. C., Fennelly, J. J., and FitzGerald, O. 1968. Homocystinuria. II. Subnormal serum folate levels, increased folate clearance and effects of folic therapy. Am. J. Med. 45:26–31.

Chanarin, I. 1969. The megaloblastic anemias. F. A. Davis Co., Philadelphia.

Chanarin, I. 1970. Folate deficiency in the myeloproliferative disorders. Am. J. Clin. Nutr. 23:855–860.

Chanarin, I., and Bennett, M. C. 1962. The plasma clearance of daily doses of folic acid in megaloblastic anaemia. Br. J. Haematol. 8:95–109.

Chanarin, I., and Rothman, D. 1971. Further observations on the relation between iron and folate status in pregnancy. Br. Med. J. 2:81–84.

Chanarin, I., Dacie, J. V., and Mollin, D. L. 1959. Folic-acid deficiency in haemolytic anaemia. Br. J. Haematol. 5:245–256.

Chanarin, I., Rothman, D., Ward, A., and Perry, J. 1968. Folate status and requirement in pregnancy. Br. Med. J. 2:390–394.

Cook, G. C., Morgan, J. O., and Hoffbrand, A. V. 1974. Impairment of folate absorption by systemic bacterial infections. Lancet ii:1416–1417.

Cowan, D. H. 1973. Thrombokinetic studies in alcohol-related thrombocytopenia. J. Lab. Clin. Med. 81:64–76.

Davis, R. E., and Smith, B. K. 1974. Pyridoxal, vitamin B_{12} and folate metabolism in women taking oral contraceptive agents. S. Afr. Med. J. 48:1937–1940.

Deller, D. J., Kimber, C. L., and Ibbotson, R. N. 1965. Folic acid deficiency in cirrhosis of the liver. Am. J. Dig. Dis. 10:35–41.

Druskin, M. S., Wallen, M. H., and Bonagura, L. 1962. Anticonvulsant-associated megaloblastic anemia. N. Engl. J. Med. 267:483–485.

Eichner, E. R., and Hillman, R. S. 1971. The evolution of anemia in alcoholic patients. Am. J. Med. 50:218–232.

Eichner, E. R., and Hillman, R. S. 1973. Effect of alcohol on serum folate level. J. Clin. Invest. 52:584–591.

Eichner, E. R., Pierce, I., and Hillman, R. S. 1971. Folate balance in dietary-induced megaloblastic anemia. N. Engl. J. Med. 284:933–938.

Elman, A., Einhorn, J., Olhagen, B., and Reizenstein, P. 1970. Metabolic studies of folic acid in non-malignant diseases. Acta Med. Scand. 187:347–352.

Farber, S., Diamond, L. K., Mercer, R. D., Sylvester, R. F., and Wolff, J. A. 1948. Temporary remissions in acute leukemia in children produced by folic acid antagonist, 4-aminopteroyl-glutamic acid (aminopterin). N. Engl. J. Med. 238:787–793.

Fleming, A. F. 1972. Urinary excretion of folate in pregnancy. J. Obstet. Gynaecol. Br. Commonw. 79:916.

Freeman, J. M., Finkelstein, J. D., and Mudd, S. H. 1975. Folate-responsive homocystinuria and "schizophrenia." N. Engl. J. Med. *292*:491–496.

Gailani, S. D., Carey, R. W., Holland, J. F., and O'Malley, J. A. 1970. Studies of folate deficiency in patients with neoplastic diseases. Cancer Res. *30*:327–333.

Gerson, C. D., Hepner, G. W., Brown, N., Cohen, N., Herbert, V., and Janowitz, H. D. 1972. Inhibition by diphenylhydantoin of folic acid absorption in man. Gastroenterology *63*:246–251.

Green, J. D. 1975. Megaloblastic anemia in a vegetarian taking oral contraceptives. South. Med. J. *68*:249–250.

Greene, H. L., Stifel, F. B., Herman, R. H., Herman, Y. F., and Rosensweig, N. S. 1974. Ethanol-induced inhibition of human intestinal enzyme activities: Reversal by folic acid. Gastroenterology *67*:434–440.

Gough, K. R., McCarthy, C., Read, A. E., Mollin, D. L., and Waters, A. H. 1964. Folic-acid deficiency in rheumatoid arthritis. Br. Med. J. *1*:212–217.

Halsted, C. H., Robles, E. A., and Mezey, E. 1971. Decreased jejunal uptake of labeled folic acid (^{3}H-PGA) in alcoholic patients: Roles of alcohol and nutrition. N. Engl. J. Med. *285*:701–706.

Halsted, C. H., Robles, E. A., and Mezey, E. 1973. Intestinal malabsorption in folate-deficient alcoholics. Gastroenterology *64*:526–532.

Hansen, H., and Rybo, G. 1967. Folic acid dosage in prophylactic treatment during pregnancy. Acta Obstet. Gynecol. Scand. Suppl. *7*:107–112.

Heinle, R. W., and Welch, A. D. 1948. Experiments with pteroylglutamic acid and pteroylglutamic acid deficiency in human leukemia. J. Clin. Invest. *27*:539a.

Herbert, V. 1962a. Experimental nutritional folate deficiency in man. Trans. Assoc. Am. Physicians *75*:307–320.

Herbert, V. 1962b. Minimal daily adult folate requirement. Arch. Intern. Med. *110*:649–652.

Herbert, V., Zalusky, R., and Davidson, C. S. 1963. Correlation of folate deficiency with alcoholism and associated macrocytosis, anemia, and liver disease. Ann. Int. Med. *58*:977–988.

Hild, D. H. 1969. Folate losses from the skin in exfoliative dermatitis. Arch. Intern. Med. *123*:51–54.

Hines, J. D. 1969. Reversible megaloblastic and sideroblastic marrow abnormalities in alcoholic patients. Br. J. Haematol. *16*:87–101.

Hines, J. D. 1975. Hematologic abnormalities involving vitamin B_6 and folate metabolism in alcoholic subjects. Ann. N. Y. Acad. Sci. *252*:316–327.

Hines, J. D., and Cowan, D. H. 1970. Studies on the pathogenesis of alcohol-induced sideroblastic bone-marrow abnormalities. N. Engl. J. Med. *283*:441–446.

Hoffbrand, A. V. 1974. Vitamin B_{12} and folate metabolism: The megaloblastic anemias and related disorders, pp. 392–472. *In* Blood and its disorders, R. M. Hardisty and D. T. Weatherall, eds. Blackwell, Oxford.

Hoffbrand, A. V., and Newcombe, B. F. A. 1967. Leucocyte folate in vitamin B_{12} and folate deficiency and in leukaemia. Br. J. Haematol. *13*:954–966.

Hoffbrand, A. V., Hobbs, J. R., Kremenchuzky, S., and Mollin, D. L. 1967. Incidence and pathogenesis of megaloblastic erythropoiesis in multiple myeloma. J. Clin. Pathol. *20*:699–705.

Hoffbrand, A. V., Chanarin, I., Kremenchuzky, S., Szur, L., Waters, A. H., and Mollin, D. L. 1968a. Megaloblastic anaemia in myelosclerosis. Q. J. Med. *37*:493–516.

Hoffbrand, A. V., Stewart, J. S., Booth, C. C., and Mollin, D. L. 1968b. Folate deficiency in Crohn's disease: Incidence, pathogenesis, and treatment. Br. Med. J. *2*:71–75.

Hogan, J. A., Maniatis, A., and Moloney, W. C. 1964. The serum *Lactobacillus casei* folate clearance test in various hematologic disorders. Blood 24:187–197.

Jimenez, C. T., Scott, R. B., Henry, W. L., Sampson, C. C., and Ferguson, A. D. 1966. Studies in sickle cell anemia. Am. J. Dis. Child. 111:497–504.

Kimber, C. L., Deller, D. J., and Lander, H. 1965. Megaloblastic and transitional megaloblastic anemia associated with chronic liver disease. Am. J. Med. 38:767–777.

Klipstein, F. A. 1964. Subnormal serum folate and macrocytosis associated with anticonvulsant drug therapy. Blood 23:68–86.

Klipstein, F. A., and Lindenbaum, J. 1965. Folate deficiency in chronic liver disease. Blood 25:443–455.

Klipstein, F. A., Berlinger, F. G., and Reed, L. J. 1967. Folate deficiency associated with drug therapy for tuberculosis. Blood 29:697–712.

Kremenchuzky, S., and Hoffbrand, A. V. 1965. Folate deficiency in polycythaemia rubra vera. Br. J. Haematol. 11:600.

Kushner, J. P., Lee, G. R., Wintrobe, M. M., and Cartwright, G. E. 1971. Idiopathic refractory sideroblastic anemia. Clinical and laboratory investigation of 17 patients and review of the literature. Medicine 50:139–159.

Lewis, F. B. 1974. Folate deficiency due to oral contraceptives. Minn. Med. 57:945–946.

Lindenbaum, J. 1965. Malabsorption during and after recovery from acute intestinal infection. Br. Med. J. 2:326–329.

Lindenbaum, J. 1974. Hematologic effects of alcohol, pp. 461–480. *In* The biology of alcoholism, Vol. 3: Clinical pathology, B. Kissin and H. Begleiter, eds. Plenum Press, New York.

Lindenbaum, J., and Klipstein, F. A. 1963. Folic acid deficiency in sickle-cell anemia. N. Engl. J. Med. 269:875–882.

Lindenbaum, J., and Klipstein, F. A. 1964. Folic acid clearances and basal serum folate levels in patients with thyroid disease. J. Clin. Pathol. 17:666–670.

Lindenbaum, J., and Lieber, C. S. 1969. Hematologic effects of alcohol in man in the absence of nutritional deficiency. N. Engl. J. Med. 281:333–338.

Lindenbaum, J., and Lieber, C. S. 1971. Effects of ethanol on the blood, bone marrow, and small intestine of man, pp. 27–53. *In* Biological aspects of alcohol, M. D. Roach, W. M. McIsaac, and P. J. Creaven, eds. University of Texas Press, Austin.

Lindenbaum, J., and Pezzimenti, J. F. 1973. Effects of B_{12} and folate deficiency on small intestinal function. Clin. Res. 21:518.

Lindenbaum, J., Whitehead, N., and Reyner, F. 1975. Oral contraceptive hormones, folate metabolism, and the cervical epithelium. Am. J. Clin. Nutr. 28:346–353.

Line, D. H., Seitanidis, B., Morgan, J. O., and Hoffbrand, A. V. 1971. The effects of chemotherapy on iron, folate, and vitamin B_{12} metabolism in tuberculosis. Q. J. Med. 40:331–340.

Lopez, R., Shimizu, N., and Cooperman, J. M. 1973. Recurrent folic acid deficiency in sickle cell disease. Am. J. Dis. Child. 125:544–548.

Lowenstein, L., Brunton, L., and Hsieh, Y.-S. 1966. Nutritional anemia and megaloblastosis in pregnancy. Can. Med. Assoc. J. 94:636–645.

Luhby, A. L., and Cooperman, J. M. 1961. Folic-acid deficiency in thalassaemia major. Lancet ii:490–491.

Lui, Y. K. 1974. Folate deficiency in children with sickle cell anemia. Am. J. Dis. Child. 127:389–393.

Lui, Y. K. 1975. Folic acid deficiency in sickle cell anaemia. Scand. J. Haematol. 14:71–79.

MacGibbon, B. H., and Mollin, D. L. 1965. Sideroblastic anaemia in man: Observations on seventy cases. Br. J. Haematol. 11:59–69.

Magnus, E. M. 1967. Folate activity in serum and red cells of patients with cancer. Cancer Res. *27*:490–497.

Maxwell, J. D., Hunter, J., Stewart, D. A., Ardeman, S., and Williams, R. 1972. Folate deficiency after anticonvulsant drugs: An effect of hepatic enzyme induction? Br. Med. J. *1*:297–299.

May, C. D., Stewart, C. T., Hamilton, A., and Salmon, R. J. 1952. Infection as a cause of folic acid deficiency and megaloblastic anemia. Am. J. Dis. Child. *84*:718–728.

Mohamed, S. D., and Roberts, M. 1965. Abnormal histidine metabolism in thyrotoxicosis in man. Lancet *ii*:933–935.

Morley, A. A., Baikie, A. G., and Galton, D. A. G. 1967. Cyclic leukocytosis as evidence for retention of normal homeostatic control in chronic granulocytic leukemia. Lancet *ii*:1320–1323.

Noronha, J. M., and Sreenivasan, A. 1959. Formate metabolism in the vitamin B_{12}-deficient rat. Biochem J. *73*:732–735.

Norris, J. W., and Pratt, R. F. 1974. Folic acid deficiency and epilepsy. Drugs *8*:366–385.

Paine, C. J., Eichner, E. R., and Dickson, V. 1973. Concordance of radioassay and microbiological assay in the study of the ethanol-induced fall in serum folate level. Am. J. Med. Sci. *266*:135–138.

Paine, C. J., Grafton, W. D., Dickson, V. L., and Eichner, E. R. 1975. Oral contraceptives, serum folate, and hematologic status. J. Am. Med. Assoc. *231*:731–733.

Pearson, H. A., and Cobb, W. T. 1964. Folic acid studies in sickle-cell anemia. J. Lab. Clin. Med. *64*:913–921.

Prasad, A. S., Lei, K. Y., Oberleas, D., Moghissi, K. S., and Stryker, J. 1975. Effect of oral contraceptive agents on nutrients. II. Vitamins. Am. J. Clin. Nutr. *28*:385–391.

Pritchard, J., Scott, D. E., and Mason, R. A. 1965. Severe anemia with hemolysis and megaloblastic erythropoiesis. J. Am. Med. Assoc. *194*:457–459.

Purugganan, G., Leikin, S., and Gautier, G. 1971. Folate metabolism in erythroid hyperplastic and hypoplastic states. Am. J. Dis. Child. *122*:48–52.

Retief, F. P., and Huskisson, Y. J. 1969. Serum and urinary folate in liver disease. Br. Med. J. *2*:150–153.

Rigas, A. N., Wilson, E. A., and Montgomery, D. A. 1968. Folic acid metabolism in thyroid disease. Ir. J. Med. Sci. *7*:255–261.

Roberts, P. D., Hoffbrand, A. V., and Mollin, D. L. 1966. Iron and folate metabolism in tuberculosis. Br. Med. J. *2*:198–202.

Rose, D. P. 1966. Folic acid deficiency in leukaemia and lymphomas. J. Clin. Pathol. *19*:29–32.

Sevitt, L. H., and Hoffbrand, A. V. 1969. Serum folate and vitamin B_{12} levels in acute and chronic renal disease. Effect of peritoneal dialysis. Br. Med. J. *2*:18–21.

Shojania, A. M. 1975. The effect of oral contraceptives on folate metabolism. III. Plasma clearance and urinary folate excretion. J. Lab. Clin. Med. *85*:185–190.

Shuster, S., Marks, J., and Chanarin, I. 1967. Folic acid deficiency in patients with skin disease. Br. J. Dermatol. *79*:398–402.

Smith, J. L., Goldsmith, G. A., and Lawrence, J. D. 1975. Effects of oral contraceptive steroids on vitamin and lipid levels in serum. Am. J. Clin. Nutr. *28*:371–376.

Stebbins, R., Scott, J., and Herbert, V. 1973. Drug-induced megaloblastic anemias. Semin. Hematol. *10*:235–251.

Sullivan, L. W., and Herbert, V. 1964. Suppression of hematopoiesis by ethanol. J. Clin. Invest. *43*:2048–2062.

Teasdale, P. R., and Pearce, J. 1972. Comparative and serial assays of folate metabolism in anticonvulsant-treated epileptics. J. Clin. Pathol. *25*:721–725.

Thomas, F. B., Caldwell, J. H., and Greenberger, N. J. 1973. Steatorrhea in thyrotoxicosis. Ann. Intern. Med. 78:669–675.

Touraine, R., Revus, J., Zittoun, J., Jarret, J., and Tulliez, M. 1973. Study of folate in psoriasis: Blood levels, intestinal absorption and cutaneous loss. Br. J. Dermatol. 89:335–341.

Van Niekerk, W. A. 1966. Cervical cytological abnormalities caused by folic acid deficiency. Acta Cytol. 10:67–73.

Vinke, B., Piers, A., and Irausquin-Cath, H. 1969. Folic acid and vitamin B_{12} deficiencies in negroid hospital patients on Curacao. Trop. Geogr. Med. 21:401–406.

Watson-Williams, E. J. 1965. The role of folic acid in the treatment of sickle-cell disease, pp. 435–443. In Abnormal hemoglobins in Africa, J. H. P. Jones, ed. Oxford, London.

Whitehead, N., Reyner, F., and Lindenbaum, J. 1973. Megaloblastic changes in the cervical epithelium. J. Am. Med. Assoc. 226:1421–1424.

Whitehead, V. M., Comty, C. H., Posen, G. A., and Kaye, M. 1968. Homeostasis of folic acid in patients undergoing maintenance hemodialysis. N. Engl. J. Med. 279:970–974.

24

Summary of
the Workshop

VICTOR HERBERT

This Workshop covered the biochemical, physiological, nutritional, gastroenterologic, hematologic, and other facets of human folate requirement. As such, it ranged across forms in which the vitamin may be ingested and mechanisms of absorption, transport, distribution, utilization, fate, and excretion.

FOLATE BIOCHEMISTRY

Folate biochemistry, from the point of view of the most recent research, was reviewed by Blakley. He noted that recent claims of methylation of biogenic amines by methylfolate appear incorrect; what appears to happen is that the methylene tetrahydrofolate reductase reaction reverses, producing tetrahydrofolate and formaldehyde, and the latter combines with the amine (such as in the methylation of dopamine to yield epinine). Recent work from the laboratory of Rabinowitz indicates that in certain bacteria folate is involved in methylation of transfer RNA bases, suggesting that investigation of this possibility is needed in humans.

277

Recent work suggests that in mammalian cells, as well as in bacterial cells, folates control their own enzymes by feedback inhibition and end product repression. Formyl folate appears to be one of the most inhibitory of the naturally occurring folate derivatives. It appears on the serosal side of everted sacs when folate is supplied on the mucosal side; Chanarin noted that the formyl form was then rapidly converted to the methyl form.

Antifolates may enhance the production of folate apoenzymes. Although it had been suggested that the rise in thymidylate synthetase produced by methotrexate may relate to accumulation of thymidine triphosphate, Hoffbrand stated that deficit rather than accumulation occurs.

In a colloquy between Blakley and Scott, it became clear that it is not yet certain whether 10-formyl folic acid is an inhibitor of or a substrate for dihydrofolate reductase; Stokstad noted it could not be inhibitory because it is as active as tetrahydrofolate.

BIOLOGICAL ROLE OF POLYGLUTAMATES

The biological role of polyglutamates was reviewed by Krumdieck. One function appears to be to reduce the ability of folate to leave cells, since ovaries of mutant Chinese hamsters that cannot make polyglutamate have very low folate levels. Some bacterial apoenzymes only function with folate polyglutamate coenzyme, but this has not yet been demonstrated in a mammalian cell.

Folate polyglutamates may activate such non-folate-requiring enzymes as cystathionine synthetase; conversely, glutamic dehydrogenase, another non-folate-requiring enzyme in mitochondria, is inhibited by both oxidized and tetrahydro- forms of folate. Polyglutamate forms up to heptaglutamate inhibit it even more.

In rapidly proliferating cells, such as those of the rat uterus, slime mold, and quail liver, high folate polyglutamate and high conjugase activity appear to run together. Hoffbrand raised the question of whether the conjugase increase could be part of a general increase in all lysosomal enzymes; Rosenberg cautioned that not all conjugase may originate from lysosomes.

DOMINANT POLYGLUTAMYL CHAIN LINKS IN MAMMALIAN CELLS

These were discussed by Scott. The amount of each polyglutamate form depends on the balance between the speeds of anabolism versus catabolism, so that, in the short term (1 day) pentaglutamate predominates, with lesser amounts of tetra- and heptaglutamates. In the long term, folate hexa- and heptaglutamates predominate. There is some evidence that increased concentrations of extracellular folate result in intracellular polyglutamates of shorter chain lengths, as shown by Stokstad.

In discussion, Scott noted that tissue polyglutamate is preserved by extraction at pH 9 because conjugase is inactive at this pH. Subsequent boiling destroys the conjugase so that pH may then be safely lowered without reducing polyglutamate chain length. Boiling in ascorbate at pH 9 appears to yield 70–100 percent extraction of radioactively labeled folate from rat liver.

DISTRIBUTION OF FOLATE FORMS IN FOOD AND FOLATE AVAILABILITY

These were reviewed by Stokstad. The main methods for determining distribution of folates are column separation of the intact folates, using Sephadex followed by DEAE, and separation of the polyglutamates after breaking them at the 9,10 position. Using the former method, Stokstad's group noted that practically all milk folate is in methyl form, whereas in soybean about 65 percent is 5-formyl. Cabbage contains a conjugase that at pH 6–7 reduces extracted chain length to triglutamate and, at more acid pH, to monoglutamate. To determine polyglutamate chain lengths in the native cabbage, it was necessary to inactivate the conjugase by exposing the cabbage to boiling ascorbate. The folic acid activity of orange juice is predominantly in the 5-methyl form, with about 30 percent being monoglutamate and most of the rest pentaglutamate.

Food folate availability must be studied in the native food rather than by using pure folates extracted from the native food. It has been known since the work of Swendseid in the late 1940's that pure heptaglutamate from yeast was absorbed as well on a molar basis as folic acid, as determined by excretion in urine in an 8-h period, but the same folate in intact yeast was only about 25 percent as available, due to the presence in yeast of conjugase inhibitor. Urinary excretion of folate does not become perceptible for a given foodstuff until the dose exceeds about 0.3 mg. The availability of folate from orange juice appeared to be about 31 percent; from lettuce about 25 percent; from egg yolk, 39 percent; and from bananas, dry lima beans, and frozen lima beans, 75 to 100 percent. Since the amount of a foodstuff that must be fed to provide 0.3 mg of folate is generally substantially higher than amounts ordinarily consumed in the diet, other methods of measuring food folate availability are needed.

The relatively low availability of orange juice folate may have been due to interference with conjugase action by the low pH of the juice.

Wagner and Rosenberg noted that binding of folate polyglutamates to protein in food may interfere with ability of conjugase to function, since pure polyglutamate appears better absorbable than food polyglutamate. Rothenberg noted that the lesser absorbability of food polyglutamate by achlorhydric persons may be because of less splitting of polyglutamates from protein. Hoffbrand noted that microbiologic assay of urine folate may yield lower than true results because of growth inhibition of the test organism by DNA and RNA; radioassay may be preferable.

Chanarin noted that normal volunteers have a wide variance in absorption of tritiated pteroylglutamic acid, ranging from 55 to about 90 percent absorption. He also noted that substantial urine folate is excreted split at the 9,10 position.

Scott noted that substantial amounts of the polyglutamates of meat may be deconjugated during autolysis when meat is stored for 1 day or more at room temperature.

SIGNIFICANCE OF FOLATE BINDERS

The significance of folate binders was reviewed by Rothenberg. Binders may be specific or nonspecific. Specific binders have a specific conformational structure between folate and binder, a high affinity of binder for folate, and saturation kinetics (i.e., a finite maximal binding capacity) and the attached folate is not dialyzable or extractable by charcoal. Nonspecific binders have a nonconformational structure, a low affinity for folate, and no saturation kinetics (50 percent of almost any amount may be bound, for example) and detached folate is both dialyzable and extractable by charcoal.

The folate binder found in chronic myelogenous leukemia leukocytes is stable to 57° C, folate dissociates from it at pH below 5, and only PGA and dihydrofolate significantly inhibit it; other folates do not. That antibody to chronic myeloid leukemia binder cross-reacts with folate binders in serum, urine, liver, milk, L-1210 leukemia, and other binders suggests a common antigenic site on all specific folate binders.

The small fraction of folate in serum that is bound appears to be oxidized rather than reduced folate; Hoffbrand suggested it may be a 10-formyl form (which Blair had reported in serum). The binders, by regulating free folate concentration, may have a regulatory function on cell metabolism and polyglutamate formation and may also have an antibacterial function.

RADIOASSAYS OF SERUM FOLATE

Serum folate radioassays were reviewed by Waxman. Commercially available beta-lactoglobulin is contaminated with a folate binder that is stable on storage and highly reproducible when used as the ligand in folate radioassay. Endogenous folate binder in serum complicates the assay; this binder may be dealt with in various ways, including boiling the serum to destroy it (as was done by Dunn and Foster), by using relatively large amounts of milk folate binder and relatively small amounts of serum, and by using as binder a milk containing a substance that splits endogenous folate from endogenous serum folate-bound binding protein, as reported by Colman and Herbert.

POLYGLUTAMATE SYNTHESIS IN HUMAN CELLS

This was discussed by Hoffbrand. After 72 h of incubation of human lymphocytes with mitogen and radiofolate, the predominant radioactive peak contained 4-, 5-, and 6-glutamates. Radiofolate concentration was highest in cytoplasm and second highest in mitochondria–lysosome fraction. Work of Sakami's group in *Neurospora crassa* and rat liver indicates that the intracellular substrate for the polyglutamate synthesizing enzyme(s) is only tetrahydrofolate, and not any of the tetrahydrofolates containing one-carbon units. Hoffbrand's studies suggest that the same is true in human lymphocytes. It appears that, in B_{12} deficiency, the methylfolate that enters cells cannot be converted to tetrahydrofolate, which is the substrate for polyglutamate synthesis, and so the methylfolate may then diffuse out of the cell; this may explain the lower intracellular folate content of B_{12}-deficient as compared to normal cells.

Hoffbrand presented evidence that folate polyglutamates in mammalian (rat liver, human lymphocyte) cells are not broken down when the cells are intact because the conjugase is entirely contained in the lysosomes, which do not break down until the cells die. Conjugase, acting as an exopeptidase, splits off glutamates one by one and is involved in folate absorption, recycling after cell death, and possibly in alteration of glutamate chain length in viable cells.

The discussion pointed out that there may be some polyglutamate synthesis from oxidized folate and from folates containing one-carbon adducts, but such synthesis is much less than that from tetrahydrofolate.

Girdwood suggested folate deconjugase as a more descriptive term than folate conjugase for the enzyme Blakley calls gamma-glutamyl carboxypeptidase. I agree.

REGULATION OF FOLATE METABOLISM BY VITAMIN B_{12}

Vitamin B_{12} regulation of folate metabolism was reviewed by Stokstad. In support of the folate trap hypothesis, methionine is generated from homocysteine in the presence of B_{12}, and the methionine is converted to S-adenosyl methionine, which by negative feedback reduces the level of the enzyme 5,10-methylenetetrahydrofolate reductase, thereby reducing the level of methyltetrahydrofolate. Via this mechanism, in the B_{12}-deficient rodent, supplying methionine reduces the abnormally elevated formiminoglutamate, formate, and aminoimidazole carboxamides. The methionine-perfused liver makes less methylfolate but more polyglutamates, since the latter are synthesized more rapidly from tetrahydrofolate than from methyltetrahydrofolate, since the conjugate synthetase substrate is tetrahydrofolate and not methyltetrahydrofolate. Like the B_{12}-deficient human, the B_{12}- and methionine-deprived rat has reduced liver folate and increased plasma folate, and the plasma folate drops on therapy with B_{12} or methionine (but both are needed to produce a rise in liver folate). The effects of methionine may be produced by lower amounts of ethionine, since it forms a very stable S-adenosyl ethionine. In the B_{12}-methionine-deficient rat, 40 percent of the urine folate is 5-methyl folate; repleting the rat with B_{12} or methionine lowers this to 13 percent. Stokstad's evidence indicated that in B_{12} deficiency methylfolate can get into rat liver cells but then leaks out rather than being incorporated into polyglutamate, which would hold the folate in the cell.

The regulatory system in bone marrow appears different from that in liver, since methionine increases methylfolate in bone marrow but decreases it in liver. This is consistent with the fact that methionine worsens the hematologic damage of B_{12} deficiency.

CHARACTERIZATION AND ROLE OF CONJUGASE IN THE ABSORPTION OF FOLATES

This was discussed by Rosenberg. He reviewed the evidence supporting the concept that available conjugase in the upper small intestine is of sufficient quantity and functionality such that any limits on folate absorption are not due to unavailability of adequate deconjugation but are rather due to limitation on the rapidity with which the deconjugated folate (i.e., pteroylmonoglutamates) could be transported across the intestinal epithelial cell. The flow rate of folate across the gut cell appears to be much lower than the hydrolysis rate of polyglutamates by conjugase, suggesting that the flow rate, rather than the amount of conjugase, may control folate transport across the gut into the mesenteric circulation. This would fit with the approximately equal absorption of folate monoglutamate and heptaglutamate in both celiac and tropical sprue. During the process of crossing the gut cell wall, a substantial portion of monoglutamate is converted to methylfolate.

Hoffbrand pointed out that Peters had shown that all lysosomal enzymes are increased in sprue, and conjugase could be expected to be increased, and thus the absorption of heptaglutamate and monoglutamate forms of folate in sprue should be (and are) about the same.

The importance of using low concentrations of PGA, or using already reduced forms of folate, to study folate absorption was noted. Such doses "slot into the physiological pathways" of absorption (Chanarin), with virtually 100 percent being reduced and methylated when it comes out the serosal side. Large doses of PGA, on the other hand, may go through the gut mucosa unaltered.

AUTOMATED MICROBIOLOGIC ASSAY FOR FOLATE

Folate automated microbiologic assay was discussed by Magnus, who also presented some data on plasma conjugase activity in various disease states in man.

In the general discussion it was brought out that, in most hands, use of the chloramphenicol-resistant strain of *Lactobacillus casei* offers no advantages, and some liabilities, as compared to the aseptic addition method using the standard *L. casei* strain.

In addition to Magnus, Krumdieck and Stokstad reported on their successful use of automated microbiologic folate assays.

MEGALOBLASTIC ANEMIA AS THE HEMATOLOGIC CONSEQUENCE OF INADEQUATE FOLATE COENZYME FUNCTION

This was reviewed by Chanarin. He noted the McBurney and Whitmore hamster ovary work as evidence that polyglutamate forms are concerned in the synthesis of thymidine, adenosine, and glycine; in rebuttal Krumdieck noted that, in his own system, only monogluta-mates were clearly coenzymes in function. He noted that the best explanation for the Hoffbrand data is the methylfolate trap hypothesis, but he also noted that his own laboratory was unable to find slow clearance of methylfolate in pernicious anemia, as would be expected if the folate trap hypothesis were correct. (However, Bertino's labora-tory did find such slow clearance in pernicious anemia.)

Chanarin also noted that children with congenital methylmalonic aciduria show no disturbed folate metabolism, suggesting there is some reversibility of the methylfolate trap (i.e., some methylfolate can be converted directly back to 5,10-methylene tetrahydrofolate; Stebbins and Silber have found some evidence to support this as the "escape hatch" from the folate trap). (Such an escape hatch had been noted to exist by Waxman, Metz, and Herbert [J. Clin. Invest. *48*:284–289, 1969].)

Chanarin reviewed the Chen and Wagner data on reduced uptake of methylfolate by the choroid plexus of the pig when PGA was added, although it must be determined if these data in fact reflect more than dilution of radioactive methylfolate with nonradioactive PGA. If con-firmed in humans, this could help explain the Reynolds observation of increase in fit frequency of epileptics otherwise controlled by Dilantin when given folic acid (an observation dramatically confirmed by But-terworth's group [Am. J. Clin. Nutr., 1975]). In a study of British alcoholics (who, unlike American skid row alcoholics, were all doing a normal day's work), Chanarin's group noted that 85 percent were macrocytic, with the macrocytosis correctable by stopping ethanol and not by giving folate; and that, of the one-third who were megaloblastic, half had normal serum, red cell, and liver folate, suggesting that the other half who were megaloblastic had this lesion because of a direct toxic effect of alcohol on the erythroblasts. (Of course, a direct effect on folate function of alcohol could also explain the megaloblastosis.) As American workers have found, Chanarin's group found those ingesting beer had higher folate levels than those ingesting whiskey.

Chanarin also reviewed the increased daily requirement for folate due to pregnancy, chronic hemolytic states, and possibly myelofibrosis (in which the increased need may be due to increased or ineffective utilization).

Chanarin also noted that PGA was 55–90 percent absorbed, but tetrahydrofolate and methyltetrahydrofolate were 90–100 percent ab-sorbed, i.e., pharmacologic forms are not as well absorbed as physio-logical forms, which are almost all practically completely absorbed when in monoglutamate form.

Blakley noted that, of the monoglutamates in reduced form, methyl-tetrahydrofolate is relatively stable to oxidation. When metabolism is increased, folates spend more time in nonmethyl forms and thus are more subject to oxidative degradation, which largely explains why the speed of folate catabolisms is related to the speed of body metabolic rate.

CELLULAR MECHANISMS OF UPTAKE OF FOLATE MONOGLUTAMATES

These were reviewed by Bertino. A number of laboratories have demonstrated that there is an energy-dependent uptake of reduced folates and methotrexate, but not of PGA, by mouse leukemia cells (and human bone marrow cells) with competition by the various reduced agents and methotrexate for the same transport site in the membrane. The laboratory of Huennekens has shown that uptake by cells of re-duced folate, but not the uptake of PGA, is inhibited by phenylmercuric borate. The agents that block dihydrofolate reductase shut down folate entry into cells. As Goldman has shown, iodoacetate or vincristine increases methotrexate uptake by blocking egress from cells; hydrocortisone (but not dexamethasone) does the opposite. Labeled methylfolate transfer of methyl groups is poor in the B_{12}-deficient cell, supporting the folate trap hypothesis. Unlike the mouse leukemia cell, active transport was demonstrable in rat gut cells, suggesting that they allow only passive absorption of folate.

INTESTINAL ABSORPTION OF FOLATE MONOGLUTAMATES

The intestinal absorption of folate monoglutamates was reviewed by Cooper. Both oxidized and reduced monoglutamyl folate are rapidly transferred from gut to portal vein, with much of the reduced folate being converted to methyl form *en route*. Conversely, a substantial portion of oxidized folate (PGA) is absorbed unchanged, and then it flushes reduced folate from the liver. The optimal pH for folate transport across the gut appears to be approximately 6, so such transport is reduced by bicarbonate. There appears to be better folate transport across jejunum than ileum. The reported cases of congenital inability to transport folate across the gut wall strongly suggest the existence of carrier-mediated folate transport across the gut wall, with the congenital defect cases being instances of inadequacy of this carrier (or binder) system. Blakley noted that these genetic data are reconcilable with either facilitated passive transport or active transport.

MECHANISMS OF INTESTINAL MUCOSAL UPTAKE OF POLYGLUTAMATES

These were reviewed by Halsted. From his most recent studies, he tentatively concluded that polyglutamates were hydrolyzed by mucosal conjugases possibly after entry into mucosal cell preparations similar to those used for folate uptake studies by Momtazi and Herbert (Am. J. Clin. Nutr. 26:23–29, 1973).

EARLY ESTIMATES OF HUMAN FOLATE REQUIREMENT

Early estimates of human folate requirement were reviewed by Darby, who noted that a reasonable estimate of adult requirement made in the late 1940's was about 500 μg daily, and, in the early 1950's, 200 μg of folate daily for infants. He noted that the usual state of scientific development after a nutrient is newly recognized as essential and identified is that requirements are approached from an initial "safe" and usually excessive therapeutic level, through later observations resulting in downward revisions of the estimate of requirement.

MODERN TABLES OF FOOD FOLATE CONTENT

Modern tables of food folate content are now being constructed in the United States and Canada, as Hoppner indicated. His group in Canada found a close correlation between folate calculated from food tables for fresh food and determined by actual analysis of prepared food. Free folate was found to be approximately half of total folate, and total daily dietary folate appeared to be in the range of 200 μg. Cooper indicated that Canadian diets in Montreal appear to yield about 200 μg of folate per day, and Chanarin indicated roughly the same was true in London (approximately 230 μg per day, of which perhaps a quarter was free folate). This information was considered of importance, since these were presumably "normal" population groups ingesting presumably "normal" diets; since they were not folate deficient on about 200 μg of total dietary folate per day, this was strong evidence that the adult RDA for folate could not be substantially greater than 200 μg and, additionally, that to provide a daily diet of more folate would involve altering dietary habits of these population groups.

DETECTING FOLATE DEFICIENCY BY NUTRITIONAL SURVEYS OF POPULATION GROUPS

Sauberlich discussed detecting folate deficiency by nutritional surveys of population groups. He summarized information from WHO and other sources on daily dietary folate intake, determined by dietary recall or by analysis in the laboratory of folate content of "typical diets," and comparing these results with recommended daily allowances. Because of uncertainties in these data, measurement of both serum and red cell folate appeared useful as guidelines in population surveys. He presented a considerable amount of previously unpublished information on serum and red cell folate in various population groups in the United States, and Cooper followed with some similar information from Canada.

There was some discussion by Hoppner and Chanarin indicating the value of liver folate levels; Chanarin found liver levels of below 1 μg/g when megaloblastic anemia was present and higher levels in the absence of megaloblastosis.

Waslien and Hoffbrand commented on relatively high red cell folates in iron deficiency and their fall with iron therapy; several papers have appeared in the literature on this subject.

It seemed clear from the INCAP guidelines of 1971, the WHO guidelines of 1968–1972, and the Ten-State Nutrition Survey that serum folate below 3 ng/ml and a red cell folate below 140–160 ng/ml were suggestive of deficiency. Some of the unpublished Ten-State Nutrition Survey data from the group of Clement Finch in the state of Washington indicated that red cell folates were higher in Caucasians than in Negroes and Hispanics and were higher in high-income than in low-income states.

The median serum folate in 20,000 Canadians surveyed in "Nutrition Canada" was 4.4 ng/ml, but Cooper found that Montreal blood donors (reasonably well-off economically) had a median serum folate of 7.5–8 ng/ml.

Hoppner noted that of 560 autopsy livers in Canada only two showed a folate below 5 μg/g, and Chanarin noted that in England symptoms appeared only when the liver folate was below 2 μg/g on biopsy.

FOLIC ACID REQUIREMENT IN CHILDREN

This was discussed by Waslien. She noted the study by Sullivan *et al.* of six children age 6–12 months with goat milk megaloblastic anemia who responded to 50 μg of folic acid daily (after 1 failed to respond to 10 and to 20 μg). The folate total from milk plus the administered PGA was 7.6–9.4 μg of folic acid per kg of body weight. The FAO/WHO report to which Waslien referred also noted the study by Velez *et al.* of seven children with megaloblastic anemia in association with protein-calorie malnutrition, who responded to 5–20 μg of PGA daily in addition to a diet calculated to contain approximately 10 μg of free folate per day. The response to PGA was complicated by simultaneous hematologic response to other nutrients supplied, making it difficult to determine how much of the anemia and response related to folate.

Ghitis and Tripathy in Colombia noted two megaloblastic children who responded to 15 and 35 μg of folic acid, corresponding to 3.7 and 5.9 μg/kg body weight.

Robinson found one child with megaloblastic anemia who responded to 15 μg micrograms of folic acid, corresponding to about 8 μg/kg of body weight.

The U.S. Navy Research Group in Cairo, Egypt, studied response of folate deficiency to folate in children with protein–calorie malnutrition. Halsted *et al.* noted restoration of normoblastic marrow in 11 such children on 75 μg of PGA parenterally superimposed on a whole-milk diet (containing 51 μg of total folate per liter; fraction of liter consumed by each child each day was unreported). Waslien *et al.* used a formula diet containing 25 μg of free and 27 μg of total folate per liter of formula. Additional folate was administered parenterally. This provided a folate intake of 9 μg/kg in those receiving 20 μg folate per day by injection. Since the intestinal mucosa is damaged in protein–calorie malnutrition, oral folate absorption may have been decreased. Reticulocyte response was noted to as little as 20 μg of PGA by injection (three out of five cases), 30 μg (four out of six), 40 μg (four out of five), and 50 μg (five out of seven). The reticulocyte peak was higher in the group receiving the 50-μg dose, and double reticulocyte response was noted after giving an additional 50 μg of PGA parenterally in each group, with not all of each group showing the second reticulocyte peak. Increase in hemoglobin to more than 11 g/100 ml was possibly more frequent with the higher doses of folic acid.

There was little clear difference between the 20- and the 50-μg PGA daily injected dose in terms of benefit. As Herbert noted, this study is limited to its own facts, i.e., applicable only to PGA superimposed on a milk diet (or a milk formula diet), and must take into account the high folate binder in milk that may render substantial amounts of its folate unabsorbable, so the folate requirement (i.e., the amount absorbed) may be less than the amount of folate fed. In children with protein–calorie malnutrition whose albumin levels have been restored, absorption of tritiated PGA appeared similar to that of normal adults: the children with clinical diarrhea absorbed 67 percent, and those without diarrhea absorbed 83 percent.

Seven Lebanese children on the formula diet plus 5 or 10 μg of oral PGA had stable serum and red cell folate and did not develop megaloblastosis over 6 to 9 months. A 100-μg dose of PGA produced marked increase in serum and red cell folate.

In summary, Waslien felt that 3.6 μg of folate per kg of body weight is adequate for the child less than 2 years of age.

Butram of the Consumer and Food Economics Institute at USDA reported that they are collecting all available analytical data on folates in food and drugs for inclusion in tabular form in the International Nutrient Data Bank being established in their institute.

FOLATE REQUIREMENTS IN ADULTS, INCLUDING PREGNANT AND LACTATING FEMALES

These were reviewed by Herbert. The minimal daily adult requirement to sustain normality appeared to be about 50 μg of PGA equivalents per day, a quantity that, administered orally or parenterally to the patient with folate deficiency uncomplicated by other systemic disease and not ingesting more than 5 μg of food folate daily, would produce a relatively rapid return toward hematologic normality.

Assuming adequate folate stores at the start of pregnancy, approximately 100 μg of PGA daily appears to sustain normality in the range of the minimal daily requirement in such pregnancy. Assuming lesser stores at the start of pregnancy, and supplementation beginning later than the start of pregnancy, this figure may rise to 200 or even 300 μg of PGA daily.

About 50 μg of folate per day is lost in the breast milk during lactation, making the minimum daily requirement for the lactating woman in the range of approximately 100 μg of PGA equivalents daily.

It should be noted that the amount of folate required to sustain normality, or the minimal daily requirement, will probably always be somewhat below the recommended dietary daily allowance (RDA), because the RDA is always set at a level sufficiently above the top of the range of normal individual human variability so as to allow a substantial margin of safety to encompass such factors as variable absorption of folates from different foodstuffs, variable inhibition of absorption by conjugase inhibitors in foodstuffs, and other factors touched on in this Workshop.

The folate cost of a one-fetus pregnancy appears to be in the range of 50 μg per day × 9 months, i.e., 13.5 mg, which exceeds the total body stores of the pregnant woman at the start of pregnancy.

Krumdieck presented data of a normal woman given labeled folic acid, which showed a half-life in her body, as measured by urinary excretion over 130 days, of 101 days. Thus, half the body folate pool may be lost in about 100 days. If the body pool is 8 mg, 4 mg may be lost in 100 days, equivalent to 40 μg per day, which is about the minimum necessary to sustain normality. Chanarin pointed out that studies of this group indicate the normal range of liver folate to be 5 to 17 μg/g, which, calculating the normal adult liver as 1,500 g, means folate stores of 7.5 to 25.5 mg in the liver, which contains only half the body folate. Thus, total body folate may be as high as 50 mg in an adult.

Krumdieck noted that in their study of the half-life of ingested radio folate they found fecal losses difficult to assess but often greater than loss in urine.

Scott noted that recent studies from his laboratory (Am. J. Clin. Nutr., 1975) suggested that tetrahydrofolate without an added 1-carbon adduct might be nutritionally inactive because it might break at the 9,10 bond prior to absorption; that 10-formyl tetrahydrofolate in the diet would probably be nutritionally active because it oxidizes to the stable 10-formyl folic acid without breaking at the 9,10 bond; and that 5-formyl tetrahydrofolate (folinic acid) was stable, but 5-methyl tetrahydrofolate may be nutritionally poor because of oxidation to 5,β-dihydrofolate, which rearranges to form an inactive compound.

FOLATE REQUIREMENT IN SITUATIONS OF INCREASED NEED

Folate requirement in situations of increased need was discussed by Lindenbaum. Increased need is defined as failure of folate deficiency megaloblastic anemia to respond to doses of PGA in the range of 50–100 μg daily in an adult, followed by response to higher doses. These situations of increased need include pregnancy and lactation, hemolytic anemias, alcohol ingestion, the presence of dihydrofolate reductase inhibitors, and possibly certain homocystinurias.

Patients with hemolytic anemia and megaloblastosis may not improve on up to 200 μg of PGA daily but respond to doses of 300 μg or more daily. About 80 percent of reported cases have additional factors adversely affecting folate balance, such as poor diet, pregnancy, infancy, administration of folate antagonists, infections, malabsorption, and alcohol ingestion.

Alcohol not only raises the folate requirement (as shown by Sullivan and Herbert) but may also cause a rapid fall in the serum folate level (as reported by Eichner and Hillman) and decrease folate polyglutamate formation (Scott *et al.*) and can reverse the ratio of bound to free folate (Hines).

Increased folate requirement has been suspected, but is so far unproved, in infection and other inflammatory disorders, myelofibrosis, sideroblastic anemias (Hoffbrand reported a case requiring more than 200 μg of folate daily, and Mollin reported two similar cases), anticonvulsant drug usage, malignancy, iron deficiency, increased folate excretion (in desquamated skin with skin disorders, in the urine in patients with congestive heart failure or liver disease, in renal dialysis, and in instances of biliary drainage), and in hyperthyroidism.

Localized folate deficiency in the cervical epithelium accompanying the use of oral contraceptives has been documented by Lindenbaum's group. In the Symposium on Oral Contraceptive Hormones in the April and May 1975 issues of the *American Journal of Clinical Nutrition*, reduction in serum and red cell folate levels in women on oral contraceptives was documented in several separate surveys in different parts of the country. Herbert's group noted that some patients on oral contraceptives may show a subnormal du suppression test, corrected to normal by folate in lymphocytes but not in bone marrow specimens. Similar selective folate deficiency in bone marrow white, but not red, cells was reported in certain patients with intestinal disorders by Hoffbrand and Newcombe (Br. J. Haematol. *13*:954–966, 1967, Figure 2). Bertino noted that hydrocortisone may depress uptake of methylfolate by human leukemia cells, as it does the uptake of methotrexate by such cells, and this may be analogous to oral contraceptive suppression of cell folate uptake.

DRUG-INDUCED FOLATE DEFICIENCY

This was reviewed by Girdwood. His paper supplemented his own 1973 review and the 1973 review from Herbert's laboratory (Semin. Hematol. *10*:235–251, 1973).

CONCLUSIONS

This Workshop addressed itself particularly to seven crucial questions posed by Dr. Butterworth, as follows:

1. What is (or should be) the recommended dietary allowance (RDA) for folate?

ANSWER: In adults, at least an amount from which is absorbed 50 μg of folate per day. This amount would not exceed 300 μg, so 300 μg was decided upon to allow a substantial safety margin. It was recognized that further research may reduce this proposed adult RDA of 300 μg/day to 250 or even to 200 μg/day. This amount is approximately doubled by pregnancy or lactation. In infants, 4 μg of folate per kg of body weight per day appears a reasonable approximation based on the available evidence.

2. What constitutes appropriate assessment of nutritional status with regard to folate?

ANSWER: Measurement of serum plus red cell folate appears to be the most practical approach. Current evidence suggests that, when serum and red cell folate are both low, other more direct indices of folate deficiency will be present (i.e., a low liver folate and a bone marrow "dU suppression" test demonstrating subnormal DNA synthesis by bone marrow cells correctable by adding folate or methylfolate *in vitro*). Measurement of tissue folate (i.e., red cell folate or liver folate) alone is not adequate because deficiency of vitamin B_{12} results in low tissue folate (but not low serum folate). Low serum folate alone is not adequate as a test for folate deficiency because it is too sensitive; i.e., serum folate is low after only 3 weeks of folate deprivation, which is months prior to exhaustion of tissue folate stores and development of biochemical folate deficiency.

3. What are the effects of folate deficiency or excess?

ANSWER: Nutrient deficiency means inadequate nutrient to sustain normal metabolism. Thus, folate deficiency produces inadequate folate metabolism manifested biochemically as inadequate transfer of 1-carbon units and clinically as the result of such inadequate transfer. The most-studied biochemical abnormality is slowed DNA synthesis, manifested by megaloblastosis in all proliferating cells, including those of the bone marrow, the gastrointestinal tract, and the cervical epithelium. Folate excess may interfere with the pharmacologic action of anticonvulsants; diphenylhydantoin (Dilantin) appears to block folate absorption from the intestine, and folic acid in large doses appears to interfere with the ability of diphenylhydantoin to suppress convulsions.

4. How can methodology and techniques for folate assays be standardized?

ANSWER: A reference laboratory should provide reference samples, and each laboratory publishing folate assay data should indicate the reading their laboratory obtains on reference laboratory samples as compared to the reference laboratory value. The reference laboratory "true value" should be derived as the mean of values obtained in a number of laboratories collaborating with the reference laboratory.

5. Is there a need to standardize procedures for determining total folate, including determining completeness of enzymic release of folate from polyglutamate forms?

ANSWER: Until an "ideal" method for determining total folate appears, each laboratory publishing "total folate" data should provide enough methodologic information so that other workers can compare their own method.

6. Is there a need for a system of biologic or nutritional equivalence of different folates?

ANSWER: Equivalence depends on destructibility, absorbability, and interchangeability. Further data on these three facets of equivalence will create an adequate system of equivalence.

7. Are the presently available tables of folate content in food adequate?

ANSWER: Values in tables obtained without ascorbate (or other reducing agent) protection of folate content against oxidative destruction are completely unsatisfactory, i.e., essentially all values obtained before 1963. Tables published in 1963 and subsequently are of limited scope in terms of foodstuffs encompassed.

Contributors

JOSEPH R. BERTINO, Departments of Pharmacology and Medicine, Yale University School of Medicine, New Haven, Connecticut

RAYMOND L. BLAKLEY, Department of Biochemistry, University of Iowa College of Medicine, Iowa City, Iowa

CHARLES E. BUTTERWORTH, JR., Director, The Nutrition Program, University of Alabama Medical Center, Birmingham, Alabama

I. CHANARIN, Department of Haematology, Clinical Research Center, Northwick Park Hospital, Harrow, Middlesex HA1 3UJ, England

BERNARD A. COOPER, Haematology Division, McGill University Medical Clinic, Royal Victoria Hospital, Montreal 112, Quebec, Canada

PHILLIP E. CORNWELL, The Nutrition Program, University of Alabama, Birmingham, Alabama

MARIA DA COSTA, New York Medical College, Flower and Fifth Avenue Hospitals, New York, New York

WILLIAM J. DARBY, President, The Nutrition Foundation, Inc., New York, New York

CRAIG FISCHER, Division of Hematology, Department of Medicine, New York Medical College, New York, New York

RONALD H. GIRDWOOD, University Department of Therapeutics, The Royal Infirmary of Edinburgh, Edinburgh, Scotland

GERALD S. GOTTERER, Department of Physiological Biochemistry, The Johns Hopkins University School of Medicine, Baltimore, Maryland

CHARLES H. HALSTED, Department of Internal Medicine, University of California, School of Medicine, Davis, California

VICTOR HERBERT, Medical Investigator and Chief of the Hematology and Nutrition Laboratory, Bronx Veterans Administration Hospital, New York, New York, and Clinical Professor of Pathology and Medicine, Columbia University College of Physicians and Surgeons, New York, New York

A. V. HOFFBRAND, Department of Haematology, Royal Free Hospital and School of Medicine, London NW3 2QG, England

K. HOPPNER, Nutrition Research Division, Bureau of Nutritional Sciences, Health Protection Branch, Department of National Health and Welfare, Ottawa, Ontario K1A 0L2, Canada

CARLOS L. KRUMDIECK, Biochemistry and Pediatrics, University of Alabama Medical Center, Birmingham, Alabama

B. LAMPI, Nutrition Research Division, Bureau of Nutritional Sciences, Health Protection Branch, Department of National Health and Welfare, Ottawa, Ontario, K1A 0L2, Canada

A. LAVOIE, Hôpital de l'Enfant-Jésus, 1401, 18 ème Rue, Quebec, G1J 1Z4, Canada

295

JOHN LINDENBAUM, Chief, Hematology, Harlem Hospital Center, and Department of Medicine, Columbia University, College of Physicians and Surgeons, New York, New York

ERIK M. MAGNUS, Spes. Indremedisin, Krohgstøtten Hospital, Oslo, Norway

A. NAHAS, Department of Biochemistry, University of Rochester Medical School, Rochester, New York

PETER F. NIXON, Department of Biochemistry, St. Lucia, Brisbane, Australia 4067

JANET PERRY, Clinical Research Centre, Northwick Park Hospital, Harrow, Middlesex HA1 3UJ, England

ANN REISENAUER, Department of Physiological Biochemistry, The Johns Hopkins University School of Medicine, Baltimore, Maryland

IRWIN H. ROSENBERG, Department of Medicine, University of Chicago, Chicago, Illinois

SHELDON P. ROTHENBERG, Division of Hematology, Department of Medicine, New York Medical College, New York, New York

HOWERDE E. SAUBERLICH, Chief, Department of Nutrition, Letterman Army Institute of Research, Presidio of San Francisco, California

CAROL SCHREIBER, Department of Medicine, Mount Sinai School of Medicine, New York, New York

JOHN M. SCOTT, Department of Biochemistry, Trinity College, Dublin 2, Ireland

Y. S. SHIN, Department of Nutritional Sciences, University of California, Berkeley, California

DOROTHY C. SMITH, Nutrition Research Division, Bureau of Nutritional Sciences, Health Protection Branch, Department of National Health and Welfare, Ottawa, Ontario, K1A 0L2, Canada

E. L. ROBERT STOKSTAD, Department of Nutritional Sciences, University of California, Berkeley, California

T. TAMURA, Department of Nutritional Sciences, University of California, Berkeley, California

RONALD W. THOMPSON, The Nutrition Program, University of Alabama, Birmingham, Alabama

E. TRIPP, Department of Haematology, Royal Free Hospital and School of Medicine, London, NW3 2QG, England

CAROL I. WASLIEN (Youssef), Department of Home Economics, Auburn University, Auburn, Alabama

SAMUEL WAXMAN, Department of Medicine, Mount Sinai School of Medicine, New York, New York

WILLIAM E. WHITE, JR., The Nutrition Program, University of Alabama, Birmingham, Alabama

Attendees

ROBERT B. BENNETT, Staff Officer, Food and Nutrition Board, National Academy of Sciences, Washington, D.C.

HEINZ BERENDES, Center for Population Research, NICHD/DHEW, Bethesda, Maryland

JOSEPH R. BERTINO, Department of Medicine and Pharmacology, Yale University School of Medicine, New Haven, Connecticut

JOHN G. BIERI, Nutrition Biochemistry Section, NIAMDD, National Institutes of Health, Bethesda, Maryland

RAYMOND L. BLAKLEY, Department of Biochemistry, University of Iowa College of Medicine, Iowa City, Iowa

HARRY P. BROQUIST, Department of Biochemistry, Vanderbilt University, Nashville, Tennessee

MYRTLE L. BROWN, Staff Officer, Food and Nutrition Board, National Academy of Sciences, Washington, D.C.

RITVA BUTRAM, ARS/USDA, Federal Building, Hyattsville, Maryland

CHARLES E. BUTTERWORTH, JR., Director, The Nutrition Program, University of Alabama Medical Center, Birmingham, Alabama

I. CHANARIN, Department of Haematology, Clinical Research Center, Northwick Park Hospital, Harrow, Middlesex HA1 3UJ, England

BERNARD A. COOPER, Haematology Division, McGill University Medical Clinic, Royal Victoria Hospital, Montreal 112, Quebec, Canada

NEVILLE COLMAN, Veterans Administration Hospital, Bronx, New York

WILLIAM J. DARBY, President, The Nutrition Foundation, Inc., New York, New York

EDWARD R. EICHNER, Department of Medicine, Louisiana State University Medical Center, Shreveport, Louisiana

RONALD H. GIRDWOOD, University Department of Therapeutics, The Royal Infirmary of Edinburgh, Edinburgh, Scotland

WILLIS GORTNER, Director, Human Nutrition Research Division, U.S. Department of Agriculture, Beltsville, Maryland

CHARLES H. HALSTED, Department of Internal Medicine, University of California, School of Medicine, Davis, California

VICTOR HERBERT, Medical Investigator and Chief of the Hematology and Nutrition Laboratory, Bronx Veterans Administration Hospital, New York, New York, and Clinical Professor of Pathology and Medicine, Columbia University College of Physicians and Surgeons, New York, New York

A. V. HOFFBRAND, Department of Haematology, Royal Free Hospital and School of Medicine, London, NW 3 2QG, England

K. HOPPNER, Nutrition Research Division, Bureau of Nutritional Sciences, Health Protection Branch, Department of National Health and Welfare, Ottawa, Ontario, K1A 0L2, Canada

297

PAUL E. JOHNSON, Executive Secretary, Food and Nutrition Board, National Academy of Sciences, Washington, D.C.

CARLOS L. KRUMDIECK, Biochemistry and Pediatrics, University of Alabama Medical Center, Birmingham, Alabama

JOHN LINDENBAUM, Department of Medicine, Columbia University, College of Physicians and Surgeons, New York, New York

ERIK M. MAGNUS, Spes. Indremedisin, Krohgstøtten Hospital, Oslo, Norway

KRISTEN MCNUTT, The Nutrition Foundation, Inc., Washington, D.C. 20006

H. N. MUNRO, Department of Nutrition and Food Science, Massachusetts Institute of Technology, Cambridge, Massachusetts

LEON PROSKY, Division of Nutrition, Food and Drug Administration, Washington, D.C.

IRWIN H. ROSENBERG, Department of Medicine, University of Chicago, Chicago, Illinois

SHELDON P. ROTHENBERG, Divison of Hematology, Department of Medicine, New York Medical College, New York, New York

HOWERDE E. SAUBERLICH, Chief, Department of Nutrition, Letterman Army Institute of Research, Presidio of San Francisco, California

JOHN M. SCOTT, Department of Biochemistry, Trinity College, Dublin 2, Ireland

RUSSELL B. STEVENS, Executive Secretary, Division of Biological Sciences, National Academy of Sciences, Washington, D.C.

E. L. ROBERT STOKSTAD, Department of Nutritional Sciences, University of California, Berkeley, California

CONRAD WAGNER, Vanderbilt University, School of Medicine, Nashville, Tennessee

CAROL I. WASLIEN (Youssef), Department of Home Economics, Auburn University, Auburn, Alabama

SAMUEL WAXMAN, Department of Medicine, Mount Sinai School of Medicine, New York, New York

V. MICHAEL WHITEHEAD, Division of Haematology, Montreal General Hospital, Montreal, Quebec, Canada

4 3 16